NEPHROLOGY AND UROLOGY

CONTEMPORARY ISSUES IN SMALL ANIMAL PRACTICE VOLUME 4

Volumes Already Published

Vol. 1 Medical Emergencies
Robert G. Sherding, D.V.M., Guest Editor
Vol. 2 Surgical Emergencies
Ronald M. Bright, D.V.M., Guest Editor
Vol. 3 Infectious Diseases
Fredric W. Scott, D.V.M., Ph.D., Guest Editor

Forthcoming Volumes in the Series

Vol. 5 Neurologic Disorders
Joe N. Kornegay, D.V.M., Ph.D., Guest Editor
Vol. 6 Oncology
Neil T. Gorman, B.V.Sc., Ph.D., Guest Editor
Vol. 7 Dermatology
Gene Nesbitt, D.V.M., Guest Editor
Vol. 8 Disorders of Exotic Animals
Elliott R. Jacobson, D.V.M., Ph.D. and
George V. Kollias, Jr., D.V.M., Ph.D.,
Guest Editors
Vol. 9 Cardiology
John D. Bonagura, D.V.M., Guest Editor

NEPHROLOGY AND UROLOGY

Edited by

Edward B. Breitschwerdt, D.V.M.

Diplomate, American College of
Veterinary Internal Medicine
Associate Professor of Medicine
Department of Companion Animal and
Special Species Medicine
School of Veterinary Medicine
North Carolina State University
Raleigh, North Carolina

Churchill Livingstone
New York, Edinburgh, London, Melbourne 1986

ISBN 0-443-08429-7

Distributed in the United Kingdom by Churchill Livingstone, Robert Stevenson House, 1-3 Baxter's Place, Leith Walk, Edinburgh EH1 3AF, and by associated companies, branches, and representatives throughout the world.

Accurate indications, adverse reactions, and dosage schedules for drugs are provided in this book, but it is possible that they may change. The reader is urged to review the package information data of the manufacturers of the medications mentioned.

Acquisitions Editor: *Gene C. Kearn*
Copy Editor: *Patricia Rind*
Production Designer: *Charlie Lebeda*
Production Supervisor: *Jane Grochowski*

Printed in the United States of America

First published in 1986

My efforts in the evolution of this volume are dedicated to my parents for emphasizing the value of collegiate education and to my wife, Anne, for facilitating the ongoing process of my medical education.

Contributors

Timothy A. Allen, D.V.M. Diplomate, American College of Veterinary Internal Medicine. Associate Professor of Medicine, College of Veterinary Medicine and Biomedical Sciences, Colorado State University, Fort Collins, Colorado

Jeanne A. Barsanti, D.V.M., M.S. Diplomate, American College of Veterinary Internal Medicine. Associate Professor of Medicine, Department of Small Animal Medicine, College of Veterinary Medicine, The University of Georgia, Athens, Georgia

Edward B. Breitschwerdt, D.V.M. Diplomate, American College of Veterinary Internal Medicine. Associate Professor of Medicine, Department of Companion Animal and Special Species Medicine, School of Veterinary Medicine, North Carolina State University, Raleigh, North Carolina

Dennis J. Chew, D.V.M. Diplomate, American College of Veterinary Internal Medicine. Associate Professor of Medicine, Department of Veterinary Clinical Sciences, College of Veterinary Medicine, The Ohio State University, Columbus, Ohio

Deborah J. Davenport, D.V.M. Assistant Professor of Medicine, Division of Agricultural and Urban Practice, Virginia-Maryland Regional College of Veterinary Medicine, Virginia Tech, Blacksburg, Virginia

Stephen P. DiBartola, D.V.M. Diplomate, American College of Veterinary Internal Medicine. Associate Professor of Medicine, Department of Veterinary Clinical Sciences, College of Veterinary Medicine, The Ohio State University, Columbus, Ohio

Daniel A. Feeney, D.V.M., M.S. Diplomate, American College of Veterinary Radiology. Associate Professor of Radiology, Department of Small Animal Clinical Sciences, College of Veterinary Medicine, University of Minnesota, St. Paul, Minnesota

Delmar R. Finco, D.V.M., Ph.D. Diplomate, American College of Veterinary Internal Medicine. Professor of Veterinary Physiology, Department of Physiology, College of Veterinary Medicine, University of Georgia, Athens, Georgia

Gary R. Johnston, D.V.M., M.S. Diplomate, American College of Veterinary Radiology. Associate Professor of Radiology, Department of Small Animal Clinical Sciences, College of Veterinary Medicine, University of Minnesota, St. Paul, Minnesota

Carl A. Osborne, D.V.M., Ph.D. Diplomate, American College of Veterinary Internal Medicine. Professor of Medicine, Department of Small Animal Clinical Sciences, College of Veterinary Medicine, University of Minnesota, St. Paul, Minnesota

Rodney L. Page, D.V.M., M.S. Assistant Professor of Medicine and Oncology, Department of Companion Animal and Special Species Medicine, School of Veterinary Medicine, North Carolina State University, Raleigh, North Carolina

David J. Polzin, D.V.M., Ph.D. Diplomate, American College of Veterinary Internal Medicine. Assistant Professor of Medicine, Department of Small Animal Clinical Sciences, College of Veterinary Medicine, University of Minnesota, St. Paul, Minnesota

Linda A. Ross, D.V.M., M.S. Diplomate, American College of Veterinary Internal Medicine. Assistant Professor of Medicine, Department of Medicine, School of Veterinary Medicine, Tufts University; Clinician, Foster Hospital for Small Animals, Tufts New England Veterinary Medical Center, North Grafton, Massachusetts

David F. Senior, B.V.Sc. Diplomate, American College of Veterinary Internal Medicine. Associate Professor, Department of Medical Sciences, College of Veterinary Medicine, University of Florida, Gainesville, Florida

Elizabeth A. Stone, D.V.M., M.S. Diplomate, American College of Veterinary Surgery. Associate Professor of Surgery, Department of Companion Animal and Special Species Medicine, School of Veterinary Medicine, North Carolina State University, Raleigh, North Carolina

Jill W. Verlander, D.V.M. Diplomate, American College of Veterinary Internal Medicine. Fellow, Division of Nephrology and Hypertension, College of Medicine, University of Florida, Gainesville, Florida

Preface

As with other areas of internal medicine, there has been rapid expansion in the quantity and quality of information in companion animal nephrology and urology. Routine use of urinalysis, patient chemistry profiles, contrast radiography, and renal biopsy has facilitated earlier detection, more complete characterization, and more effective management of diseases of the urinary tract. Despite this progress, there is an obvious need for more exacting information to allow earlier recognition of renal dysfunction, to enhance our understanding of the pathophysiologic mechanisms of renal disease, and to allow the appropriate use of diet, drugs, and surgery in the management of canine and feline urinary tract diseases.

The authors of the chapters in this volume have contributed significantly to recent progress in veterinary nephrology and urology. Each has attempted to consider his or her subject in a complete but concise manner. Information is presented in a forum that is clinically relevant, yet provides the reader with the author's assimilation of available scientific documentation of the subject.

I am deeply grateful to the contributing authors for their cooperation and exceptional effort. It is our hope that this volume, despite deficiencies in current knowledge, will assist those colleagues confronted with the challenges of patient management.

Edward B. Breitschwerdt, D.V.M.

Contents

1 Canine Urolithiasis

David F. Senior

The ability to concentrate and dilute urine is an evolutionary adaptation to terrestrial life. In healthy dogs, normal food and water intake necessitates production of hypertonic urine to maintain osmolar balance. When producing hypertonic urine, water is reabsorbed in the collecting tubules, the final urine is supersaturated with respect to a number of salts, and crystalluria is frequently observed. Crystalluria would be a clinically unimportant biological phenomenon if the precipitated solid particles in urine always moved at the same rate as the urine in which they form. However, the solid particles sometimes move at a different velocity from the urinary stream, and stone disease occurs.[1] Stone disease becomes clinically important when solid particles grow and fail to pass spontaneously, either through the ureter (in the case of renal pelvic and ureteral stones) or the urethra (in the case of bladder and urethral stones). In dogs, urinary stones are composed of a major mineral component, which may vary, and a minor organic matrix component, which appears to remain relatively constant.[2]

EPIDEMIOLOGY

The incidence of stone disease has been cited as 0.4 to 2.0 percent of all dogs receiving veterinary care.[3–5] In all surveys, struvite was the most common stone type, while oxalate, ammonium urate, and cystine stones varied in frequency (Table 1-1). Because qualitative chemical methods were used to identify mineral composition in many surveys, the number of calcium oxalate stones recorded in these studies may have been falsely low, as such methods often fail to detect this mineral.[6] However, one survey where stones were analyzed by x-ray diffraction also demonstrated a low prevalence of calcium oxalate stones.[7] Differences in prevalence between surveys may be due to geographical variations. A relatively high prevalence of cystine stones (37 percent) was

Table 1-1. Incidence of Different Types of Urinary Stones in the Dog

Study	Year	Total No. Examined	Struvite	Urate	Cystine	Oxalate	Other
Brodey[57]	1955	52	42	10	—	—	—
White[5]	1966	350	211	18	67	54	—
Finco[3]	1970	73	62	6	5	0	—
Weaver[58]	1970	100	53	13	20	14	—
Clark[10]	1974	110	49	2	24	35	—
Brown[9]	1977	438	307	21	95	12	3
Hicking[7]	1981	299	151	16	37	4	18[a]
Bovee[6]	1984	272	187	19	9	27	30[a]
Total		1694	1062	105	257	146	51
(Percent)			(63%)	(6%)	(15%)	(9%)	(3%)

Studies by Brodey[57], Finco[3], Brown[9], and Bovee[6] were done in the United States.
Studies by White[5], Weaver[58], and Clark[10] were done in the United Kingdom.
The study by Hicking[7] was done in West Germany.
[a] These surveys used accurate crystallographic or x-ray diffraction methods of stone analysis.

recorded in Germany, where the dachshund, a breed afflicted by inherited cystinuria, is popular.[7] Silicate renal calculi were observed in 53 percent of wild dogs in Kenya, where a special environmental setting may predispose to such precipitation.[8]

Most stones in dogs are located in the bladder or urethra, with less than 10 percent found in the kidney.[3,5,9] Occasionally, calculi occur simultaneously at a number of different anatomical locations.

Calculi may be diagnosed at almost any age, from suckling puppies 3 weeks old to very old dogs. Most cases are diagnosed at between 3 and 7 years of age, with the average age at diagnosis about 5.5 years.[3,9,10]

Some dog breeds appear to be predisposed to calculi. Many surveys do not correct for the popularity of breeds, so it is often difficult to accurately determine whether a true breed predisposition exists. In a recent survey, the miniature schnauzer, Welsh corgi, Lhasa apso, Yorkshire terrier, Pekingese, and pug appeared to have a higher than average probability of stone disease.[6] Struvite stones have been observed very commonly in some families of miniature schnauzers.[11] Cystine stones have been seen in the dachshund, basset hound, bulldog, Yorkshire terrier, Chihuahua, Irish terrier, and mix breeds. A high prevalence of ammonium urate stones has been observed in dalmatians, and this appears to be a real breed predisposition.[6] Ammonium urate stones frequently occur secondary to portosystemic vascular anomalies.[12] Thus, breeds commonly affected by vascular shunts, such as the Yorkshire terrier, miniature poodle, and miniature schnauzer, may have a high incidence of this stone type. Recently, miniature schnauzers were reported to have a predisposition to calcium oxalate stones also.[6]

Struvite stones occur more commonly in female dogs, whereas ammonium urate stones have been observed more commonly in males.[3,5,9,10] Cystine stones occur almost exclusively in male dogs, because cystinuria appears to be a sex-linked recessive trait.[13,14]

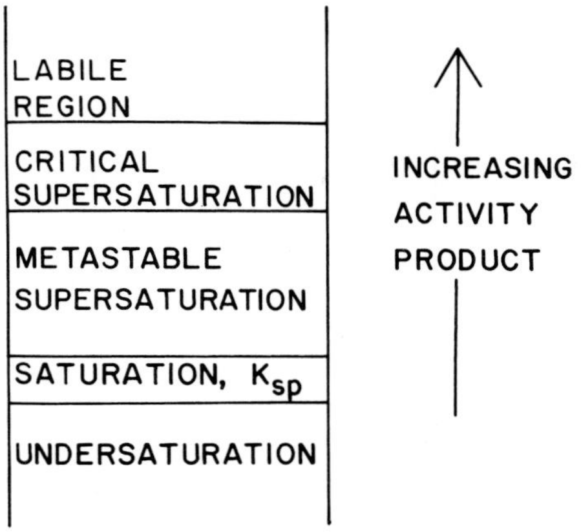

Fig. 1-1. The effect of increasing activity product on solution saturation. (Nancollas GH: The kinetics of crystal growth and renal stone-formation. In Fleisch, Robertson, Smith, et al (eds): Urolithiasis. Plenum Press, 1976.)

PATHOPHYSIOLOGY—GENERAL

Stone formation in the urinary tract depends upon three independent variables[15]:

1. The degree of urinary supersaturation. More concentrated solutes have a greater tendency to precipitate, and crystalline particles tend to grow faster.
2. The presence or absence of inhibitors and promoters of crystal aggregation and growth. Surface-acting inhibitory substances have been identified in calcium stone systems.
3. Urinary particle retention. Crystalline particles retained in the urinary stream for a long time grow larger.

Urinary Supersaturation and Precipitation

In normal dogs, urine in the renal pelvis at the end of the concentration process is supersaturated for a number of salts. Supersaturated urine has a potential energy driving force or "free energy" of precipitation which causes crystal formation. With a higher degree of supersaturation, the driving force is greater, precipitation will tend to occur more readily, and formed crystals will tend to grow faster.

Not all supersaturated solutions spontaneously form precipitates. Two ranges of supersaturation are recognized, metastable and labile (Fig. 1-1). Labile supersaturation leads to spontaneous precipitation (nucleation) of dissolved solute, without the need for a preformed surface. Metastable supersaturation does not result in nucleation unless a preexisting surface for crystallization, a nidus, is available. Although crystallization in urine may form on a preexisting surface, the nature of the nidus is not clear. When wettable foreign bodies are retained in the lumen of the bladder (e.g., silk sutures), they soon become coated by a mineral encrustation.[16] Cellular debris, bacteria, mucoprotein, and other crystals have all been suggested; however, there is no definitive evidence that they are involved in nidus formation, because such structures are not commonly found in the middle of stones.

Once precipitation has occurred, crystalline particles may increase in size by additional solute deposition on the crystal surface or by aggregation of many crystals. Crystal growth is relatively slow, whereas crystal aggregation can result in a rapid increase in particle size. The driving force for crystal growth is supersaturation, and the rate of crystal growth depends on the degree of supersaturation. The factors that control aggregation are not well understood.

Inhibitors and Promoters of Crystallization

Inhibitors of calcium oxalate crystal growth and aggregation have been identified in human and canine urine. In human urine, citrate, pyrophosphate, chondroitin sulfate, RNA, and glycosaminoglycans have all been shown to inhibit crystallization of calcium salts,[17] but the relative importance of each is not entirely clear. It is not known whether similar inhibition occurs in dogs, although the canine bladder appears to produce a calcium oxalate crystallization inhibitor.[18] When inhibitory activity is reduced, crystalline particles can increase in size more rapidly, and stone disease is more likely. Thus, the risk of calcium oxalate stones in humans who have normal anatomy (no increased particle retention time) is determined by the balance between supersaturation and inhibition. In the dog, inhibitors of ammonium urate colloidal sol flocculation have been described in urine, but similar inhibitors have not been identified in other systems.[19]

Promoters of crystallization may also be present in urine. It has been suggested that stone organic matrix may act as a promoter of initial crystallization.[2] The role of matrix in stone formation is controversial and remains to be clarified.

Urinary Particle Retention

Under most circumstances, the urine stream moves fast enough to wash out all formed particles, irrespective of their growth rate. Conditions which delay the movement of formed particles through the urinary tract allow growth to continue and predispose to stone disease. Crystalline particles normally do not adhere to the uroepithelial surface, but epithelial damage caused by necrosis and infection may lead to crystal adherence.[20] In an atonic bladder, failure to completely void all urine may leave a sludge of formed crystalline material in the ventral portion.

DISSOLUTION

Just as supersaturation sets up potential free energy of crystallization, undersaturation results in potential free energy of dissolution. When a solution is very undersaturated with respect to an immersed crystal, the free energy of dissolution will be large and the rate of dissolution will tend to be fast. The dissolution rate of a crystal is proportional to the surrounding solution's degree of undersaturation. However, not all minerals dissolve rapidly when immersed in an undersaturated solution, because a number of other factors also determine crystal dissolution rate.

Inhibitory substances may coat the crystal and partially prevent exposure to the surrounding undersaturated solution. The electrical charge on the surface of the crystal may bind water molecules very tightly and prevent free exchange of solute between the crystal and the solution. A high lattice energy in the crystal may hold molecules together avidly and reduce the rate of stone dissolution. Stones with a large exposed surface area tend to dissolve rapidly. A rough, jagged stone will present a higher surface area to the surrounding solution than a smooth-surfaced stone of the same size.

A matrix diffusion barrier may reduce the rate of dissolution. Stones suspended in undersaturated solutions in vitro tend to dissolve more slowly as dissolution progresses.[21–23] As stones dissolve, organic matrix remains and the distance from matrix surface to mineral surface increases. The matrix acts as a diffusion barrier, slowing stone dissolution. This may explain the observation that struvite stones in the renal pelvis tend to dissolve more slowly than similar-sized bladder stones when dogs are placed on dissolution protocols. Bladder stones tend to move around in the bladder with each urination, so that any remaining undissolved stone matrix would erode from the surface of the stone.

Struvite bladder stones in dogs readily dissolve when urine is made undersaturated with respect to struvite,[24,25] and there is preliminary evidence that ammonium urate stones may do the same.[26] Uric acid and cystine stones in man can also be dissolved readily if urine is made undersaturated with respect to these minerals.[27,28] It is not known whether calcium oxalate stones can be dissolved in a similar manner.

In this discussion of crystallization and dissolution, two important concepts arise: it is thermodynamically impossible (1) for stones to form and grow in undersaturated urine, and (2) for stones to dissolve in supersaturated urine.

CLINICAL SIGNS

Stones cause uroepithelial irritation, predispose to urinary tract infection, and induce ureteral and urethral obstruction. The clinical signs may vary. Infected renal stones may destroy the affected kidney and cause chronic renal failure if the disease is bilateral. Stones in the upper urinary tract may cause renal and ureteral colic, although this has been reported infrequently. Bladder stones usually cause signs of lower urinary tract inflammation, with pollakiuria, dysuria, tenesmus, and hematuria. Urethral obstruction is common in male dogs with stone disease. Pollakiuria, dysuria, tenesmus, hematuria, incontinence, and a distended bladder are usually observed, and this syndrome constitutes a medical emergency.

Table 1-2. Prediction of the Mineral Composition of Stones from the Age, Breed, and Sex of the Patient Based on Epidemiologic Data

Age, Sex, and Breed	Stone Type (%)			
	Struvite	Oxalate	Urate	Cystine
All age females (all breeds)	97	1–2	1–2	0
All age dalmations	23	0	77	0
Immature males (not dalmation)[a]	97	1	1	1
Mature males (basset, bulldog, Chihuahua, Irish and Yorkshire terrier, dachshund)	25	10	5	60

[a] Except young animals with portosystemic shunts, which usually have ammonium urate stones.

(Modified from Lewis LD, Morris ML, Jr: Small Animal Nutrition. 2nd Ed. Mark Morris Associates, Topeka, KS, 1984.)

DIAGNOSIS

Renal stone disease does not always cause overt clinical signs, and stone disease is often recognized as an incidental finding when working up a patient for another disease. Vague malaise or increased water consumption may be the only presenting complaints. Advanced bilateral renal stones associated with infection can lead to loss of renal function until chronic renal failure becomes apparent. Renal and ureteral colic have not been frequently recognized.

Bladder stones usually cause lower urinary tract inflammation with pollakiuria, tenesmus, and hematuria. The differential diagnoses with these signs include urinary tract infection and neoplasia. Bladder stones may be palpable as firm masses in the caudal abdomen if they are large enough, and crepitus may be felt if more than one stone is present.

Acute urethral obstruction with stones induces post-renal uremia with tenesmus, a full bladder, and overflow incontinence. Urethral stones may be found when they obstruct passage of a urethral catheter, and crepitus may be felt through the catheter.

Abdominal radiographs are usually sufficient to confirm a diagnosis of stone disease. Most stones in dogs are sufficiently radiopaque to be visible on plain radiographs, but the more radiolucent stones—ammonium urate and cystine—may only be seen after good patient preparation with fasting and enemas or contrast radiography. Intravenous pyelography can determine whether mineralized densities in the kidney are intraluminal or extraluminal.

To use dietary dissolution strategies, it is necessary to estimate the most likely mineral component of a stone prior to treatment. Direct analysis of previously removed or spontaneously passed stones determines composition without doubt. Unfortunately, stone material is not available for analysis in most cases, but several epidemiological and clinical clues can help to establish mineral composition with a fair degree of accuracy.

1. The patient's age, breed, and sex may suggest a certain mineral type (Table 1-2).
2. The stone's anatomical location may help, because about 75 percent of renal and ureteral stones are composed of struvite.

3. The radiographic density of stones may provide clues to their composition. Calcium oxalate stones are always very radiopaque, whereas struvite stones may vary from moderate to very radiopaque. Cystine and ammonium urate stones are usually the least radiopaque, and on rare occasions, ammonium urate stones may be radiolucent.

4. Examination of urine is usually rewarding. Urine pH tends to be alkaline with struvite stones, acidic with cystine stones, and either alkaline or acidic with ammonium urate and oxalate stones. Characteristic struvite, cystine, ammonium urate, or calcium oxalate crystals may be present in the urine sediment. Evidence of bacterial infection with a urease-producing organism such as *Staphylococcus intermedius* or *Proteus* sp. is consistent with a struvite stone. However, previously infected struvite stones may become sterile after antibiotic treatment, struvite stones may form in the absence of infection, and urease-producing infections can develop in patients with a stone type other than struvite. In one survey, 55 percent of dogs with ammonium urate stones had concurrent urinary tract infection.[6]

If stones are spontaneously passed or removed at surgery, they must be accurately analyzed for mineral composition. A chemical kit (Oxford Stone Analysis Set for Urinary Calculi, Oxford Laboratories, 1149 Ches Drive, Foster City, CA 94404) is available, but it may fail to identify the presence of oxalate and falsely identify urate in cystine calculi.[6] Accurate analysis can be obtained at a number of laboratories: Urolithiasis Laboratory, PO Box 25375, Houston, TX 77005; Louis C. Herring and Co., PO Box 2191, Orlando, FL 32707; Urinary Stone Analysis Laboratory, Department of Medicine, School of Veterinary Medicine, University of California, Davis, CA 95616.

TREATMENT

Conventional surgical treatment of stone disease and urethrohydropropulsion in the dog have been described elsewhere.[29–31] In human medicine, there is a major recent trend toward percutaneous extraction and shock wave destruction for renal stones, instead of open surgery. The cost of these methods precludes their routine use in veterinary medicine; however, some of the techniques are readily applicable to dogs. Nephrostomy tract dilatation using concentric dilators can simplify resection of renal stones during laparotomy. In female dogs, cystoscopy may be an alternative treatment for bladder stones.[32] Stone baskets may be introduced through a cystoscope to snare and remove stones.[32] If stones are too large for such extraction, electrohydraulic shock wave lithotripsy has been used to fragment stones so that smaller pieces may be flushed out, spontaneously passed, or snared and extracted with a stone basket.[32] Ultrasonic lithotriptors can also be passed into the bladder via a cystoscope. During ultrasonic fragmentation, small stone fragments are rapidly broken off the stone and sucked out of the bladder through the ultrasonic probe.

Only the most powerful models can fragment smooth canine struvite stones, which tend to be relatively resistant to this form of fragmentation.

For struvite stones, nonsurgical strategies to induce dissolution are currently practiced, and similar approaches may be available soon for other stones. All stones require post-treatment preventive measures with long-term management and follow-up. Dissolution and prevention protocols must be based on an understanding of the pathogenesis of the stone type involved.

STRUVITE/APATITE STONES

Pathogenesis

Most urinary stones in dogs are composed of struvite, $MgNH_4PO_4 \cdot 6H_2O$. Struvite stones often contain minor quantities of carbonate-apatite, $Ca_{10}(PO_4 \cdot CO_3OH)_6(OH)_2$. The urine of most dogs is supersaturated with respect to struvite, provided they are eating a normal diet, and struvite crystals are commonly observed in the urine sediment of healthy dogs.

A number of factors determine the degree of supersaturation of struvite in urine. At metabolic equilibrium, the daily dietary intake (gastrointestinal absorption) of a substance must be matched by the daily excretion. Most canine diets contain abundant animal protein which is rich in magnesium and orthophosphate. As both of these are primarily excreted in the urine, gastrointestinal absorption is matched by urinary output. However, urinary orthophosphate exists in four different forms, and only the trivalent form (PO_4^{3-}) is incorporated into the struvite crystal lattice. The concentration of urinary trivalent phosphate varies with urinary pH. At a pH of 8.0 there is about 100 times more trivalent phosphate present than at a pH of 6.0.

$$H_3PO_4 \rightleftarrows H^+ + H_2PO_4^- \quad pKa = 2.1$$

$$H_2PO_4^- \rightleftarrows H^+ + HPO_4^{2-} \quad pKa = 7.2$$

$$HPO_4^{2-} \rightleftarrows H^+ + PO_4^{3-} \quad pKa = 12.7$$

Ammonia and ammonium constitute a major urinary buffer system.[33] Tubular secretion of ammonia is stimulated by secretion of hydronium ion (H^+) and prevents a drop in tubular fluid pH (Fig. 1-2). The amount (and therefore concentration) of ammonium ion in urine varies with the amount of acid excreted.

From the above, it is apparent that ammonium and trivalent phosphate concentrations in urine are dependent on pH, and the relationship is reciprocal. When urine pH is high, the amount of ammonium excreted will be low and more orthophosphate will be in the trivalent form. When urine pH is low, the amount of ammonium excreted will be high and less orthophosphate will be in the trivalent form. In this manner, extreme urinary supersaturation with respect to struvite is prevented in the normal dog.

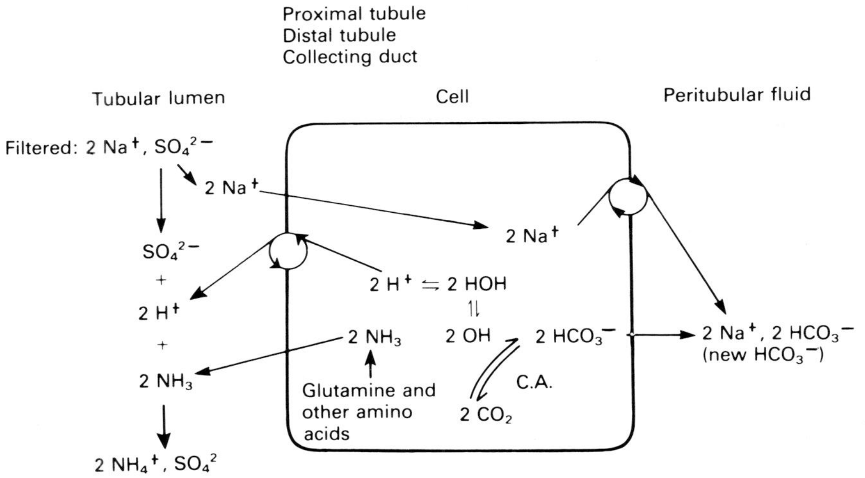

Fig. 1-2. Mechanism for the renal excretion of ammonium. (Valtin H: Renal Function. Mechanisms preserving fluid and solute balance in health. 2nd Ed. Little, Brown and Co., 1983.)

Most struvite stones in dogs form in the presence of a urease-producing urinary tract infection. Bacterial urease hydrolyzes urea as follows:

$$NH_2\text{–}CO\text{–}NH_2 + H_2O \xrightleftharpoons{\text{urease}} 2NH_3 + CO_2$$

Further hydrolysis yields

$$NH_3 + H_2O \rightleftharpoons NH_4^+ + OH^- \qquad pKa = 9.03$$

$$CO_2 + H_2O \rightleftharpoons H_2CO_3 \rightleftharpoons H^+ + HCO_3^- \qquad pKa = 6.33$$

$$HCO_3^- \rightleftharpoons H^+ + CO_3^{2-} \qquad pKa = 10.1$$

The urinary concentration of ammonium and carbonate increases, and as the urine pH becomes alkaline, the proportion of orthophosphate in the trivalent form increases. Thus, urine develops extreme supersaturation with respect to struvite and, to a lesser extent, carbonate-apatite, and the likelihood of stone formation is markedly increased.

At any given daily output of magnesium, ammonium, and trivalent phosphate, the concentration of all ions in urine depends on urine volume. Humans can concentrate urine to about 1,200 mOsm/kg H_2O, and struvite stones rarely, if ever, form if a urease-producing infection is absent. Cats can concentrate urine to 3,000 mOsm/kg H_2O, and struvite stones almost always form in the absence of detectable infection. Dogs may be intermediate in this respect, as they can concentrate urine to about 2,400 mOsm/kg H_2O. A urease-producing infection is usually present, but not always.[6] The pathogenesis of sterile struvite

Table 1-3. Protocol for Struvite Stone Dissolution

1. S/D prescription diet
2. Antibiotic treatment
3. Urease inhibitor treatment: acetohydroxamic acid 12.5 mg/kg bid (optional)
Aim: $U_{sp\ gr} \leq 1.015$; $U_{pH} \leq 6.0$; $P_{urea} < 10$ mg/dl
Urine culture—negative
4. Reradiograph every 4–6 wk
5. Continue until 4–6 wk after stones are undetectable on radiographs

stone formation in dogs is not known. Perhaps sterile struvite stones form in dogs that drink less and concentrate their urine more. Normal dogs vary considerably in their water intake, but most dogs on a high-protein diet tend to produce relatively concentrated urine.

Management: Dissolution

Struvite stones may be treated surgically or dissolved in situ by dietary manipulation. Dissolution strategies are aimed at reducing urinary concentrations of ammonium, magnesium, and trivalent phosphate, so urine becomes very undersaturated with respect to struvite. The following protocol has been advocated to induce struvite stone dissolution in the dog (Table 1-3):

1. Feed S/D prescription diet (Hills Pet Products, Inc., Topeka, KS 66601) exclusively. When fed to provide the daily energy requirements (45 to 75 cal/kg/d), dogs have reduced intake of protein, phosphate, and magnesium and a high intake of sodium. This results in reduced urinary magnesium and orthophosphate output, yields a net acidic metabolite load, and causes the production of acidic urine so the proportion of orthophosphate in the trivalent form is further reduced.

Dogs fed S/D drink large volumes of water and produce very dilute urine. This large water consumption appears to be due to the combination of low protein and high sodium levels in the diet. Low-protein diets reduce plasma urea levels and may reduce the development of medullary interstitial hypertonicity. High-sodium diets induce a solute diuresis. The diet may also affect thirst directly, but at present this is unclear. Increased urine volume reduces the concentration of all solutes in urine. The extremely low protein intake of dogs fed S/D results in reduced hepatic urea production and less urinary urea output. Reduced urea levels in urine may inhibit bacterial urease production.

When feeding S/D, absolutely no other food should be given, and adequate fresh water should be available at all times.

Dogs with infected struvite bladder stones form urine undersaturated with respect to struvite, and their stones dissolve slowly when they are fed S/D alone and given no other treatment.[24,34]

2. Treat any urease-producing infection. The degree of undersaturation is greater and the rate of dissolution of infected struvite stones is faster if the urine of dogs fed S/D is rendered bacteriologically sterile with antibiotic treatment.[26,34] Antibiotics should be chosen on the basis of sensitivity testing. If

the urine is culture negative and there is no evidence of infection in the urine sediment, antibiotic treatment is unnecessary.

3. Treatment to inhibit urease activity in urine may be useful when antibiotic resistance precludes long-term antibacterial sterilization of urine. Direct urease inhibition prevents conversion of urea to ammonia, even though bacteria may continue to survive. When a urease inhibitor was given to dogs fed a calculolytic diet, the struvite stone dissolution rate was greater than in dogs on the diet alone.[35] Acetohydroxamic acid (Lithostat, Mission Pharmacal Company, San Antonio, TX 78296) is the only urease inhibitor currently available. The recommended dose is 12.5 mg/kg po bid. Hemolytic anemia has been observed in dogs given higher doses.[36]

The first two strategies, diet and antibiotic treatment, are essential for reasonably fast struvite stone dissolution, whereas the third strategy, urease inhibition, is optional. The dissolution protocol should be continued for 4 weeks after radiographs have shown no evidence of remaining mineral densities in the urinary tract. Complete dissolution requires 8 to 20 weeks with an average of 14 weeks.[37] Stones that fail to reduce in size after 8 weeks are probably not composed of struvite and should be treated another way.

The choice between surgical and medical treatment may not be clear-cut. Owner compliance, patient acceptance of the diet, practice philosophy, and a knowledge of the indications and contraindications are necessary to make a decision. If stone dissolution is prolonged or fails, it may be more costly than surgical treatment. The following precautions are suggested to avoid problems with medical treatment.

Before starting medical dissolution, perform a physical examination, complete blood count, serum chemistry panel (including creatinine, urea, phosphate, calcium, albumin, SALT, and SAP), urinalysis, urine culture and sensitivity, abdominal radiographs, and blood pressure measurement, if possible. Contraindications include heart failure, edema, ascites, pleural effusion, hypertension, hepatic failure, renal failure, and hypoalbuminemia. Base the choice of antibiotic on the sensitivity results, and use the abdominal radiograph for baseline measurement of stone size.

After 4 weeks of treatment, another physical examination should be performed, with the same studies repeated. The dissolution diet may have to be discontinued if any of the above contraindications have developed; however, a degree of hypoalbuminemia can be expected and usually is well tolerated. Owner compliance is readily determined. When the protocol has been adhered to, the following results can be anticipated: urine pH ≤ 6.5; urine specific gravity (sp gr) ≤ 1.015; serum urea ≤ 10 mg/dl. The urine culture should be negative, and there should be minimal evidence of infection in the urine sediment. The radiographs should be compared with the previous ones for stone size.

Management: Prevention

Once surgical or medical treatment is complete, a preventive program (Table 1-4) to avoid development of extreme urinary supersaturation with respect to struvite can begin.

Table 1-4. Protocol for Struvite Stone Prevention

1.	Eliminate urease-producing urinary tract infections
2.	Maintain acidic urine, pH <6.5 (administer 200 mg/kg NH_4Cl or an equivalent acidifier, if necessary)
3.	Check pH of first voided urine before feeding weekly
4.	If pH > 7.0, return to veterinarian for urinalysis and culture
5.	Feed low-phosphate, low-magnesium, acid-ash diet (K/D[a]) (optional)

[a] Hills Pet Products, Inc., Topeka, KS 66601.

1. Reduce the concentration of the major struvite solutes in urine. Prescription diets U/D or K/D (Hills Pet Products, Inc., Topeka, KS 66601) lower urinary phosphate, magnesium, and urea output and may prevent struvite stone formation.[38]

2. Maintain an acidic urine pH. The degree of supersaturation with respect to struvite is exquisitely sensitive to changes in pH between 6.0 and 7.0 because the third dissociation of phosphoric acid to form trivalent phosphate has a pKa of 12.7. At pH 6, the proportion of orthophosphate in the trivalent phosphate form is extremely small. Dogs only form struvite stones when the urine pH rises above this level.

Urease-producing infections should be eliminated. Each week, owners should check the pH of the first voided urine in the morning after an overnight fast. Morning collection avoids confusion caused by the postprandial alkaline tide. The urine pH will be acidic in most dogs fed a normal diet, and provided it remains acidic, struvite stone formation should be prevented. If alkaline urine is detected, the patient should return for urinalysis and urine culture, and further treatment if infection is present.

When dogs are fed some commercial diets, the pH of the first voided urine in the morning can be alkaline, even though infection is not present. Urinary acidifiers may be mixed with the evening meal to produce acidic urine in the morning so that owners are not confused. The smallest effective dose should be used, and acidifiers should not be continued if the urine pH remains alkaline.

3. Increase urine volume. Salt added to the diet (1 g ($\frac{1}{6}$ tsp) per 5 kg daily), or water mixed with the food will increase urine volume. This dilutes all solutes in urine, and a urine sp gr of $\leq$ 1.025 is thought to indicate adequate dilution.

Although each proposed prevention strategy reduces urinary supersaturation with respect to struvite and therefore represents a step in the right direction, there are no known methods which definitely prevent struvite stones.

CYSTINE STONES

Pathogenesis

Dogs with cystinuria, a renal tubular amino acid reabsorption defect, form stones composed almost entirely of the amino acid cystine. Normal dogs reabsorb about 97 percent of the filtered load of cystine, while affected dogs reab-

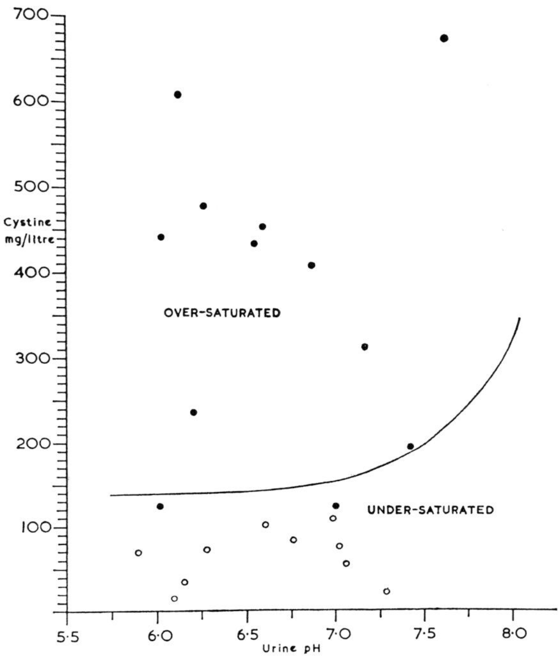

Fig. 1-3 The solubility curve for cystine versus pH in dog urine. The cystine content of specimens of dog urine is plotted against pH. (●) cystine-stone disease urines; (○) noncystine-stone disease urines. (Reprinted with permission from J Small Anim Pract 7:536, Treacher RJ: Uroliathiasis in the dog. II. Biochemical aspects. 1966, Pergamon Press, Ltd.)

sorb a much smaller proportion and may even exhibit net cystine secretion.[39] Reabsorption defects for the dibasic amino acids—lysine and others—also may be present, but they are clinically insignificant. Only cystine is so insoluble that it precipitates in urine and forms stones. Despite excessive urinary loss of cystine in cystinuric patients, plasma cystine levels remain the same as in normal dogs,[40] implying increased hepatic synthesis of cystine, probably from methionine.

Cystinuria is thought to be inherited as a sex-linked trait in Irish terriers and possibly also in other breeds.[13,14] Cystinuria occurs almost exclusively in male dogs, although two instances have been reported in female dogs, with only one developing cystine stones.[9] The defect has been reported in the dachshund, basset hound, bulldog, Chihuahua, Yorkshire terrier, Irish terrier, and mix breeds.

Cystine is relatively insoluble, and its concentration in urine depends on urine pH. Cystine dissociates to the more soluble cystinate with a pKa of about 8.0, so in more acidic solutions, a greater proportion of the total cystine (cystine and cystinate) is in the poorly soluble undissociated cystine form. At a urine pH of less than 7.0, only about 150 μg/ml total cystine can be dissolved, but solubility increases rapidly when the urine pH exceeds 7.5 (Fig. 1-3).[41] Dogs fed diets based on animal protein tend to pass acidic urine, so extreme cystine supersaturation develops. Colorless hexagonal crystals typically are observed in concentrated, acidic urine.

Table 1-5. Protocol for Cystine Stone Prevention

1. Reduce cystine concentration in urine
Give penicillamine (Cuprimine) 15 mg/kg po bid (with meals)
Increase urine volume with $U_{sp\ gr} \leq 1.025$
Add water to food
Add salt to food 1 g ($\frac{1}{6}$tsp)/5 kg daily (water ad lib)
2. Reduce cystine solubility
Alkalinize the urine ($U_{pH} \geq 7.5$)
Add $NaHCO_3$ to food 1 g ($\frac{1}{4}$tsp)/5 kg tid

Management

In human medicine, cystine stone dissolution has been reported after vigorous treatment with water diuresis, urinary alkalinization, and disulfide exchange therapy. Although the same strategies are recommended for canine cystine stone prevention, similar successful dissolution has not been reported.

In dogs, cystine stones should be surgically removed, the mineral content of the stone confirmed by analysis, and strategies to prevent recurrence instituted. As cystinuria in the dog is a life-long defect of tubular reabsorption, there is no cure. Cystine stones tend to recur within 12 months without post-surgical preventive management, and often they recur despite attempts at prevention.[9]

It is not known whether dietary protein restriction affects cystinuria in the dog. Although methionine supplementation increased urinary cystine output in dogs,[42] low-methionine diets were unreliable in decreasing urinary cystine output in humans.[43,44] Furthermore, methionine intake cannot be restricted for long because it is an essential amino acid.

The aim of preventive treatment is to reduce urine to an undersaturated state or at least to only minimal supersaturation with respect to cystine. The solubility of cystine in canine urine at pH 7.8 is twice that at 6.5 (Fig. 1-3). Strategies for prevention should aim to keep the plot of cystine concentration against pH below and to the right of the solubility curve in Fig. 1-3. Thus, treatment to prevent stone recurrence should reduce the concentration of cystine in urine and alkalinize the urine (Table 1-5).

The concentration of cystine in the urine is lowered by lowering cystine output and increasing urine volume, as follows. First, reduce cystine output with disulfide exchange substances. Penicillamine (Cuprimine, Merck Sharp

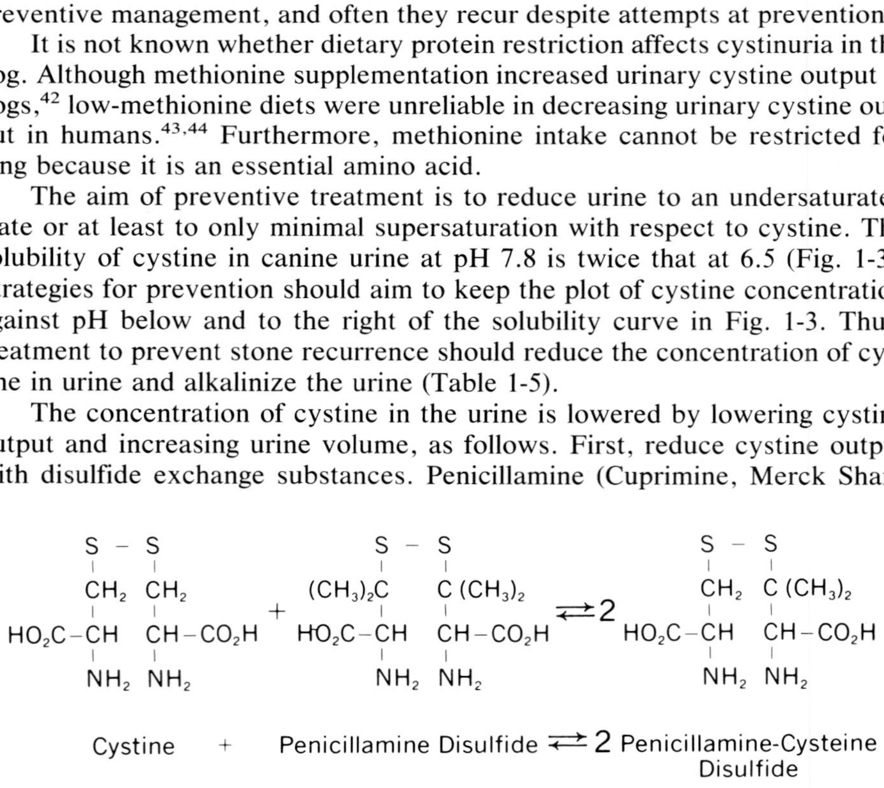

Fig. 1-4. Disulfide exchange reaction.

and Dohme, West Point, PA 19486) significantly reduces cystine output by reacting with cystine by exchange at the disulfide bridge to form penicillamine–cysteine, which is 50 times more soluble than cystine (Fig. 1-4).[45] The recommended dose in dogs, 15 mg/kg po bid, is said to reduce cystine excretion and prevent stone disease.[46] Unfortunately, about 40 percent of dogs treated with this dose exhibit anorexia and vomiting. The vomiting can be partially resolved in some dogs by giving the medication with meals, first at a reduced dose and then slowly building up to the recommended level. However, severe dose reduction or complete withdrawal is often necessary to resolve gastrointestinal side-effects. Second, increase urine volume by mixing water with the food, or by adding salt to the diet at 1 g ($\frac{1}{6}$ tsp)/5 kg daily. The urine volume should be doubled, and the effectiveness can be monitored by checking urine specific gravity (sp gr $\leqslant$ 1.025).

Increase cystine solubility by alkalinizing the urine. It can be seen from Figure 1-3 that the urine should be alkalinized to pH $\geqslant$ 7.5 by adding sodium bicarbonate at 1 g ($\frac{1}{4}$ tsp)/5 kg tid to the diet.[41]

Provided urine volume is doubled and the urine pH is maintained above 7.5, most cystinuric dogs will pass urine only slightly supersaturated or undersaturated for cystine.[41] Then only relatively small doses of penicillamine may be necessary to achieve 24-hour undersaturation for cystine.

If a dog has cardiac disease, hepatic disease, renal disease predisposing to sodium retention and edema, or hypertension, treatment with sodium chloride and sodium bicarbonate may be contraindicated. In these cases, urine volume should be increased by adding water to the diet.

URATE STONES

Pathogenesis

Most urate stones in dogs are composed of ammonium urate, although uric acid and sodium urate have been described.[6,7] In normal dogs, almost all urate formed from degradation of nucleic acids is metabolized by hepatic uricase to allantoin (Fig. 1-5), which undergoes renal excretion and is very soluble. In dalmatians, hepatic uricase activity is reduced and only 30 to 40 percent of uric acid is converted to allantoin, compared with about 90 percent in other breeds.[47] Their 24-hour urinary uric acid excretion is 400 to 600 mg, compared to approximately 60 mg in non-dalmatian dogs of similar size.[48,49] Dogs with portosystemic vascular anastomoses also tend to develop ammonium urate stones.[12]

Hepatic conversion of urate to allantoin probably is reduced in these patients as well.

Ammonium acts as a tubular buffer for secreted hydronium ion (H^+), and ammonium excretion is enhanced when an acid load is excreted.[33] Dalmatians fed a diet high in animal protein excrete a net acid load in the urine, and urinary ammonium output is increased. In dogs with portosystemic vascular anasto-

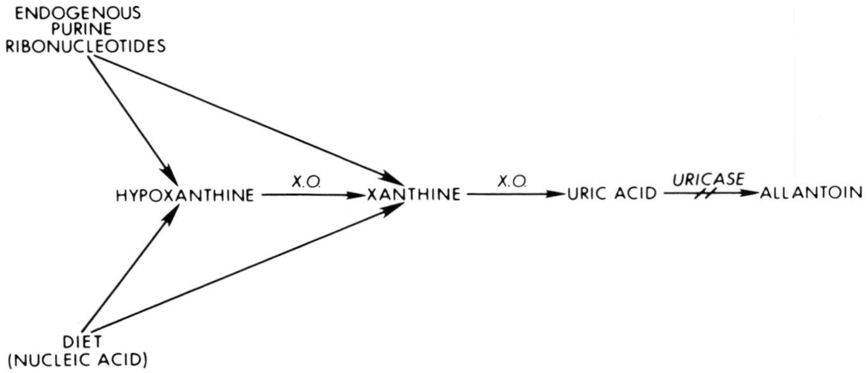

Fig. 1-5. Reactions leading to uric acid and allantoin formation. Uricase activity is greatly reduced in dalmatian dogs in vivo. X.O. = xanthine oxidase.

mosis, increased urinary ammonium output may be partially due to the increased filtered load of ammonia because plasma levels of ammonia tend to be elevated.

Ammonium urate is extremely insoluble, and most dogs probably produce supersaturated urine.[50] However, precipitation does not usually occur, because the urate salts adopt a colloidal form. In the colloidal state, the urate salt particles, composed of multiples of single urate salt molecules, are not large enough to settle out under the action of gravity, so they harmlessly pass out with the urine. However, colloidal particles can rapidly coalesce to form larger particles, with subsequent precipitation, in a process called flocculation. Brown spherulitic aggregates of ammonium urate form in urine, and these are commonly seen in the urine sediment of dalmatian dogs. Excessive flocculation leads to the formation of ammonium urate stones.

Although flocculation of ammonium urate particles is sensitive to all cations in urine, it is most sensitive to ammonium ion and hydrogen ion. As the concentration of ammonium, hydrogen ion, and urate increases in urine, ammonium urate colloidal particles flocculate (Figs. 1-6, 1-7).[51] Glycosaminoglycans in urine seem to prevent flocculation by coating individual colloidal particles and preventing further coalescence.[19,52] It is not known whether changes in urinary glycosaminoglycans may cause or prevent ammonium urate stone formation in the dog.

Management

Many dalmatians with ammonium urate stones present with urethral obstruction, and initial emergency care involves immediate relief of obstruction by catheterization, stone removal by urethral hydropropulsion, or urethrostomy. Medical dissolution of ammonium urate stones may be possible by using low-protein diets to reduce urinary urate output and by inducing alkaluria to

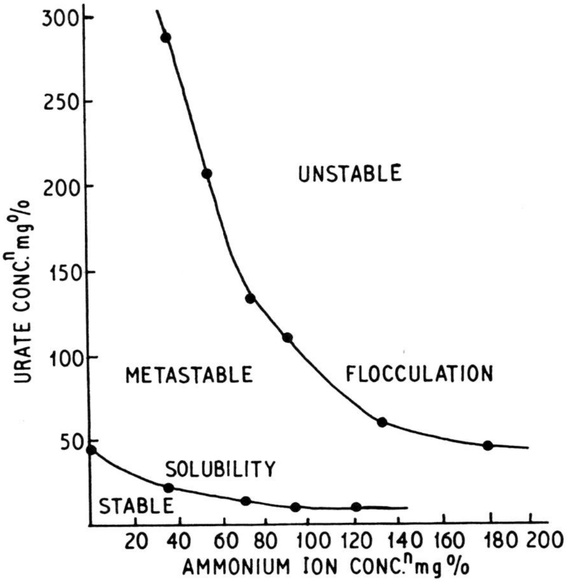

Fig. 1-6. Flocculation and solubility curves for ammonium urate over the normal range of urinary ammonium ion concentration. (Porter P: Physio-chemical factors involved in urate calculus formation. II. Colloidal flocculation. Res Vet Sci 4:592, 1963.)

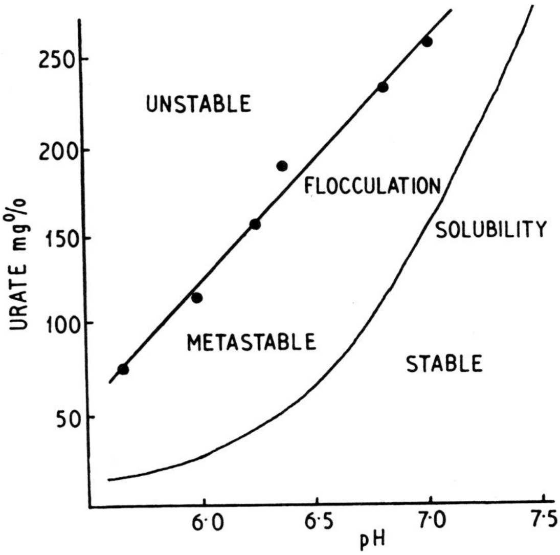

Fig. 1-7. Flocculation of lyophobic urate colloids over the range of physiologic pH. (Porter P: Physio-chemical factors involved in urate calculus formation. II. Colloidal flocculation. Res Vet Sci 4:592, 1963.)

Table 1-6. Protocol for Ammonium Urate Stone Prevention

1. Reduce urinary urate output
Give allopurinol (Zyloprim) 7 mg/kg po tid
2. Reduce urinary ammonium output
Add $NaHCO_3$ to food 1 g ($\frac{1}{4}$tsp)/5 kg tid ($U_{pH} \geq 7.0$)
Feed vegetable/rice diet (optional)
3. Increase urine volume ($U_{sp\ gr} \leq 1.025$)
Add water to food
Add salt to food 1 g ($\frac{1}{6}$tsp)/5 kg daily (water ad lib)

reduce urinary ammonium output. Treatment with the xanthine oxidase inhibitor allopurinol can further reduce urinary urate output, and enhanced fluid intake and urine volume would further reduce urinary ammonium and urate concentration. Extreme undersaturation should be possible, and preliminary results for dissolution are encouraging. Similar strategies are employed to prevent further ammonium urate stone formation.

Prevention strategies aim to reduce the concentration of ammonium and urate in urine to levels unlikely to induce flocculation (Table 1-6). The combined values should plot to the left and below the flocculation curve shown in Figure 1-6 and to the right and below the flocculation curve in Figure 1-7.

The first goal is to reduce urinary urate output. Allopurinol (Zyloprim, Burroughs Wellcome Co, Research Triangle Park, NC 27709) given at 3 to 10 mg/kg po tid provides significant xanthine oxidase inhibition. As a result, the nucleic acid metabolite load is excreted as a combination of xanthine, hypoxanthine, uric acid, and allantoin, rather than almost entirely as uric acid (Fig. 1-5). Allopurinol ribonucleotide may also cause negative feedback inhibition of de novo synthesis of nucleotides and further reduce urate production.[53] The effect of allopurinol on reducing urinary urate output is variable. Urate levels should be measured, and the dose may have to be increased if they are still high or if stone formation persists.

The second goal is to reduce urinary ammonium output. Alkalinization of the urine to pH $\geq$ 7 minimizes renal ammonia production. This can be achieved by administering $NaHCO_3$ 1 g ($\frac{1}{4}$ tsp)/5 kg po tid with food.

The third goal is to increase urine volume to reduce the concentration of all dissolved solutes in urine by adding salt—1 g ($\frac{1}{6}$ tsp)/5 kg daily—to the diet, or by mixing water with food so that the urine sp gr $\leq$ 1.025.

If a dog has cardiac disease, hepatic disease, renal disease predisposing to sodium retention and edema, or hypertension, treatment with sodium chloride and sodium bicarbonate may be contraindicated, and urine volume should be increased by adding water to the diet.

The proposed strategies were developed for use in dalmatians with reduced hepatic uricase activity but an otherwise normal liver. They may not be safe for use in dogs with portosystemic vascular anastomosis, because such animals tend to develop hypoalbuminemia, edema, and ascites when fed a low-protein diet. The safety of allopurinol in this setting has not been established. Alkalinization can predispose to hepatoencephalopathy because of increased gastrointestinal absorption of dietary protein metabolites.

Very low protein diets also may substantially reduce daily urinary urate output, so a dietary approach may achieve the same goals as allopurinol in this respect. For many years dalmatian breeders have advocated feeding a sodium-rich vegetable protein diet to prevent ammonium urate stone formation. The diet results in formation of high-volume, alkaline urine which substantially reduces the urinary concentration of ammonium and urate. The diet is theoretically sound and may be of some practical value.

CALCIUM OXALATE

Pathogenesis

Calcium oxalate stones, the most common type in humans in Western countries, usually develop in the renal pelvis. They are less common in dogs, occurring mostly in older animals in the bladder. Most of the information concerning calcium oxalate stones comes from extrapolation of data in humans. A normal person's urine is supersaturated for calcium oxalate, and on a theoretical basis, stone disease is observed only when supersaturation becomes extreme, when crystallization inhibitors are depleted, or when there is a delay in particle movement through the urinary tract.[15]

In humans, extreme urinary supersaturation for calcium oxalate can be attributed to factors causing hypercalciuria and to factors causing hyperoxaluria (Table 1-7).

Most stone-formers fall into the idiopathic group, and there is no clear understanding of the reason calcium is hyperabsorbed or of the nature of the "renal calcium leak." Enteric hyperoxaluria appears to result from increased colonic permeability to oxalate due to bile acid malabsorption. Fatty acid malabsorption may also bind intestinal fat to calcium and thus increase oxalate absorption.

It is not clear how hyperuricosuria predisposes to calcium oxalate stones. Precipitation of calcium oxalate may occur on preformed uric acid crystallites, or sodium urate may interact with and deplete a urinary inhibitor of calcium oxalate crystallization.[52,54,55]

In patients with no detectable metabolic abnormality, urinary calcium oxalate saturation can be normal and stone formation may result from an absence of urinary inhibitors of calcium oxalate crystallization. Ribonucleic acid, glycosaminoglycans, magnesium, citrate, and pyrophosphate have all been identified as calcium oxalate crystallization inhibitors.[56] A calcium oxalate crystal growth inhibitor, possibly a glycosaminoglycan, appears to be added to dog urine in the bladder.[18] Anatomical defects may induce stone disease by retaining particles and allowing increased time for particle growth.

Table 1-7. Causes of Calcium Oxalate Stone Disease in Humans

Hypercalciuria
Increased intestinal calcium absorption
Vitamin D intoxication
Milk-alkali syndrome
Sarcoidosis
Rapid resorption of calcium from bone
Immobilization
Hyperparathyroidism (5.8%)[a]
Hyperthyroidism
Renal tubular acidosis (0.4%)[a]
Idiopathic
Hyperabsorptive (54.3%)[a]
Renal calcium leak (8.3%)[a]
Hyperoxaluria
Primary hyperoxaluria
Enteric hyperoxaluria (2.1%)[a]
Ileal disease
Small bowel bypass or resection
Pancreatectomy
Excessive oxalate and oxalate precursor intake
Spinach and other vegetables
ascorbic acid
ethylene glycol
Hyperuricosuria (8.7%)[a]
No metabolic abnormality (10.8%)[a]
Anatomical defects
Medullary sponge kidney

[a] Refers to the percentage of human calcium oxalate stone patients in each etiological category.

(Data from Breslau NA, Pak CYC: Metabolic evaluation. p. 168. In Roth RA, Finlayson B (eds): Stones: Clinical Management of Urolithiasis. Williams & Wilkins, Baltimore, 1983.)

Management

Some of the causes listed in Table 1-7 may be involved in calcium oxalate stone formation in dogs, but at this time none have been described. Information concerning normal calcium excretion rates of dogs during fasting, calcium loading, and feeding of a standard diet would enable a reasonable workup of calcium oxalate stone-formers, but such information currently is unavailable.

A routine workup should include serum calcium, phosphate, bicarbonate, and chloride to investigate the possibility of hyperparathyroidism and renal tubular acidosis. Calcium oxalate stone dissolution by medical means has not yet been established, and current treatment is surgical removal followed by preventive strategies (Table 1-8). A protocol for prevention may include:

1. Reducing urinary calcium output by administration of thiazide diuretics. Hydrochlorothiazide (Thiuretic, Parke-Davis, Morris Plains, NJ 07950) given at 2 to 4 mg/kg po bid reduces calcium excretion, probably by decreasing ECF volume and GFR and enhancing fractional Ca^{2+} reabsorption in the prox-

Table 1-8. Protocol for Calcium Oxalate Stone Prevention

1. Reduce urinary calcium output
Hydrochlorothiazide (Thiuretic) 2–4 mg/kg po bid
2. Reduce intestinal calcium absorption and increase urinary calcium oxalate solubility
Potassium citrate (UrocitK) to effect ($U_{pH} \simeq 7.0–7.5$)
3. Increase urine volume
Add water to food ($U_{sp\,gr} \leq 1.025$)
(do not supplement food with NaCl)

imal tubule. Long-term thiazide therapy may also diminish intestinal calcium absorption.

2. Reducing intestinal calcium absorption and increasing urinary calcium oxalate solubility. Alkalinizing agents may reduce gastrointestinal calcium absorption by converting a greater percentage of ingested calcium into the non-ionized form which is less readily absorbed. Furthermore, in alkaline urine, urinary citrate levels are increased; citrate inhibits stone formation by complexing with calcium ions and reducing calcium oxalate supersaturation. Citrate also inhibits crystal growth by blocking growth sites on the crystal surface. Potassium citrate (Urocit-K, Mission Pharmcal Company, San Antonio, TX 78296) given at 5 to 20 mEq po tid to achieve a urine pH between 7.0 and 7.5 is a suitable alkalizer for this purpose although safety has not been established in the dog.

3. Increasing water consumption by adding water to the food or by flavoring the drinking water so that urine sp gr ≤ 1.025. Salt should not be added to the diet to increase water consumption, because increased sodium intake offsets the effect of thiazide diuretics on calcium excretion and enhances hypercalciuria.

The above guidelines represent extrapolation from experience with calcium oxalate stone formation in humans, and the author has limited experience with their effect on calcium oxalate stone prevention in the dog.

REFERENCES

1. Finlayson B: Where and how does urinary stone disease start? An essay on the expectation of free and fixed particle urinary stone disease. In van Reen R (ed): Idiopathic Urinary Bladder Stone Disease. Fogarty International Center Proceedings. No. 37. p. 7. Department of Health Education and Welfare Publication. No (NIH) 77–1063, Washington, DC, 1977
2. Wickham JEA: The matrix of renal calculi. p. 323. In Chisholm GD, Williams DI (eds): Scientific Foundations of Urology. 2nd Ed. Year Book Medical Pubs Inc, Chicago, 1982
3. Finco DR, Rosen E, Johnson KH: Canine urolithiasis: A review of 133 clinical and 23 necropsy cases. J Am Vet Med Assoc 157:1225, 1970
4. White EG, Treacher RJ, Porter P: Urinary calculi in the dog. I. Incidence and chemical composition. J Comp Pathol Ther 71:201, 1961

5. White EG: Symposium on urolithiasis. I. Introduction and incidences. J Small Anim Pract 7:529, 1966
6. Bovee KC, McGuire T: Qualitative and quantitative analysis of uroliths in dogs: Definitive determination of chemical type. J Am Vet Med Assoc 185:983, 1984
7. Hicking W, Hesse A, Gebhardt M, Vahlensieck W: Analytiche untersuchungen an harnsteinen von saugetieren. p. 40. In Vahlensieck W, Gasser G (eds): Harnsteinsymposien Bonn-Wien. Darmstadt Steinkopff Verlag, 1981
8. Brodey RS, Thomson R, Sayer P, Eugster B: Silicate renal calculi in Kenyan dogs. J Small Anim Pract 18:523, 1977
9. Brown NO, Parks JL, Greene RW: Canine urolithiasis: Retrospective analysis of 438 cases. J Am Vet Med Assoc 170:414, 1977
10. Clark WT: The distribution of canine urinary calculi and their reoccurrence following treatment. J Small Anim Pract 15:437, 1974
11. Klausner JS, Osborne CA, O'Leary TP, et al: Experimental induction of struvite uroliths in miniature schnauzer and beagle dogs. Invest Urol 18:127, 1980
12. Marretta SM, Pask AJ, Greene RW, Liu S: Urinary calculi associated with portosystemic shunts in six dogs. J Am Vet Med Assoc 178:133, 1981
13. Brand E, Cahill GF, Kassell B: Canine cystinuria. V. Family history of two cystinuric Irish terriers and cystine determinations in dog urine. J Biol Chem 133:431, 1970
14. Kirk RW (ed): A catalogue of congenital hereditary disorders of dogs (by breed). p. 1225. In Small Animal Practice. Current Veterinary Therapy, Vol. 8. WB Saunders, Philadelphia, 1983
15. Burns JR, Finlayson B: Why some people have stone disease and others do not. p. 3. In Roth RA, Finlayson B (eds): Stones: Clinical Management of Urolithiasis. Williams & Wilkins, Baltimore, 1983
16. Vermeulin CW, Goetz R: Experimental urolithiasis VIII: Furadantin in treatment of experimental *Proteus* infection with stone formation. J Urol 72:99, 1954
17. Breslau NA, Pak CYC: Urinary saturation, heterogeneous nucleation, and crystallization inhibitors in nephrolithiasis. p. 13. In Coe FL (ed): Nephrolithiasis. Churchill Livingstone, New York, 1980
18. Smith LH, Martin X, Opgenorth T, Werness PG, Romero JC: Influence of the bladder on calcium oxalate crystal growth inhibition in dogs. Kidney Int 25:177, 1984, abstract.
19. Porter P: Colloidal properties of urates in relation to calculus formation. Res Vet Sci 7:128, 1966
20. Chang SY, Gill WB, Vermeulen CW: Povidone-iodine bladder injury in rats and protection with heparin. J Urol 130:383, 1983
21. Pawelchak J, Flanagan DR, Simonelli AP: Rates and mechanisms of dissolution of renal calculi. I. Rates and mechanism of pure calcium oxalate monohydrate in acid and EDTA solution. p. 539. In Smith LH, Finlayson B, Robertson WG (eds): Proceedings of the Fourth International Symposium on Urolithiasis Research. Plenum Press, New York, 1981
22. Pawelchak J, Flanagan DR, Simonelli AP: Rates and mechanisms of dissolution of renal calculi. II. Development and discussion of potential models for dissolution of oxalate calculi. p. 545. In Smith LH, Finlayson B, Robertson WG (eds): Proceedings of the Fourth International Symposium on Urolithiasis Research. Plenum Press, New York, 1981
23. Pawelchak J, Flanagan DR, Simonelli AP: Rates and mechanisms of dissolution of renal calculi. III. Mechanisms and rates of dissolution of simulated oxalate calculi

in acid and EDTA solutions. p. 551. In Smith LH, Finlayson B, Robertson WG (eds): Proceedings of the Fourth International Symposium on Urolithiasis Research. Plenum Press, New York, 1981
24. Abdullahi S, Osborne CA, Leininger JR, et al: Evaluation of a calculolytic diet in female dogs with induced struvite urolithiasis. Am J Vet Res 45:1508, 1984
25. Griffith DP, Bragin S, Musher DM: Dissolution of struvite urinary stones. Experimental studies in vitro. Invest Urol 13:351, 1976
26. Osborne CA, Abdullahi S, Polzin DJ, Leininger JR, Kruger JM: Current status of medical dissolution of canine and feline uroliths. p. 53. In van Marthens E (ed): Proc. The Seventh Annual Kal Kan Symposium for the Treatment of Small Animal Diseases. Kal Kan Foods Inc, Vernon, CA, 1984
27. Thomas J, Landier JF, Charpentier C, Steg A: Cystinic lithiasis and its treatment. p. 248. In Roth RA, Finlayson B (eds): Stones: Clinical Management of Urolithiasis. Williams & Wilkins, Baltimore, 1983
28. de Vries A: Clinical management of uric acid lithiasis. p. 228. In Roth RA, Finlayson B (eds): Stones: Clinical Management of Urolithiasis. Williams & Wilkins, Baltimore, 1983
29. Bojrab MJ (ed): Current Techniques in Small Animal Surgery. Lea & Febiger, Philadelphia, 1975
30. Osborne CA, Abdullahi S, Klausner JS, Johnston GR, Polzin DJ: Nonsurgical removal of uroliths from the urethra of female dogs. J Am Vet Med Assoc 182:47, 1983
31. Piermattei DL, Osborne CA: Nonsurgical removal of calculi from the urethra of male dogs. J Am Vet Med Assoc 159:1755, 1971
32. Senior DF: Electrohydraulic shock-wave lithotripsy in experimental struvite bladder stone disease. Vet Surg 13:143, 1984
33. Pitts RF: Physiology of the kidney and body fluids. 3rd Ed. Year Book Medical Pubs, Chicago, 1974
34. Senior DF, Thomas WC Jr, Gaskin JM, Finlayson B: Relative merit of various nonsurgical treatments of infection stones in dogs. p. 589. Urolithiasis and Related Clinical Research. New York, Plenum Press, 1985
35. Osborne CA, Klausner JS, Krawiec DR, Griffith DP: Canine struvite urolithiasis: Problems and their dissolution. J Am Vet Med Assoc 179:239, 1981
36. Krawiec DR, Osborne CA, Leininger JR: Effect of acetohydroxamic acid on dissolution of canine struvite uroliths. Am J Vet Res 45:1266, 1984
37. Osborne CA, Abdullahi S, Krawiec D, Klausner JS, Lipowitz A, Gaudet D, Griffith DP: Strategy for nonsurgical removal of canine struvite uroliths. Sci Proc Am Anim Hosp Assoc Meeting, South Bend, IN, 1982
38. Lewis LD, Morris ML, Jr: Small Animal Nutrition. 2nd Ed. Mark Morris Associates, Topeka, KS, 1984
39. Bovee KC: Genetic and metabolic diseases of the kidney, p. 339. In Bovee KC (ed): Canine Nephrology. Harwal, Philadelphia, 1984
40. Treacher RJ: The aetiology of canine cystinuria. Biochem J 90:494, 1964
41. Treacher RJ: Urolithiasis in the dog. II. Biochemical aspects. J Small Anim Pract 7:537, 1966
42. Thier SO, Segal S: Cystinuria. p. 1579. In Stanbury JB, Wyngaarden JB, Fredrickson DS (eds): The Metabolic Basis of Inherited Diseases 4th Ed. McGraw-Hill, New York, 1978
43. Kolb FO, Earll JM, Harris HA: Disappearance of cystinuria in a patient with prolonged low methionine diet. Metabolism 16:378, 1967

44. Zinneman HH, Jones JE: Dietary methionine and its influence on cystine excretion in cystinuric patients. Metabolism 15:915, 1966
45. Lotz M, Potts, JT, Jr, Holland JM, et al: D-penicillamine therapy in cystinuria. J Urol 95:257, 1966
46. Bovee KC: Urolithiasis. p. 355. In Bovee KC (ed): Canine Nephrology. Harwal, Philadelphia, 1984
47. Porter P: Urinary calculi in the dog. II. Urate stones and purine metabolism. J. Comp Pathol 73:119, 1963
48. Kuster G, Shorter RG, Dawson B, et al: Uric acid metabolism in Dalmatians and other dogs. Arch Intern Med 129:492, 1972
49. Lemieux G, Plante GE: The effect of starvation in the normal dog including the Dalmatian coach hound. Metabolism 17:620, 1968
50. Porter P: Physico-chemical factors involved in urate calculus formation. I. Solubility. Res Vet Sci 4:580, 1963
51. Porter P: Physico-chemical factors involved in urate calculus formation. II. Colloidal flocculation. Res Vet Sci 4:592, 1963
52. Robertson WG, Knowles CF, Peacock M: Urinary acid mucopolysaccharide inhibitors of calcium oxalate crystallization. p. 331. In Fleisch H, Robertson WG, Smith LH, Vahlensieck W (eds): Urolithiasis Research. Plenum Press, New York, 1976
53. Wyngaarden JB, Kelley WN: Gout. p. 916. In Stanbury JB, Syngaarden JB, Fredrickson DS (eds): The Metabolic Basis of Inherited Diseases 4th Ed. McGraw-Hill, New York, 1978
54. Coe FL, Lawton RL, Goldstein RB, Tembe V: Sodium urate accelerates precipitation of calcium oxalate in vitro. Proc Soc Exp Biol Med 149:926, 1975
55. Pak CYC, Barilla DE, Holt K, et al: Effect of oral purine load and allopurinol on the crystallization of calcium salts in urine of patients with hyperuricosuric calcium urolithiasis. Am J Med 65:593, 1978
56. Robertson WG, Peacock M: Risk factors in the formation of urinary stones. In Chisholm GD, Williams DI (eds): Scientific Foundations of Urology 2nd Ed. Year Book Medical Pubs, Chicago, 1982, p 267
57. Brodey RS: Canine urolithiasis. J Am Vet Med Assoc 126:1, 1955
58. Weaver AD: Canine urolithiasis. Incidence, chemical composition and outcome of 100 cases. J Small Anim Pract 11:93, 1970
59. Breslau NA, Pak CYC: Metabolic evaluation. p. 168. In Roth RA, Finlayson B (eds): Stones: Clinical Management of Urolithiasis. Williams & Wilkins, Baltimore, 1983

2 Canine Prostatic Disease

Jill W. Verlander

The frequency of prostatic disease in the intact, mature male dog makes it of great importance in small animal practice. Depending on the nature of the problem, prostatic disease can result in chronic medical care, surgical therapy, loss of breeding potential, morbidity, or even death. At times it presents a diagnostic or therapeutic challenge.

Cats also may suffer from prostatic disease, although it is rare. Of the few published feline reports, prostatic neoplasia has been the predominant diagnosis.[1]

In the following pages, the normal structure and function of the prostate, the spectrum of prostatic disease, diagnostic procedures, and therapeutic options are discussed.

NORMAL STRUCTURE AND FUNCTION OF THE PROSTATE

The prostate is an accessory sex gland, the only one in the dog, and its function is to produce seminal fluid, which serves as a transport and life support medium for sperm. In the normal mature dog, the gland is retroperitoneal and bilobed. It encircles the proximal urethra and neck of the bladder. In addition to the discrete gland, a small amount of prostatic tissue is present in the wall of the urethra. The cat also has a discrete prostate gland and disseminated prostatic tissue.[2]

Microscopically, the prostate consists of glandular acini supported by a stroma of connective tissue and smooth muscle. The secretions of the acini are transported via excretory ducts lined with transitional epithelium and are emptied into the prostatic urethra. The rate of fluid production and secretion is increased during erection and ejaculation, but even under resting conditions, seminal fluid is continuously produced and secreted into the proximal urethra, often resulting in reflux of prostatic fluid into the bladder.[3] The pH of prostatic fluid in normal dogs has been reported to range from 6.0 to 7.4, but numerous studies indicate that canine prostatic fluid is consistently acidic, pH 6.0 to 6.4, both in normal animals and in dogs with experimentally induced bacterial prostatitis.[3–6] This may be an important consideration in the choice of an antibiotic for the treatment of prostatitis, and will be discussed later.

The prostate depends upon the presence of androgens to maintain its size and function. An alteration in the level of androgens or in the relative amounts of androgens and estrogens can contribute greatly to the generation of a disease state. Similarly, manipulation of sex hormone levels by surgical or medical means can have marked effects on the prevention, progression, or elimination of prostatic disease.

THE SPECTRUM OF PROSTATIC DISEASE

Prostatic disorders fall within three categories—hyperplasia, inflammation, and neoplasia. These categories can be subdivided as follows:

1. Hyperplasia
   a. Benign prostatic hyperplasia
   b. Cystic hyperplasia
2. Inflammation
   a. Acute prostatitis
   b. Chronic prostatitis
   c. Prostatic abscess
3. Neoplasia
   a. Primary prostatic neoplasia
   b. Metastatic neoplasia

Any of the disorders listed can exist as isolated entities but frequently occur in combination, with two or three disease processes at work simultaneously. In such cases, overt disease may obscure the signs of an occult problem. For example, if prostatic neoplasia coexists with acute bacterial prostatitis, the inflammatory component may be readily diagnosed, but the neoplastic condition may be inapparent unless extensive diagnostic procedures are done initially or after there is less than the expected response to appropriate therapy for the inflammatory disease.

In addition, paraprostatic cysts are often covered in discussions of prostatic disease. These structures are thought to develop from remnants of the müllerian duct rather than the prostate, and will not be discussed.

PROSTATIC HYPERPLASIA

Prostatic hyperplasia is unquestionably the most common prostatic disease in the dog. It is reported to be present in 60 to 80 percent of intact male dogs over five years of age.[7] Prostatic hyperplasia is thought to be a result of an imbalance of androgen and estrogen levels. The most common form is glandular hyperplasia, which is due to an absolute or relative androgen excess. Unlike the disease in humans, there is diffuse involvement of the gland rather than nodular hyperplasia, with an increase in the size of the acini and no formation of new acini or ducts.[8] Hyperplasia can also be due to fibromuscular proliferation and squamous metaplasia as a result of an absolute or relative estrogen excess, such as in dogs with a Sertoli cell tumor or in those subjected to exogenous estrogen therapy.[9–11] Cyst formation is often present with this form of prostatic hyperplasia and may predispose the animal to prostatitis, presumably due to stasis of flow of prostatic fluid, resulting in diminished protection from ascending bacterial infection.[10,11]

In uncomplicated prostatic hyperplasia of either form, clinical signs are usually absent. Occasionally there may be constipation or hematuria without signs of inflammation. Only rarely is dysuria noted, in contrast to the situation in man, where dysuria is a frequent complication of prostatic hyperplasia. The difference can be explained by the relative absence of prostatic tissue in the urethral wall of the dog. Perineal hernias are associated with prostatic hyperplasia, particularly with the fibromuscular form.[7] The development of perineal hernias may be due in part to mechanical stresses created by partial obstruction of the pelvic canal by the enlarged prostate and subsequent tenesmus. However, the association of perineal hernias with fibromuscular hyperplasia suggests that estrogen excess may play a direct role in the weakening of perineal soft tissue structures.

Typically, physical examination of the dog with uncomplicated prostatic hyperplasia reveals a prostate that is enlarged (often over the pelvic brim), symmetrical, firm, smooth or slightly irregular, movable, and painfree.

PROSTATIC INFLAMMATION

Inflammatory disease of the prostate is also a common entity and is often seen in conjunction with prostatic hyperplasia, particularly cystic hyperplasia, or with neoplasia. The inflammation may be acute or chronic, with or without abscessation.

The infectious agent usually reaches the prostate by an ascending route from the urethra, although hematogenous infection does occur. The most common organisms isolated are *Mycoplasma* spp., *E. coli, Proteus* spp., *Pseudomonas* spp., *Staphylococcus* spp., and *Streptococcus* spp.[3,12] *Brucella canis* is sometimes the cause of prostatitis in the breeding animal, and mycotic prostatitis is occasionally diagnosed.[3] Although sterile prostatitis is well recognized in humans, it has not been documented in dogs.[8]

Prostatic abscesses may be small or large, single or multiple, and closed or open. Open abscesses usually drain into the prostatic urethra, but occasionally abscesses rupture and drain into the abdomen, with disastrous consequences.

The pathogenesis of prostatitis is not well understood, but it is logical to assume that infection of the gland occurs as a result of increased exposure to an infectious agent, decreased host resistance to infection, or a combination of both. Increased exposure of the prostate to an infectious agent would result from urinary tract infection or septicemia. Decreased host resistance may be caused by many factors. There may be a defect in the cellular or humoral immune system or an alteration in the composition of the prostatic fluid causing a reduction in its antibacterial properties. In particular, in bacterial prostatitis in man there is a reduction in the amount of a low molecular weight zinc compound present in prostatic fluid. This has been implicated as a cause of diminished antibacterial activity.[6,10]

Stasis of flow of prostatic secretions may reduce resistance to infection. Fluid stasis may be caused by a reduction in the volume of prostatic fluid produced, which may occur with prostatic hyperplasia of either form or with exogenous estrogen administration.[13] Prostatic fluid stasis may also result from partial or total obstruction of excretory ducts, as seen with squamous metaplasia or neoplasia. It is easy to see why prostatitis often accompanies prostatic hyperplasia or neoplasia.

The clinical signs of prostatitis vary considerably and are determined to a large extent by the severity and time course of the inflammation. In acute prostatitis there may be fever, anorexia, depression, tenesmus, constipation, and painful defecation. Urinary tract signs may include dysuria due to concurrent urethritis or cystitis, hematuria, pyuria, urinary incontinence, or a bloody or purulent urethral discharge. The dog may be reluctant to rise from recumbency, may stand with its back arched or abdomen tensed, and may move with a stiff, guarded gait.

The clinical signs of chronic prostatitis are more subtle. The most frequent sign is recurrent urinary tract infection, but constipation, tenesmus, and urethral discharges may also be noted.

Although prostatic abscessation is most often associated with chronic or recurrent prostatic infection, it is usually not recognized until signs of acute inflammation are apparent.

Physical examination of the dog with acute prostatitis reveals an enlarged prostate that is usually symmetrical, smooth, bilobed, movable, and often painful. The prostate of the dog with chronic prostatitis is also usually enlarged, symmetrical, bilobed, and movable. However, in chronic prostatitis, palpation rarely elicits a painful response, and the surface or texture of the gland may be irregular due to scar formation from previous episodes of inflammation.

If a prostatic abscess is present, the physical findings vary with the size and location of the abscess, in addition to the degree of inflammation of the prostatic parenchyma. The prostate is usually asymmetrical and painful. If the abscess is large or near the surface of the gland, the examiner may feel a fluctuant area. If the abscess is open and draining into the prostatic urethra, a hemorrhagic or purulent urethral discharge is often seen after palpation.

PROSTATIC NEOPLASIA

Prostatic neoplasia is uncommon in the dog in comparison to man. However, it is not a rare event, as was once thought. The increased frequency of identification of prostatic cancer is probably a result of improved diagnostic methods, although the possibility of an increase in the actual incidence of the disease, for whatever reason, cannot be discounted.

The cause of prostatic cancer in dogs, as in man, has not been elucidated. The role of androgens in the pathogenesis of the disease has not been determined. Similarly, the effect of estrogens in control of prostatic neoplasia remains controversial.

The tumor type most often seen in dogs is adenocarcinoma.[14] Leiomyosarcoma and transitional cell carcinoma, arising within the prostate or invading from a primary urethral tumor, are occasionally seen.

Clinical signs of prostatic neoplasia may be absent in the early stages of the disease. However, extensive local invasion of the tumor or concurrent prostatitis or prostatic abscessation can produce signs similar to acute prostatitis. Common signs are hematuria, dysuria, a hemorrhagic or purulent urethral discharge, and signs related to pain in the caudal abdomen and pelvis (constipation, painful defecation, arching of the back, stiffness of gait, reluctance to rise, and tensing of the abdomen). Occasionally, the tumor may cause partial or total obstruction of the urethra or ureters, which, in addition to dysuria, may cause renal failure and associated signs.

In some cases, dogs with prostatic neoplasia manifest signs produced by metastasis of the tumor to distant sites. Probably the most frequent such sign is lameness or pain due to bony metastases. Pulmonary metastases severe enough to cause signs of respiratory distress are rarely seen.

Hypercalcemia has been reported as a paraneoplastic condition related to prostatic adenocarcinoma in humans.[15] The possibility of prostatic neoplasia should be considered by the veterinarian when unexplained hypercalcemia is observed.

Physical examination findings vary with the severity of the disease, as would be expected. In the early stages, results of examination may be normal. In advanced stages, the prostate is often asymmetrical and irregular in texture, with obliteration of the median fissure. The gland is usually enlarged and is often far over the brim of the pelvis, so that it can only be palpated abdominally, rather than per rectum. Palpation of the gland often elicits a painful response or a hemorrhagic urethral discharge.

Local invasion may cause the gland to be fixed to the floor of the pelvis, and urethral or ureteral obstruction may cause a palpable distension of the urinary bladder or renomegaly due to hydronephrosis. Regional lymph node involvement may result in palpable sublumbar lymphadenopathy.

DIAGNOSTIC PROCEDURES

The diagnostic procedures applicable to the identification of prostatic disease are many and varied. The choice of particular procedures appropriate for an individual case depends on the clinical impression gained from the history and physical exam and on the wishes of the owner. For example, an intensive investigation would be inappropriate in the case of an asymptomatic animal with symmetrical prostatomegaly, unless the owner desired substantiation of a clinical diagnosis of benign prostatic hypertrophy. Similarly, an animal with clinical signs suspicious of prostatic neoplasia deserves a thorough investigation unless the owner wishes to limit the diagnostic efforts.

The following diagnostic procedures are pertinent to the diagnosis of prostatic disease in small animal practice.

Urinalysis/Urine Culture

Urinalysis, including examination of the urine sediment, and bacterial culture of the urine are helpful, particularly in the diagnosis of acute prostatitis. As a result of reflux of prostatic fluid into the urinary bladder, pyuria and hematuria, with or without bacteriuria, are usually found in acute prostatitis or an open prostatic abscess.[16] It is preferable to obtain the urine sample by cystocentesis to avoid contamination of the sample or the urinary bladder by organisms or cellular elements present in the distal urinary tract.

In addition, urinalysis and urine culture are helpful in the diagnosis of chronic prostatitis, since the most frequent sign of chronic prostatitis is recurrent urinary tract infection. Although the combination of a history of recurrent episodes of dysuria, documentation of urinary tract infection, and physical findings of prostatomegaly is not definitive evidence of chronic bacterial prostatitis, it should at least lead the clinician to pursue this possibility by means of further procedures. Cytologic examination and culture of an ejaculate or prostatic wash or observation of the animal's response to appropriate therapy for chronic prostatitis is indicated.

In benign prostatic hypertrophy uncomplicated by inflammation, the sediment from a urine sample obtained by cystocentesis usually contains normal elements or red blood cells only. Similarly, in the early stages of neoplasia, hematuria alone is a frequent finding, but the urinalysis may be normal.[16]

Prostatic Wash

A prostatic wash for cytologic examination and bacterial culture is often the most useful procedure in the diagnosis of prostatic disease. The procedure has been well described and is outlined in Table 2-1. The procedure requires little equipment and rarely requires chemical restraint. However, patient cooperation is not necessary, since it can be done successfully with the animal under sedation or anesthesia.

Prostatic washes are reserved for the animal with signs suggestive of in-

Table 2-1. Procedure for Prostatic Wash

Using aseptic technique:

1. Empty bladder by allowing the dog to void or by catheterization if there is residual urine.
2. Pass urinary catheter into bladder, if not already done.
3. Rinse bladder with 5 ml sterile physiologic saline or lactated Ringer's solution. Be sure the solution does not contain a bacteriostatic agent.
4. Aspirate this fluid from the bladder and save it. This is the pre-prostatic massage sample (PM-1).
5. Withdraw the urinary catheter until the tip is just caudal to the prostate. This is determined by rectal palpation.
6. Massage the prostate per rectum for 1 min.
7. Slowly infuse 5 ml sterile physiological saline or lactated Ringer's solution through the catheter while occluding the urethral orifice to prevent reflux of the solution.
8. Aspirate while advancing the catheter into the bladder. The fluid recovered is the post-prostatic massage sample (PM-2).
9. Reserve samples of PM-1 and PM-2 for bacterial culture.
10. Centrifuge remainder of PM-1 and PM-2 and examine sediments for cytology using a Wright's stain.

(Modified from Barsanti JA, Shotts EB, Prasse K, et al: Evaluation of diagnostic techniques for canine prostatic diseases. J Am Vet Med Assoc 177:160, 1980.)

flammation or neoplasia. Usually, bacterial cultures of prostatic fluid washings are negative in animals with benign prostatic hyperplasia, and cytologic examination shows hemorrhage at most.

A difference between the pre-prostatic massage sample (PM-1) and the post-prostatic massage sample (PM-2) (Table 2-1) is often apparent by gross examination in animals with acute prostatitis or an abscess draining into the prostatic urethra. In such cases, the PM-2 contains more cellular material than the PM-1 and appears more opaque or blood-tinged. There may be flocculent material in the PM-2 as well. In this instance, the expense of culture and cytologic evaluation of the PM-1 may be avoided. Microscopic examination of the PM-2 will reveal numerous leukocytes, erythrocytes, and sometimes bacteria. A thorough search for glandular cells should be made, since overt inflammation may mask underlying neoplasia. However, hyperplastic glandular cells are not diagnostic of neoplasia, since hyperplastic cells may be exfoliated in severe inflammation alone. The opinion of a veterinary cytologist should be obtained when the question of hyperplasia versus neoplasia arises, and confirmation of the diagnosis should be sought by means of additional diagnostic procedures.

In cases where prostatic involvement in urinary tract infection is not readily apparent, a comparison of the sediments and cultures of the PM-1 and PM-2 can be helpful. This is particularly true in the case of chronic prostatitis. It has been suggested that a single dose of ampicillin be given before the prostatic wash when the urinalysis shows signs of infection, since this antibiotic is concentrated in the urine and does not penetrate the prostate very well.[5] In this way, if prostatitis is present, elimination of the urinary tract infection at the time of the prostatic wash will increase the difference between the cytology and culture results from the PM-1 and PM-2 and will more clearly implicate the prostate as a source of infection. Quantitative cultures of PM-1 and PM-2 are desirable in order to make an accurate comparison.

It should be remembered that *Mycoplasma* spp. were the most frequently isolated organisms in one clinical study.[12] Since these organisms will not grow in routine aerobic culture conditions, a special request for culture of the sample on a pleuropneumonia-like organism agar plate may be indicated in chronic cases.

Ejaculation

Collection of the latter part of an ejaculate also will provide prostatic fluid for cytology and culture. The advantages of this technique over a prostatic wash are that it is noninvasive, eliminating the possibility of contaminating the urinary tract by catheterization and that it provides an undiluted sample of prostatic fluid, allowing measurement of the pH. However, the procedure cannot be done on fractious or unresponsive animals, and contamination of the sample by the testicular portion of the ejaculate, the urethral contents, or preputial material results in more false positive cultures than does the prostatic wash technique. Cytologic examination of an ejaculate is more sensitive than the prostatic wash for the diagnosis of prostatic inflammation, but the prostatic wash appears to be more helpful for identification of neoplasia.[16] This may be due to exfoliation of neoplastic cells by the prostatic massage or lack of response to the stimulus to ejaculate in animals that are painful from prostatic neoplasia.

Needle Aspiration or Biopsy Techniques

Needle aspiration of the prostate gland is simple, useful, and safe in most instances. A 20- to 22- gauge $1\frac{1}{2}$-inch needle is used, and an aspirate of the gland is obtained for cytology and culture. The procedure can be done with or without chemical restraint, depending on the patient. The placement of the needle can be random, guided only by palpation, guided by fluoroscopy if the prostate is not readily palpable, or guided by ultrasound in order to specifically sample areas of abnormal sonic density. The approach is usually transabdominal, but a transperineal approach has been used by some.

Direct sampling of the prostate provides material for cytology and culture not contaminated by urine or by urethral or preputial elements. The hazards of this technique include rupture of a prostatic abscess (creating local or generalized peritonitis), hemorrhage, and perforation of the rectum or urethra. However, complications are rare when the procedure is done cautiously.

A limitation of needle aspiration is the small area of the gland represented in the material obtained. Focal lesions are easily missed. Multiple aspirations from various areas of the gland may increase the accuracy of the procedure but also increase the risk of complications.

Similarly, needle biopsy, providing a core of tissue for histopathology as well as cytology and culture, increases the amount of information gained but also increases the hazards of the procedure. In some cases, a laparotomy and wedge biopsies are indicated. Numerous tissue samples should be obtained from suspicious areas of the prostate and the sublumbar lymph nodes to improve the chance of an accurate histopathologic diagnosis.

Needle aspiration of enlarged sublumbar lymph nodes, when possible, is an excellent technique for the diagnosis of prostatic neoplasia. There is no chance of confusion of hyperplastic glandular cells with neoplastic cells when the lymph node is sampled, since only carcinomatous cells will metastasize to the nodes. The needle placement is guided by palpation, fluoroscopy, or ultrasound. Risks include hemorrhage or perforation of the colon. However, in a study of fine-needle sublumbar lymph node aspiration in men, there were no complications from the procedure, and a definitive diagnosis of carcinoma was made on the basis of cytology in 54 percent of the patients in which metastatic prostatic adenocarcinoma was suspected.[17] These patients were spared open biopsies as a result of this procedure.

Complete Blood Count

An elevation of the absolute count of mature or immature neutrophils is often seen in acute prostatitis or abscessation. Occasionally the total neutrophil count is low early in these diseases, presumably due to sequestration of neutrophils in the gland before enough time has elapsed for the bone marrow response to be evident in the peripheral blood.

In some cases of prostatic neoplasia, chronic hemorrhage or chronic systemic disease results in anemia. The duration and severity of the blood loss or systemic disease determines the type of anemia.

Serum Chemical Analyses

Serum chemistries are rarely helpful in the diagnosis of prostatic disease in the dog, except as part of preoperative assessment, particularly in aged animals, or as an aid to identification of diffuse involvement or unrelated concurrent disease in systemically ill animals. The serum creatinine and urea nitrogen levels are useful when ureteral or urethral obstruction is present. Also, as mentioned earlier, the development of hypercalcemia has been noted in some cases of prostatic adenocarcinoma in humans.

Radiographs

Radiographic procedures, whether survey or contrast studies, often provide little or no more significant information than does a thorough physical examination. They are useful in determining the size and symmetry of the prostate when a thorough palpation of the gland is not possible. However, important information may be gained by radiography when prostatic neoplasia is present. The radiographic signs of prostatic neoplasia that may be found on survey radiographs are prostatomegaly (often asymmetrical), sublumbar lymph node enlargement, periosteal proliferation along the ventral aspects of the caudal lumbar vertebrae or in the pelvic canal, osteolytic lesions (particularly in

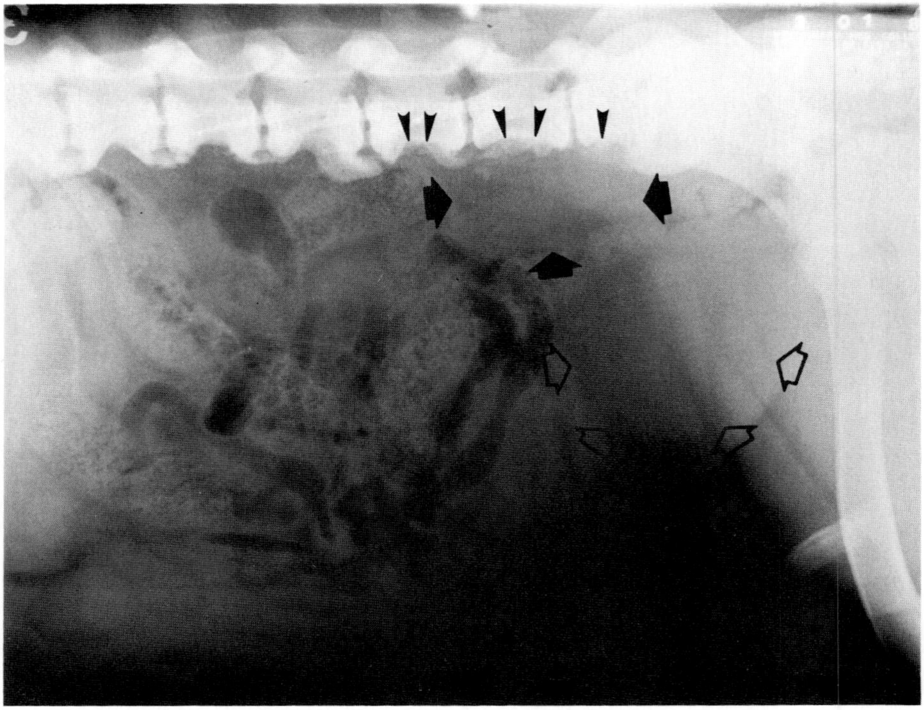

Fig. 2-1. Survey radiograph of a dog with prostatic adenocarcinoma. Note enlarged prostate (open arrows), enlarged sublumbar lymph nodes (closed arrows), and periosteal proliferation along the ventral aspects of the caudal lumbar vertebrae (arrowheads). This dog also has marked spondylosis deformans, which should not be confused with the periosteal proliferation.

long bones), and pulmonary metastases.[18] Several of these signs are illustrated in Figure 2-1.

Contrast studies may be useful at times. Retrograde urethrocystography may identify a prostatic abscess if it is open to the urethra. Neoplasia may also be demonstrated if there is involvement of the urethra or urinary bladder creating a filling defect. Reflux of contrast material into the prostate is no indication of current disease. In fact, urethroprostatic reflux was demonstrated in 21 of 24 normal beagles.[19] Excretory urography may be used to determine whether ureteral obstruction from a prostatic tumor is present, bearing in mind the problems associated with systemic administration of iodinated contrast material to an azotemic animal.

Ultrasound

Although ultrasound units are not available in most veterinary practices, increasing numbers of veterinarians, particularly those in large animal or mixed practices, have access to two-dimensional ultrasound devices. The prostate is

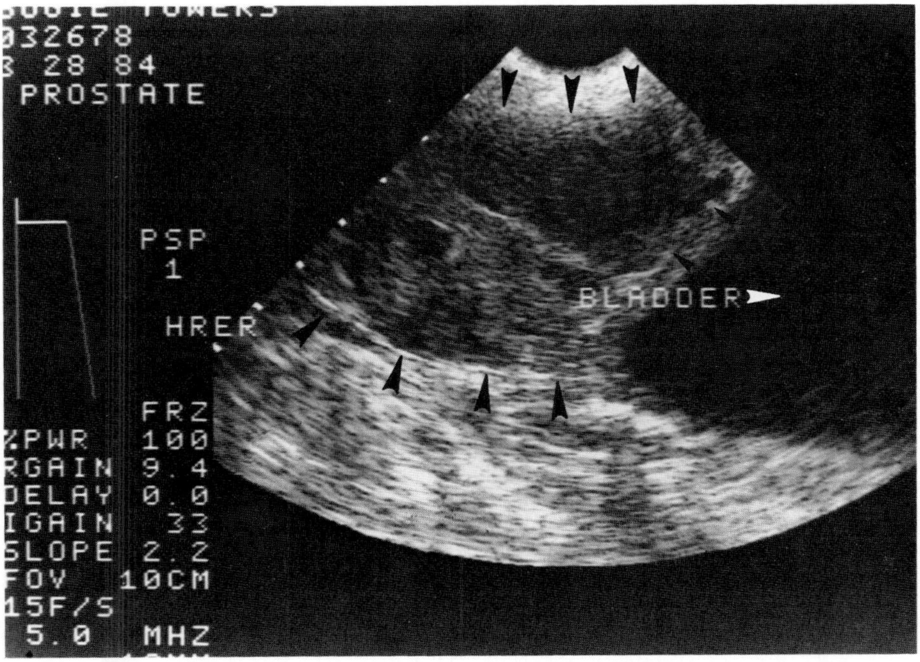

Fig. 2-2. Two-dimensional sonograph of a dog with prostatic abscesses. The large echolucent (black) structure on the right is the fluid-filled urinary bladder. The prostate (arrowheads) is enlarged with many echolucent, or fluid-filled, areas within the parenchyma. Needle aspirates of these areas, under ultrasonic guidance, confirmed the clinical suspicion of abscessation.

ideally suited to ultrasonic examination for the following reasons: the diseased prostate is frequently enlarged and at least partially or totally abdominal in location, there are few structures between the skin and the gland, and the urinary bladder may be used as a landmark. Most animals can be examined with minimal restraint, either standing or in lateral or dorsal recumbency. Usually patient preparation consists of shaving the inguinal area, at most. The procedure is safe in that neither the patient nor the examiner is exposed to ionizing radiation.[20]

Ultrasonography of the prostate provides information regarding the consistency of the parenchyma, in addition to the size and shape of the gland. Abscesses or cysts in the parenchyma are seen as echolucent (black) areas (Fig. 2-2), since the transmitted sound waves pass through fluid-filled structures and are only reflected back to the transducer by tissue interfaces. Although the nature of the fluid in the cavity cannot be determined sonographically, the device can be used to guide a needle directly into the cavity and aspirate fluid for cytology and culture. In addition, the size of an abscess can be accurately measured, which can help determine the need, or the immediacy of the need, for a laparotomy and surgical drainage.

In humans, a transrectal approach with the ultrasonic transducer is used most often. A tumor appears as an abnormally echolucent or echogenic area within the parenchyma. Localization of a suspicious area is followed by guided needle aspiration or biopsy and positive cytology or histopathology results provide a definitive diagnosis.[21,22] Perhaps similar techniques will be developed to this level of sophistication in veterinary medicine, providing a means of early diagnosis of neoplasia and improved chances of survival of affected dogs.

Acid phosphatase. Acid phosphatases are present in numerous tissues, including blood, bone, spleen, kidney, liver, intestine, and prostate. In the prostate, acid phosphatase activity is limited to the epithelial cells, and, unlike most tumors, prostatic carcinoma cells have been shown to be high in acid phosphatase activity.[23] In recent years, numerous investigators have attempted to refine both immunoassays and enzymatic assays for the prostatic isoenzyme and to establish parameters for the use of a serum acid phosphatase assay as a means of detecting or staging prostatic adenocarcinoma in man. However, the initial wave of enthusiasm has waned because of the low specificity of the enzyme elevation for prostatic neoplasia or metastasis. It is currently accepted that the usefulness of acid phosphatase assays lies in following response to therapy in patients with prostatic adenocarcinoma and high serum acid phosphatase levels before treatment.[24]

The role of serum acid phosphatase in the diagnosis, staging, or monitoring of prostatic adenocarcinoma in dogs has yet to be established.

TREATMENT OF PROSTATIC DISEASE

At present, the options for the therapy of prostatic disease in dogs are limited. Currently accepted treatment involves either manipulation of sex hormone levels by castration or administration of estrogens, administration of antibiotics, or surgical drainage or removal of the prostate gland. Symptomatic or supportive therapy is indicated in some instances.

Hormonal Manipulation

Castration is by far the best means of hormonal control of prostatic disease, except when general anesthesia is contraindicated or when the patient is a breeding animal. Castration permanently removes the source of androgens (or estrogens in Sertoli cell tumor), which are essential to the development of prostatic hyperplasia. Since prostatic hyperplasia is a major contributing factor in the pathogenesis of prostatic infection, castration is indicated not only in the treatment of symptomatic benign prostatic hypertrophy but also in cases or chronic, recurrent, or severe prostatitis. Subsequent atrophy of the prostate and appropriate antibiotic therapy, when indicated, usually result in rapid regression of clinical signs of prostatic disease and prevent recurrence. Exceptions include cases where prostatic neoplasia, abscessation requiring drainage, or severe squamous metaplasia are present.

It should be mentioned here that although *early* castration prevents the development of prostatic hyperplasia and prostatitis, the prostate gland should still be examined in castrated dogs. First, there are no studies to support or refute the hypothesis that early castration leads to a decreased risk of prostatic carcinoma in dogs.[25] Second, castration of a dog with preexisting prostatic disease does not resolve the problems mentioned above, that is, neoplasia, surgical abscesses (or cysts), and squamous metaplasia. Prior castration should be taken into account when interpreting the results of physical examination—rapid atrophy of the prostate follows castration, and what is considered normal size for the prostate of an intact dog should be considered abnormally large for a castrated dog.

The second method of hormonal manipulation for treatment of prostatic disease is administration of exogenous estrogens. The routine use of such agents should be discouraged, particularly in patients in which there are no absolute contraindications to castration. The known systemic side effects of exogenous estrogens include feminization and nonregenerative anemia, which may be either dose-related and reversible or idiosyncratic and irreversible. Although exogenous estrogens will cause glandular cell atrophy in the prostate by suppressing pituitary gonadotrophin release and testosterone production, they also cause fibromuscular hypertrophy, squamous metaplasia, and decreased prostatic fluid production and flow, predisposing the animal to cyst formation and infection.[7,10,26] In cases where castration is contraindicated, it is better to rely on symptomatic or antibiotic therapy for the management of prostatic hyperplasia or bacterial prostatitis, remembering that chronic medical treatment will be necessary in the intact dog.

The role of castration or estrogen therapy in the treatment of prostatic adenocarcinoma has not been elucidated. There may be a direct effect of sex hormones on the behavior of the neoplastic cells. Also, castration or estrogen therapy may be palliative when hyperplasia or infection coexist with prostatic neoplasia, since these benign processes often compound the clinical manifestations of neoplasia. When palliation of the disease is desired, the risks and benefits of hormonal manipulation should be considered on an individual basis.

Antibiotics

The three major considerations in the selection of an antibiotic for the treatment of bacterial prostatitis are the bacterial culture and antibiotic susceptibility results, the status of the "blood–prostate barrier," and the pH of the prostatic fluid.

The choice of an antibiotic in any case should be limited to the agents indicated by the culture and susceptibility testing of prostatic fluid obtained by prostatic massage, ejaculation, or needle aspiration of the prostate, or of urine if prostatic fluid is not obtained.

The ability of the antibiotic to cross the blood–prostate barrier should be considered. In the normal animal, the concentration of most antibiotics in prostatic fluid is low due to the absence of active transport of these drugs into the prostate and the low rate of diffusion of most antibiotics across the lipid cell membranes.[10]

In acute prostatitis, epithelial cell permeability is increased and higher tissue levels of antibiotics are achieved than in normal animals. Therefore, the selection of a drug indicated by the culture results is generally adequate, assuming that the drug and dose chosen will produce high blood and urine levels.[26]

In chronic prostatitis, the epithelial cell permeability is not significantly increased, and the lipid solubility of the antibiotics effective against the particular organisms present should be considered. Lipid solubility is determined by a number of factors, including the ionization, size and shape, and protein binding of the molecule. Of these, ionization is probably the most important.[10]

Since most antibiotics are weak acids or weak bases, the pH of the fluid medium in which they are dissolved determines the degree of ionization of the drug. Since blood is usually slightly alkaline, drugs that are weak acids (e.g., penicillin derivatives, cephalothin, sulfas) are ionized in the blood and are unable to cross lipid membranes, resulting in low levels of the drug in the prostatic parenchyma. However, drugs that are weak bases (e.g., trimethoprim, erythromycin, oleandomycin, rosaramicin) are not ionized in blood and are relatively lipid soluble. Moreover, after diffusion across the cell membranes, these drugs become ionized in the acidic environment of the prostate and are trapped within the parenchyma. Of the four drugs mentioned, trimethoprim and rosaramicin have broader ranges of activity and are generally preferred over erythromycin and oleandomycin. In addition, tetracycline, being amphoteric, and chloramphenicol have adequate lipid solubility to achieve effective concentrations within the prostate.[10,26]

Although the pH of prostatic fluid was consistently acidic in recent studies of both normal dogs and dogs with experimentally induced bacterial prostatitis, others have reported alkaline prostatic fluid in men and dogs with bacterial prostatitis.[4,5,7,10] With this in mind, measurement of the pH of prostatic fluid obtained by ejaculation or needle aspiration is advised. If the prostatic fluid is alkaline, slightly acidic antibiotics are trapped more effectively than basic antibiotics and may achieve higher prostatic tissue concentrations. It should be kept in mind that the testicular portion of the ejaculate is normally alkaline, and contamination of the prostatic portion with it will give a spuriously high pH.

The minimum duration of antibiotic treatment for acute bacterial prostatitis recommended by various authors ranges from 2 to 3 weeks.[10,26] In the treatment of chronic prostatitis, a minimum of 8 weeks has been advised, with prostatic fluid cultures at 4 weeks to assure control of the infection.[26] After the treatment period, the animal should be reevaluated by physical examination, and prostatic fluid should be cultured at least twice, at 3 to 4 week intervals. This is particularly important in the animal with chronic prostatitis, in order to allow early detection of recurrence.

Surgical Treatment

Surgery, other than castration, is most often indicated for treatment of large prostatic abscesses or cysts. Various techniques to provide drainage of such lesions have been described, including marsupialization, drainage with a

Foley catheter, or placement of Penrose drains through the abscessed prostate.[11,27] Currently, the most popular method is that involving the use of Penrose drains. Small abscesses can sometimes be resolved by percutaneous drainage and medical therapy.[11]

Subtotal or total prostatectomy has been recommended by some authors for the treatment of abscesses, chronic prostatitis, or prostatic neoplasia.[26,27] Total prostatectomy is an extremely difficult procedure and is not recommended, except when done by an experienced surgeon and as a salvage procedure. Transurethral prostatectomy is an easier and less traumatic procedure, and it is hoped that the technique will be more widely used in veterinary medicine in the years to come.

Whenever prostatic surgery is done, multiple tissue samples of the prostate and sublumbar lymph nodes should be obtained and submitted for histopathology in an attempt to detect occult neoplasia.

Radiation Therapy

Both external beam irradiation and interstitial irradiation, alone or in combination, have been used in humans for the treatment of prostatic carcinoma. Radiation of either form is suitable only for nonmetastatic neoplasia. Longer follow-up times are necessary to determine if radiation therapy of any kind provides a better survival time than the natural course of the disease or other modes of therapy.[28]

Radiation therapy has been used at some veterinary institutions, but there are no published reports of efficacy.

Chemotherapy

There is evidence that single-agent or combined chemotherapy is beneficial in men with advanced prostatic carcinoma that is not responsive to hormonal therapy.[29] It remains to be seen if chemotherapy is helpful in the management of canine prostatic carcinoma.

Supportive and Ancillary Care

Supportive measures, such as fluid therapy, are often needed when systemic illness coexists with prostatic disease, as in patients with renal failure, septicemia, or toxemia secondary to prostatic neoplasia or infection. Laxatives are indicated when constipation results from prostatomegaly or pain. Analgesics should be given when needed, particularly in cancer patients where palliation of the disease is the goal. Zinc supplementation has been suggested in the treatment of prostatitis, since zinc levels are low in the prostatic fluid of men with prostatic infection. However, despite the fact that prostatic zinc levels increase with supplementation, no improvement in response to therapy or recurrence rate has been demonstrated when compared with antibiotic therapy alone.[26]

PROGNOSIS

Although prostatic disease is a problem frequently encountered in small animal practice, most cases can be managed successfully or even cured when appropriate diagnostics and therapeutics are instituted. The exception is prostatic carcinoma, in which case, due consideration should be given to the *quality* of life to be expected with any form of therapy, since at present the prognosis is poor for survival or comfort, regardless of the treatment.

REFERENCES

1. Hawe RS: What's your diagnosis? J Am Vet Med Assoc 182:1257, 1983
2. Ellenport CR: Carnivore urogenital apparatus. p. 1576. In Getty R (ed): The Anatomy of the Domestic Animals. 5th Ed., Vol. 2. WB Saunders Co, Philadelphia, 1975
3. Barsanti JA, Finco DR: Canine bacterial prostatitis. Vet Clin North Am: [J Small Anim Pract] 9:679, 1979
4. Barsanti JA, Shotts EB, Prasse K, et al: Evaluation of diagnostic techniques for canine prostatic diseases. J Am Vet Med Assoc 177:160, 1980
5. Barsanti JA, Prasse KW, Crowell WA, et al: Evaluation of various techniques for diagnosis of chronic bacterial prostatitis in the dog. J Am Vet Med Assoc 183:219, 1983
6. Fair WR, Cordonnier JJ: The pH of prostatic fluid: a reappraisal and therapeutic implications, J Urol 120:695, 1978
7. Greiner TP, Johnson RG: Diseases of the prostate gland. p. 1459. In Ettinger SJ (ed): Textbook of Veterinary Internal Medicine: Diseases of the Dog and Cat. 2nd Ed, Vol. 2. WB Saunders Co, Philadelphia, 1983
8. McNeal JE: The prostate gland: Morphology and pathobiology. Monog Urol 4:3, 1983
9. Eaton CL, Pierrepoint CG: Epithelial and fibroblastoid cell lines derived from the normal canine prostate. II. Cell proliferation in response to steroid hormones. Prostate 3:493, 1982
10. Klausner JS, Osborne CA: Management of canine bacterial prostatitis. J Am Vet Med Assoc 182:292, 1983
11. Zolton GM, Greiner TP: Prostatic abscesses—a surgical approach. J Am Anim Hosp Assoc 14:698, 1978
12. Ling GV, Branam JE, Ruby AL, et al: Canine prostatic fluid: techniques of collection, quantitative bacterial culture, and interpretation of results. J Am Vet Med Assoc 183:201, 1983
13. Wheaton LG, deKlerk DP, Strandberg JD, et al: Relationship of seminal volume to size and disease of the prostate in the beagle. Am J Vet Res 40:1325, 1979
14. Hargis AM, Miller LM: Prostatic carcinoma in dogs. Comp Cont Ed Pract Vet 5:647, 1983
15. Mahadevia PS, Ramaswamy A, Greenwald ES, et al: Hypercalcemia in prostatic carcinoma. Report of eight cases. Arch Intern Med 143:1339, 1983

16. Barsanti JA, Finco DR: Evaluation of techniques for diagnosis of canine prostatic diseases. J Am Vet Med Assoc 185:198, 1984
17. von Eschenbach AC, Zornoza J: Fine needle percutaneous biopsy: A useful evaluation of lymph node metastasis from prostatic cancer. Urology 20:589, 1982
18. Thrall DE: Radiographic aspects of prostatic disease in the dog. Comp Cont Ed Pract Vet 3:718, 1981
19. Feeney DA, Johnston GR, Osborne CA, et al: Maximum-distention retrograde urethrocystography in healthy male dogs: Occurrence and radiographic appearance of urethroprostatic reflux. Am J Vet Res 45:948, 1984
20. Cartee RE, Rowles T: Transabdominal sonographic evaluation of the canine prostate. Vet Radiol 24:156, 1983
21. Harada K, Igari D, Tanahashi Y: Gray scale transrectal ultrasonography of the prostate. J Clin Ultrasound 7:45, 1979
22. Fritzsche PJ, Axford PD, Ching VC, et al: Correlation of transrectal sonographic findings in patients with suspected and unsuspected prostatic disease. J Urol 130:272, 1983
23. Henneberry MO, Engel G, Grayhack JT: Acid phosphatase. Urol Clin North Am 6:629, 1979
24. Fair WR, Heston WDW, Kadmon D, et al: Prostatic cancer, acid phosphatase, creatinine kinase-BB and race: A prospective study. J Urol 128:735, 1982
25. Evans JE, Zontine W, Grain E: Prostatic adenocarcinoma in a castrated dog. J Am Vet Med Assoc 186:78, 1985
26. Barsanti JA, Finco DR: Treatment of bacterial prostatitis. p. 1101. In Kirk RW (ed): Current Veterinary Therapy. Small Animal Practice, Vol. 8. WB Saunders, Philadelphia, 1983
27. Knecht CD: Diseases of the canine prostate gland (part II): Surgical techniques. Comp Cont Ed Pract Vet 1:426, 1979
28. Stamey TA: Cancer of the prostate. Monogr Urol 3:67, 1982
29. Slack NH, Murphy GP: A decade of experience with chemotherapy for prostate cancer. Urology 22:1, 1983

3 Feline Urologic Syndrome

Jeanne A. Barsanti
Delmar R. Finco

The term *feline urologic syndrome* (FUS) has been used by different authors in different ways. This necessitates that each author define his usage. Unfortunately many authors have used the term without definition, leading to considerable confusion in interpreting their findings. Also the existence of variable definitions makes it imperative for the reader to critically evaluate each article dealing with FUS rather than to extrapolate the findings to the reader's own definition.

Currently, FUS is usually defined in one of three ways. It may be used to include all cases of hematuria and dysuria with or without urethral obstruction in cats of both sexes. Some authors have tried to extrapolate these signs to a single cause, such as crystalluria or urolithiasis,[1] or viral infection.[2] Other authors have pointed out that such signs can occur with any type of lower urinary tract disease, and thus the term FUS is merely a shortened way to say feline lower urinary tract disease.[3,4] Causes of such signs would include infection (bacterial, viral, mycoplasmic), trauma, toxins, neoplasia, and neurologic dysfunction. The first type of definition attributes all cases with similar signs to one cause, which is unlikely. The other type of definition is so broad that the fact that most cats with such signs have no easily identifiable cause is lost.

A third type of definition is one of exclusion. With this definition, FUS refers to idiopathic lower urinary tract disease of cats. Any definitive cause of the signs of hematuria, dysuria, and urethral obstruction is ruled out by appropriate laboratory testing. This definition recognizes that cats do have other urinary tract diseases that result in hematuria, dysuria, and obstruction, such as bacterial cystitis, urolithiasis, neoplasia, or trauma, but also recognizes that a large percentage of cats with these signs have no such identifiable cause. This definition does not imply that the unknown cause is always the same, but rather that further work is needed on this subset of cats to define the causes. Use of this definition puts a burden on the author to define exactly the subset of cats to which he or she is referring. It necessitates some laboratory work (at least urinalysis and perhaps urine culture and survey and contrast radiography) to rule out identifiable causes of the same signs. This definition is flawed in that it defines FUS by what it is not. It would be better to know all the causes of hematuria and dysuria in cats. Much further research is needed to accomplish this goal.

This chapter will use the exclusionary definition of FUS as often as possible and will try to identify references where a different definition of FUS has been used. Thus, other causes of hematuria and dysuria, such as bacterial cystitis, urolithiasis, neoplasia, trauma, and neurologic dysfunction, will be covered only briefly. However, it is very important for the reader to recognize that such diseases do occur in cats, and diagnostic efforts are indicated, both so that cats with persistent signs are correctly managed and so that trials of treatment efficacy deal with a characterized population of cats.

The relationship of urolithiasis to FUS is controversial because of the different definitions of FUS. Some authors use the terms synonymously.[1,5] We prefer to differentiate FUS from urolithiasis, since hematuria and dysuria without obstruction has not been proven to be caused by microcrystalluria, and since urethral obstruction in male cats is more frequently due to urethral plugs than to true uroliths. Urethral plugs are disorganized precipitates composed of variable amounts of crystalline material (primarily struvite) in a colloidal matrix, whereas uroliths are concretions with organized crystalline structure. The proportions of crystalline material to matrix vary, with some plugs being completely matrix[5,6] and other being more sabulous.[3,7,8] This chapter will deal only with urethral plugs and not with urolithiasis except where noted.

INCIDENCE

In most studies of incidence, FUS has been defined as hematuria, dysuria, and/or urethral obstruction. In spite of being evaluated at different times in different countries, incidence has been consistently about 0.6 percent.[9–12] No evidence of increasing incidence with time was found in one limited study,[10] in spite of claims of increasing incidence.[1] Although incidence studies were not conducted prior to the 1970s, it is of interest to note that one veterinarian writing in 1958 considered urethral obstruction of the male domestic cat to be common.[13] Studies reporting an "incidence" of up to 10 percent are actually referring to proportional morbidity,[14] Incidence refers to the risk of the entire population, while proportional morbidity refers to risk in a hospital population. Proportional morbidity does not necessarily reflect incidence and should not be used as such, since it refers only to a select population.

An effect of the season of the year on incidence has been reported. An increased risk was found in winter[11,12,14–18] and spring,[19,20] However, some studies have shown no relationship to season.[21,22] The difference between these studies may be related to the measurement of proportional morbidity rather than true incidence.

ETIOLOGY

Causes of hematuria and dysuria with or without urethral obstruction are multiple. These signs indicate a lower urinary tract disease but are not specific for a particular disease. Causes of hematuria and dysuria without obstruction include bacterial cystitis and urethritis, neoplasia, trauma, irritant cystitis or urethritis, and urolithiasis. Causes of urethral obstruction include uroliths, neoplasia, strictures due to connective tissue, prostatic lesions, extraluminal masses, inflammatory swelling, and possibly a functional urethral obstruction such as reflex dyssynergia.[3] All of these causes occur in cats as well as other species. However, cats also seem to have a large idiopathic category. This may be due to a lack of looking for a cause or the occurrence of one or several causes which are difficult to identify.

Cats with these signs have been investigated to some extent. Most cats (72 to 98 percent, depending on the survey) with lower urinary tract signs do not have bacterial cystitis when the criterion for diagnosis is bacterial culture of a properly collected urine sample.[23–26] Urine samples for bacterial culture should be collected by cystocentesis to avoid contamination with the normal bacterial flora of the urethra and vagina or prepuce. If catheterized samples are used, quantitative culture must be performed to accurately assess the results. Up to 1,000 organisms per milliliter can be found in catheterized urine samples as a result of urethral contamination in cats.[27] Since expressed or voided urine samples can be contaminated by greater than 100,000 organisms per milliliter, such samples should not be used for culture.

Neoplasia usually affects old cats, whereas most cats with FUS are young. Neoplasia should be considered in cats with persistent signs and in older cats. Trauma should be ruled out by careful history and physical examination. The incidence of true uroliths (as defined above) in cats with lower urinary tract signs is unknown. A prospective study including control cats utilizing contrast radiographs is warranted to determine how often uroliths or other anatomic urologic abnormalities can be identified in cats with these signs.

Because readily identifiable causes such as those above have not been found in most cats with these signs, much effort has been directed to finding another cause. This effort has been directed in three major areas: an infectious agent, diet, and epidemiologic surveys. Each of these will be reviewed separately.

Infectious Agents

As described above, bacterial infection is an uncommon cause of lower urinary tract signs in cats. Nonroutine culture methods to identify anaerobes, fastidious organisms requiring feline urine or tissue to grow, spirochetes, or mycoplasma have also been negative.[3,23,28] Bacteria were also not seen on scanning electron microscopy of urinary sediment from cats with FUS.[23]

The relationship of viral infections to naturally occurring lower urinary tract disease remains controversial. The supporting data have all originated from one laboratory and have not been duplicated elsewhere. In the original studies, urethral obstruction was induced in experimental cats by injecting urine from a cat with naturally occurring urethral obstruction.[29,30] In spite of efforts in other laboratories, obstruction has not been produced again by urine transfer,[23,26,31–33] even with the use of glucocorticoids as immunosuppressants.[26] Also, viruses have not been recovered from urine of affected cats in any higher proportion than from urine of normal cats.[23,26,28,31] The original investigators attribute these failures to their finding that the picornavirus originally isolated from urine, as well as a syncytial virus also isolated from urine of affected cats, cannot cause disease alone. A cell-associated herpesvirus which can be recovered from urinary tract tissue but not urine presumably is required for disease, with the other viruses acting only to accentuate clinical signs.[2,34,35]

The cell-associated herpesvirus was initially isolated from kidney tissue from normal kittens.[34] The only isolation from a spontaneous case was from a 4.5-month-old experimental kitten with urethral obstruction.[35] In this kitten the virus was isolated from kidney but not lower urinary tract tissue. This herpesvirus alone was found to induce urethral obstruction in specific pathogen free (SPF) cats secondary to urethral swelling, and to induce hematuria either intermittently or persistently.[2,36] Hemorrhages, as well as crystalline material and calculi, were found in the bladder and urethra.[2] The virus could be reisolated from affected cats.

In spite of the experimental induction of cystitis in SPF cats with the cell-associated herpesvirus, the virus has not been isolated from tissues of naturally affected cats.[23,26,28] Although inappropriate laboratory methods were blamed for such failure,[2,35] comparison of reported methods indicate that studies have been conducted with adequate methods to isolate a cell-associated herpesvirus.[26,28] Also, in spite of laboratory evidence for horizontal and vertical transfer,[2,36] one case control study showed no association of urethral obstruction with multiple cat households and thus no evidence for an easily transmitted infectious agent as a cause of feline urethral obstruction.[37] Since this virus induces intra- and extracellular lipid deposition in tissue culture,[38] the presence of increased lipid droplets in urine of natural cases has been cited as evidence for viral infection of natural cases.[2,39] However, the only reference to increased lipid in urine of clinical cases is an unpublished observation.[2] One clinical study found fat globules in 30 percent of cats with hematuria and dysuria.[40] However, fat droplets are generally considered normal and common in cat urine because of the presence of large amounts of lipid in cats' proximal convoluted tubules.[8,41–43]

The finding that the herpesvirus can induce extracellular crystal formation in tissue culture has been cited as evidence that this virus can induce crystals which could then cause obstruction.[2] However, feline syncytial virus induces similar crystals even though it is no longer considered related to FUS.[44] Also, the crystals induced in largest quantity were cholesterol, not struvite.[2,38]

Thus, although the cell-associated herpesvirus can induce lower urinary tract disease in SPF cats, there is no evidence that this virus is involved in natural cases. Further research in this area should be directed toward reproducing the original studies in a different laboratory and toward natural cases, both in regard to viral isolation and to antibody titers. Studies of antibody titers alone must be conducted with appropriate controls and may be difficult to interpret, since infection can be present without antibody production[2,45] and since an antibody titer might be present from previous exposure without current infection.

Diet

Many aspects of diet have been associated with FUS in cats. These include mineral content, water content, caloric content, digestibility, and frequency of feeding. This section will review these factors.

The relationship of the mineral content of the diet to urethral obstruction has received the most attention experimentally. Studies from different laboratories have confirmed that urethral obstruction can be induced in previously normal male cats by increasing the magnesium concentration of the diet. The minimum amount of Mg on a dry weight basis which resulted in obstruction was reported to be 0.3 percent.[46] Other calculogenic diets have varied from 0.4 percent Mg in a dry diet to 0.75 or 1.0 percent Mg in a canned diet.[47–49] In most of these studies, uroliths (including renoliths) formed and often caused obstruction.[48,50] The mineral components of these induced uroliths were initially reported to be magnesium and phosphate,[49,50] and urine from cats with uroliths was often alkaline.[49] The relationship of this experimental form of urolithiasis to naturally occurring lower urinary tract disease in cats has been questioned, as natural cases are not often associated with uroliths, renoliths are uncommon in cats,[51] the crystals associated with natural cases are magnesium ammonium phosphate (struvite), and urine from cats with naturally occurring obstruction is usually acidic at the time of obstruction. One study with 1 percent Mg produced obstruction with mucoid material and crystals similar to naturally occurring cases in 7 of 16 experimental cats; however, the crystals could only be identified to be struvite in one cat.[47,52]

In one recent study, urethral obstruction with dense deposits of struvite crystals was observed in cats fed 0.45 percent Mg in a dry diet (six of eight cats) or 0.5 or 0.72 percent Mg in a moist diet (six of eight cats in each group).[53] In addition, one of four cats fed 0.15 percent Mg in a dry diet developed urethral obstruction. Struvite calculi were also found in cats fed 0.72 percent Mg. One difference between this study and those done previously was that the alkalinity induced by the supplemental MgO was corrected prior to feeding the cats the experimental moist food. The failure of earlier studies to mitigate the alkalinizing effect of MgO or analytical error may have been the reason why no ammonium was found in the calculi produced. The type of obstruction was not identical to that seen in natural cases, since no mucus or mucoid plugs were identified.

Commercial cat foods contain less Mg than has been added to produce calculogenic diets, with the exception of one of four experimental cats which developed urethral obstruction on 0.15 percent Mg.[53] However, this experimental diet induced consistently alkaline urine (pH $>$ 7.0), which may have been the result of the alkalinity of the diet. In commercial diets in the United States, the mean Mg concentration on a dry weight basis is 0.03 to 0.15 percent for canned foods, 0.07 to 0.16 percent for semimoist, and 0.15 to 0.16 percent for dry.[54,55] The range for dry diets is 0.06 to 0.21 percent. The amount of minerals in commercial foods was found to be fairly consistent from lot to lot.[56] In one study, feeding the 0.16 percent Mg found in commercial dry foods did not produce obstruction in normal experimental cats.[46]

Examining only the Mg concentration on a dry weight basis can be misleading. The amount of other minerals such as calcium and phosphorus affects the calculogenic characteristics of a diet.[49] The amount of magesium that must be excreted in the urine also depends on how much magnesium is consumed and its intestinal absorption. Thus, the caloric density, palatability, and digestibility of a diet may be as important as the amount of Mg on a dry weight basis in determining the amount of Mg that must be excreted.[57] Cats eating 0.45 or 0.15 percent Mg in a dry diet were found to consume as much Mg as those eating 0.72 or 0.5 percent Mg, respectively, in a canned diet in one study in which food intake was carefully monitored.[53] The cats ate more of the dry diet, apparently because of its lower caloric content, and thus ingested more magnesium. In spite of similar Mg intake, urine Mg concentration was less on the experimental dry diet than on the moist, probably due to decreased Mg absorption associated with the high Ca content of the dry diet. This study points out that the Mg concentration of food is not a valid index of the Mg concentration of urine. Although increased rates of urethral obstruction were observed when high magnesium diets were fed, urine magnesium concentration was not the only factor involved in obstruction, since some cats remained obstruction-free even when consuming amounts of magnesium associated with obstruction of others.[53]

One question arising from these experimental studies is whether cats with naturally occurring FUS have higher than normal urine Mg concentration, either because of diet, intestinal hyperabsorption, or renal hyperexcretion. One study in England in the early 1970s found that cats eating one type of dry cat food had similar concentrations of urine Mg to cats eating a high-Mg "stone-forming" diet.[58] However, in the United States, one study has found that cats with naturally occurring FUS had markedly lower urine Mg concentrations than those fed high-Mg experimental diets.[53] Cats with naturally occurring hematuria and dysuria without obstruction had urine Mg concentrations similar to experimental cats fed the low-Mg control diet. Another investigator also found that a cat with recurrent episodes of FUS had low concentrations of urine Mg compared to control cats.[59] Thus, most naturally occurring cases of FUS are not due to increased intestinal absorption or increased urinary excretion of Mg. Urine Mg concentration in normal cats was similar (<7 mg/dl) whether cats were fed dry, semimoist, or canned commercial diets, or prescription diet c/d.[47,53]

Water intake on different diets has been studied because of the relationship of urine volume to mineral concentration. Some studies have only measured water intake or water intake and urine volume, while others have examined total water balance, which includes measuring urine and fecal water output and extrapolating to estimate insensible water loss. Studies of water intake alone cannot be extrapolated to conclusions about urine volume, since fecal water loss is an important excretory pathway that can vary with factors such as diet.[31] One English study has shown a decreased urine volume on dry foods.[46] Average urine specific gravity on dry foods was approximately 1.050, whereas specific gravity on canned foods was 1.034.[46] A marked change in urine volume occurred with a sudden change between canned and dry foods. This marked difference in urine output between dry and canned foods was not supported by studies in the United States, which found an average urine specific gravity of 1.056 on dry food and 1.051 on canned food.[47,60] Part of this difference in results might be attributed to different formulations of diets in England versus the United States.[61] Another study has shown that urine versus fecal water loss varies with the type of dry food.[62] The best conclusion from these differing results is that merely looking at canned versus dry food in general is too simplistic. Climatic conditions and ventilation in the laboratory, specific components of the diets, the age of the experimental cats, the means of providing water and food, and the degree of stress may all affect such studies.[63] For the clinician, the urine specific gravity of specific cases is more important in measuring the degree of urine concentration than determining whether diet is canned or dry. When water balance was compared between male cats with a history of urethral obstruction and normal male cats matched by age and body weight, no significant difference was found, although affected cats were more variable in regard to the percent water in feces or urine.[8,25,63,64] One study in the United States showed increased water intake and urine output on semimoist food, as compared to dry or canned food.[47]

Since struvite crystals are less soluble as pH increases, the relationship of diet to urine pH has also been studied. Ingestion of most foods causes secretion of alkaline urine immediately after eating. The degree of this postprandial alkaline tide varies with the diet.[1,65] The frequency of feeding may also affect urine alkalinity. Once-a-day feeding causes a more alkaline urine pH than ad libitum feeding,[66] but the duration of alkalinity may be less. Urine pH seems to remain fairly constant but elevated above fasting levels throughout the day with ad libitum feeding.[66] The relationship of the postprandial alkaline tide to natural cases of FUS is unknown. Epidemiologic studies comparing frequency of feeding to FUS incidence have been conducted. Results have been inconsistent, with some showing increased risk if cats are fed more than four times[11,67] but not if they are fed ad libitum.[11] Another study has shown no relationship.[9] After urethral obstruction develops, urine pH in clinical cases is usually acidic.[8,24,25,40,64] But the urine pH just prior to obstruction is unknown.

The site of formation of the crystals found in urethral plugs is still speculative. One study found microcrystals inside renal tubules and postulated that crystals form in the kidneys.[40] This result could not be duplicated in a recent study of cats obstructing on experimental high-magnesium diets.[53]

Cat owners are often confused about the relationship of dietary ash content to FUS. This confusion has been fostered by some cat food manufacturers. Ash refers to all noncombustible components of a diet and thus includes most of the mineral content, without designation of quantities of specific elements. Thus, ash content is not necessarily related to Mg concentration. The study of Dickinson and Scott,[68] which is often quoted as support that ash content is not related to FUS, is a good example. The diet used was 30 percent ash but only 0.03 percent Mg, and no urinary tract signs developed.

Despite all experimental efforts with calculogenic diets, water balance, and urine pH, the association of these factors with hematuria, dysuria, and urethral obstruction in clinical cases remains unanswered. One theory is that struvite crystals irritate the lining of the urinary tract, causing cystitis and urethritis.[1] However, limited studies have shown no difference in urine struvite concentration[25,64] or in urine Mg concentration[53] between affected and unaffected cats. In another study, 21 of 44 affected cats had few or no struvite crystals in their urine at the time of clinical signs.[24] Thus, there is currently no conclusive evidence that these signs are related to any dietary factor in naturally occurring cases. However, most cats with these signs have not been studied in relation to identifying a cause other than an infectious agent. The incidence of uroliths is considered to be low on the basis of clinical impression but not on the basis of a prospective clinical study. One study[63] in which three cats with hematuria and dysuria were necropsied found a struvite calculus in one. Unfortunately, no other diagnostic testing was reported, so it is unknown whether this case would have been identified by bacterial urinary tract infection or survey radiography.

The relationship of diet to spontaneous urethral obstruction is also not established. The clinical impression is that obstruction is usually due to an unorganized accumulation of struvite crystals in a mucoid matrix. In one study of cats euthanatized within 48 hours of urethral obstruction, crystalline material was found in the bladder of 6 of 10, and urethral calculi were identified in 3 of 10.[63] Microcalculi were identified as the cause of obstruction in one carefully studied case.[69]

The relationship of urethral plugs to true uroliths is not known. Most urethral plugs in cats contain struvite as the major mineral component. More than 85 percent of plugs contained more than 80 percent struvite.[5,6,51,70] Other plugs have been found to be all matrix with no minerals[6,70] or matrix with various other minerals such as ammonium acid urate, calcium phosphate, or calcium oxalate.[5,51] Whether the mineral or the matrix formed first is not known. Matrix is suspected because of the unorganized nature of the crystalline material. There is no known relationship between diet and matrix composition, although the biochemical composition of the matrix has received only limited study.[48] Although dense accumulations of crystals have been shown to produce obstruction in cats, the experimental conditions may not mimic naturally occurring disease. One study involved high-Mg diets with a higher urine Mg concentration than is found in clinical cases,[53] and another involved injecting crystals into the bladder in four times the amount found in clinical cases.[25]

Epidemiologic Studies

Epidemiologic studies have been widely used in the hope that etiologic factors could be identified. A major drawback has been the lack of definition of the population studied. Most studies have relied only on owners' history or retrospective studies of case diagnoses and have focused only on clinical signs of hematuria, dysuria, and/or urethral obstruction. The populations have not been defined by any diagnostic criteria such as urinalysis, urine culture, radiographs, or urine mineral excretion. Thus, these studies are limited in that they are considering all lower urinary tract disease rather than any one disease. The general conclusion that lower urinary tract disease (which is equivalent to FUS as defined by these studies) is multifactorial is not unexpected.

In general, these studies have found an increased risk of lower urinary tract disease in cats that are older than 2 years, neutered, overweight, and "lazy."[5,9,11,16,17,67] Peak age range was 2 to 6 years.[17] The activity level of cats was determined subjectively, based on the owner's impression[9,11] or on whether the cat was kept indoors or allowed outdoors.[11,16] Another interpretation of this data would be that outdoor or active cats are at less risk because the problem is less likely to be detected with outdoor and unobserved urination. The risk associated with castration was unassociated with age of neutering,[11,14] and also could not be associated with decreased urethral size.[5,71,72] However, the effect of castration on urethral compliance has not been studied, and an increase in fibrocyte numbers in the urethra has been found which might cause a decrease in urethral distensibility.[71] Risk for urethral obstruction is much greater in males, but risk for signs of cystitis is equal in both sexes.[16] One investigator noted an increased risk in Persian cats and a decreased risk for Siamese cats.[16,17]

Not all studies have confirmed these findings. One study that matched cats by age found no association with castration,[22] as did another early study.[21]

Some studies have found an association with cats that eat dry food and seem to drink less.[9,11,16,73] Data on water consumption must be interpreted cautiously, though, as only owners' estimates were used. One more specific study found an increased incidence of urethral obstruction in cats that consumed greater than 50 percent dry food and stayed indoors.[37] Data on food eaten must also be interpreted cautiously, since this study as well as others indicated that most owners feed their cats a variety of food types, rarely dry food alone.[9]

An increased frequency of feeding was associated with increased risk in some studies,[9,11] regardless of diet fed. However, risk was less for ad libitum feeding than for meal feeding.[11]

No association has been found with multiple-cat households, making an infectious agent such as an easily transferred virus unlikely.[9,37] Miscalculation of data was found to be the reason for an association with multiple-cat households in one study.[11,14]

Congenital Defects

Bladder diverticula associated with a urachal remnant have been identified in cats with lower urinary tract signs.[74,75,76] One study of 735 cats used for anatomy dissections indicated that 22 percent of males and 26.5 percent of females had identifiable urachal remnants.[74] Comparing this to the incidence of FUS (0.6 percent) suggests that most cats with urachal remnants do not have signs of lower urinary tract disease. However, an incidence study of cats with lower urinary tract disease matched with normal cats has not been conducted. One study concluded that surgical removal of urachal remnants in cats with lower urinary tract disease reduced recurrence of clinical signs, as compared to a similar group of cats not treated surgically.[74] This study should be extended, since limited diagnostic work was performed on affected cats and since it is difficult to understand how a persistent congenital defect could cause intermittent clinical signs of hematuria and dysuria or urethral obstruction.

PATHOPHYSIOLOGY AND LABORATORY FINDINGS

Hematuria and Dysuria without Obstruction

As discussed previously, this complex of clinical signs can be caused by several different disease processes in the lower urinary tract. Examples are urolithiasis, bacterial infection, neoplasia, and trauma. These cause hematuria by damage to blood vessels and dysuria via tissue irritation. However, a population of cats exists in which no predisposing cause of hematuria and dysuria can be identified. Pyuria (>5 WBC/hpf) is absent or mild. The clinical course usually is a spontaneous resolution of clinical signs within a week,[4,77] with recurrence at a later date. It is not known whether subclinical abnormalities persist between episodes, but one limited study of six cats indicated persistence of microscopic hematuria.[61] Since the hematuria and dysuria are not life threatening and since signs generally resolve, few cats with this syndrome have been studied in depth. In one research colony, three cats with dysuria and hematuria without any history of obstruction were killed to examine their urinary tracts.[63] Unfortunately, diagnostic work prior to euthanasia was not reported. On necropsy, one cat had struvite calculi in the bladder, one had struvite crystals in the bladder and all three had a thickened hemorrhagic bladder wall. Histologic examination of lesions in the bladder revealed epithelial hyperplasia, perivascular accumulation of lymphocytes, muscular degeneration and regeneration, mucosal sloughing and necrosis, and focal to severe mural hemorrhage. No lesions were found in the urethra. This limited study suggests that the bladder rather than the urethra is the site of hemorrhage in this subpopulation of cats. The cause of the hemorrhage is unknown. As discussed in the section on etiology, one theory has been irritation from struvite crystals.[1] However, there is no experimental or clinical evidence to support this theory at the present time.

Feline Urethral Obstruction

As discussed previously, there are many potential causes of urethral obstruction in cats, including urethral plugs, uroliths, strictures, and extraluminal masses including the prostate, neoplasia, and possibly inflammation or spasm. The clinical impression is that the most common cause of obstruction in cats is urethral plugs. However, few prospective case studies have been done. In one study of 32 cases, the cause of obstruction was considered to be aggregates of crystals in 23 and organic matrix in 9.[40] However, this differentiation was made largely by subjective opinion of "texture" when a catheter was passed.

The site of obstruction appears most often to be the distal penile urethra. However, the feline urethra narrows just caudal to the bulbourethral glands at the ischial arch.[5,78] One author postulated that microcalculi and matrix plugs would lodge at this site, while plugs primarily of struvite crystals could be found at any site in the urethra.[5] A study of the anatomy of the pelvic urethra in cats indicated that the preprostatic urethra was narrower than the postprostatic urethra.[79] The actual site of obstruction in most clinical cases is not determined. In one report of two cats, obstruction in one was in the musculomembranous (intrapelvic) urethra and in the other was in the penile and preprostatic urethra.[5] Obstruction in both was due to plugs of crystalline/mucoid material. In another clinical case, obstruction with microcalculi was found just caudal to the prostate, at the bulbourethral glands and at the tip of the penis.[69]

Obstruction is much more common in male than in female cats. This has been related to sex differences in urethral length, diameter, and distensibility.[78] Others have suggested a role for the prostate gland or urethral mucous glands in matrix production.[4]

Regardless of the cause, obstruction to urine outflow leads to predictable clinical and biochemical changes which vary with the duration and degree of obstruction. With complete urethral obstruction, the bladder will gradually become distended. The rate at which the bladder distends depends on rate of urine flow, bladder capacity, and previous bladder injury. The pressure associated with overdistention will result in ischemia, edema, hemorrhage, loss of epithelium, and infiltration of neutrophils around blood vessels.[69,80,81] The urethra proximal to the obstruction will have similar injuries, with desquamation of epithelium, edema, and infiltration of neutrophils around blood vessels and in the lamina propria and muscle layer.[69] The increased pressure will be transmitted up the ureters to the kidneys, causing the kidneys to appear somewhat swollen and congested.[69]

Azotemia (an increase in BUN and serum creatinine) results from inability to excrete urine. In part, azotemia may be due to reabsorption of compounds across the damaged bladder wall into capillary beds.[69,82] The more important mechanism for azotemia is the obstructive nephropathy which results. Obstructive nephropathy is defined as the functional and biochemical alterations which occur in the kidneys as a result of obstruction to urine outflow. Obstruction causes a decrease in renal blood flow (RBF) and glomerular filtration rate (GFR) and changes in reabsorption of solutes and water.[83] The mechanisms for these changes continue to be studied.[83] With increased intraluminal pressure in the bladder and ureters, intratubular pressure increases at a rate dependent on the rate of urine flow at the time of obstruction. The increased intratubular pressure opposes glomerular capillary hydrostatic pressure and leads to a decreased effective filtration pressure and a decreased GFR. Preglomerular vasoconstriction also contributes to the decrease in GFR and RBF. Most nephrons apparently stop filtering completely, while others continue but at a markedly reduced rate.[83] If the period of obstruction is short (less than 36 hours), GFR gradually increases to normal over a period of about 1 week in experimental rats. If the obstruction persists for longer than 96 hours, the loss of renal function is permanent.[83]

Physical findings in cats with urethral obstruction are related to uremia, hyperkalemia, and possibly acidemia. Signs include anorexia, depression, weakness, vomiting, hypothermia, and dehydration. Such signs occur in most experimentally obstructed cats 48 hours after obstruction; longer times are required for signs to develop in some cats.[84,85] Signs associated with hyperkalemia include bradycardia and ventricular arrhythmias. Lack of P waves, a widened QRS interval, and spiked T waves can be found by electrocardiography.[86] These signs develop when serum K concentrations are approximately 10 mEq/L or greater.[86] However, bradycardia is not a consistent finding in cats, even with marked hyperkalemia.[86] Thus, the absence of this sign does not eliminate the possibility of severe hyperkalemia. Hyperkalemia affects the heart by depressing conduction rate and contractility.[86] The acidemia associated with uremia may exacerbate the effects of hyperkalemia on the myocardium.[86] Hyperkalemia also causes generalized muscle weakness. In cats with experimental obstruction, serum potassium increased after the development of uremia.[84,85] From 48 to 96 hours of complete urethral obstruction were required for severe hyperkalemia (serum $K > 8$ mEq/L) to develop.

Laboratory changes associated with complete urethral obstruction include azotemia (increased BUN and serum creatinine) and hyperphosphatemia, both related to decreased GFR. Another change is hypocalcemia, which affected four of nine cats in one survey (serum $Ca < 7.8$ mg/dl).[86] The hypocalcemia has been attributed to hyperphosphatemia, causing the $Ca \times P$ solubility product to be exceeded and Ca to be precipitated in tissues. Serum Ca concentration is usually greater than 7 mg/dl. Since acidemia causes a greater percentage of serum calcium to be ionized (active), hypocalcemia usually causes no adverse clinical signs. Hyperkalemia probably develops because of cessation of renal K excretion and intracellular efflux of K associated with acidemia. It may also occur because K sequestered in the urinary bladder prior to anuria may be reabsorbed as the bladder wall is damaged by intracystic pressure. Acidemia also occurs due to retention of acidic metabolic waste products. Once uremia develops, dehydration can result from vomiting and lack of water intake. The acidemia, dehydration, and hyperkalemia are probably responsible for death in untreated cats with urethral obstruction. Mild hyperglycemia also develops in cats with urethral obstruction, probably secondary to epinephrine and/or glucocorticoid release from stress and perhaps secondary to peripheral inhibition of insulin by uremic toxins. This hyperglycemia may be associated with glucosuria.[8] A few cats have glucosuria with normoglycemia, and the glucosuria may persist for several days after relief of obstruction.[8,87] This may result from proximal tubular cell injury leading to decreased glucose reabsorption. In some obstructed cats, a positive finding of glucose in the urine was found due to a false positive reaction due to an oxidizing substance other than glucose.[87]

Hematuria is the principal finding on urinalysis. The cause of the hematuria is unknown, as discussed under cats without obstruction. In cats with obstruction, the hematuria may also be secondary to bladder wall injury from distention. It is usually not known whether the hematuria and, perhaps, inflammation precedes or follows urethral obstruction. Urine is usually acidic and concentrated at the time of obstruction.

DIAGNOSIS

As discussed above, FUS is by definition a syndrome, not a disease entity. By our definition, this is a syndrome of hematuria and dysuria with or without urethral obstruction, which is not associated with bacterial UTI or with another readily defined cause such as true urolithiasis, neoplasia, or trauma. In order to use this definition correctly, diagnostic procedures beyond physical examination are mandatory.

At the present time, there is no way to predict which cats will be prone to this problem, even though there seems to be a population of cats subject to frequent recurrence.[14] A study of a group of these cats between episodes of clinical signs is indicated to determine any subclinical abnormalities. In one study, 14 of 35 asymptomatic cats that previously had a perineal urethrostomy for urethral obstruction had hematuria.[89] However, the possibility of iatrogenic trauma during urine collection could not be excluded.

Affected cats with or without obstruction often have a history of urinating in unusual places (such as the sink or bathtub) as well as hematuria and dysuria. Frequent attempts to urinate may be mistaken by the owner for constipation. Frequent licking of the penis with discoloration and congestion is common in males, especially with obstruction.

The first diagnostic step, when presented with a cat with hematuria and dysuria, is to determine whether urethral obstruction is present. This can usually be done by physical examination. Finding a distended, tense bladder which may cause discomfort when palpated is suggestive of urethral obstruction. Finding a small, possibly firm bladder which may spasm when palpated is indicative of lower tract disease without obstruction.

Urethral Obstruction

When urethral obstruction is suspected on the basis of physical examination, the rest of the patient's history and physical examination will help to determine the duration and severity of the obstruction. Signs such as anorexia, vomiting, depression, dehydration, and hypothermia indicate that complete obstruction has been present for at least 48 hours.[85] Signs of hyperkalemia such as generalized weakness, cardiac arrhythmias, and/or bradycardia indicate a longer duration of complete obstruction. The combination of uremia and hyperkalemia can become life-threatening, and any diagnostic effort other than collecting blood and urine in patients with such signs should be postponed until treatment is instituted and the cat's condition is stabilized. Some data can be collected, though, as treatment is begun. As one tries to remove the obstruction by catheterization, a note should be made as to the location and texture of the obstructing material. If any obstructing material is obtained, it should be saved for analysis, by micrscopy if it is a mucoid plug and by crystallography if it is a microcalculus. Urine should be obtained for at least a complete urinalysis. Cystocentesis has been recommended prior to restoring urethral patency with reverse flushing solutions, in order to avoid altering results of urinalysis by these solutions, to immediately decompress the overdistended bladder to halt the adverse effects of obstructive uropathy, and to reduce intravesicular pressure to make repulsion of the obstructing material into the bladder easier.[90] Potential adverse effects of cystocentesis are extravasation of urine into the abdominal cavity and further injury to the bladder wall. However, these are not common if most of the urine is removed from the bladder.[90] The technique of cystocentesis has been well reviewed recently.[90] If cystocentesis is not used, then urine obtained after catheterization should be used for urinalysis. If the urinalysis indicates pyuria or bacteriuria in addition to hematuria or if the client wishes optimal medical care without regard to cost, then urine should be cultured for aerobic bacteria. Normal feline urine contains less than 5 WBC/hpf.[27] Significant bacteriuria (>100,000/ml) can be present even if bacteria are not seen on urine sediment examination.[27] Despite these limitations in using urinalysis to suggest infection, our rationale for not doing a urine culture on all patients on the initial visit is one of cost efficiency, since we have found significant bacteriuria in only one of 48 nonobstructed cats in a prospective study.[23] If culture is desired on a sample obtained by catheterization, numbers of organisms should be quantitated, since contamination by urethral organisms can occur.[27] Contamination with urethral organisms has been found to result in counts of up to 1,000 organisms per milliliter.[27] A blood sample should also be obtained for complete blood count, serum urea nitrogen and/or serum creatinine, and electrolytes. This blood sample will be an additional indicator of the severity of the cat's condition and will help to determine the type and efficacy of therapy.

Although radiographic contrast procedures such as urethrography have been recommended for cats with urethral obstruction,[91,92] there has been no study of the benefits versus patient risk or cost. Until such a study is done, it is difficult to recommend contrast radiographs on all cats during the first episode of obstruction. Such procedures are more easily justified if the cat has any evidence of UTI or any possibility of trauma, is older (presenting the possibility of neoplasia), is a female, has suffered repeated episodes of obstruction, or is to undergo perineal urethrostomy.[91,92] However, there are no data to help predict how often radiography would alter the decision as to whether perineal urethrostomy is indicated in male cats to try to prevent future obstruction. Techniques for performing radiographic contrast studies of the lower urinary tract in cats have been recently reviewed.[92]

Nonobstructed Cats

If there is no evidence of obstruction and the cat is bright, alert, and active, our diagnostic plan on the initial visit includes only a urinalysis in addition to the history and physical examination. Urine is collected, preferably by cystocentesis, and an aliquot is saved for bacterial culture if the urinalysis indicates pyuria and/or bacteriuria in addition to hematuria. Since cystocentesis can be difficult to accomplish in affected cats who tend to void frequently, a voided sample can be used for urinalysis if attempts at cystocentesis fail. If pyuria or bacteriuria are evident, a cystocentesis is essential to obtain a sample for culture, since a voided sample is often contaminated by urethral organisms.[27] To assist in obtaining a sample for culture, we administer either a diuretic such as furosemide or subcutaneous fluids to stimulate bladder filling. Hematuria unassociated with bacteriuria and with pyuria mild or absent is typical of cats with FUS. The possibility that blood in a urine sample was introduced iatrogenically during collection must be considered if the sample was obtained by cystocentesis or catheterization.

If a cat is reexamined because of persistent or recurrent hematuria and dysuria without urethral obstruction, our diagnostic plan is expanded to include a second urinalysis, a urine culture, survey radiography of the entire urinary tract, and contrast radiography of the lower urinary tract, especially the bladder. Carbon dioxide rather than air should be used for pneumocystography in cats with hematuria, because of the risk of fatal venous air embolism.[93,94] If these tests also reveal no cause and if episodes of recurrence are frequent, an exploratory cystotomy is recommended. Cultures of the urine for bacteria and of the bladder wall for the cell-associated herpesvirus are performed, and samples of bladder wall are collected for histology. One study of 14 clinical cases of hematuria and dysuria indicated the fallibility of contrast radiographs.[40] Of the 14 cats, nine were thought to have a thickened bladder wall on penumocystography. At surgery, seven of these had the thickening confirmed whereas two were normal. The only cat that was taken to surgery with a bladder wall considered normal on radiography had inflammation of the bladder with hemorrhage and necrosis. This study[40] suffers from being apparently retrospective, with criteria for case selection being poorly defined, and from having other questionable conclusions. A prospective study of the accuracy of cystography in cats is indicated.

The question arises as to whether mineral excretion should be studied in cats with FUS. In an initial study, no increase in urinary mineral concentration was found in cats with naturally occurring FUS, whether obstructed or unobstructed.[53] However, a few cats did have urinary Mg concentrations comparable to cats on calculogenic diets. Whether these cats represent a subpopulation of FUS cats with an abnormality in mineral excretion which might be helped by a low Mg diet remains unanswered.

TREATMENT

Since the cause of FUS as we have defined it is not known, no specific treatment is possible. Supportive therapy for the obstructed cat is fairly well defined, although some controversy exists even in the management of these cats. No therapy has been proven efficacious to date in managing the unobstructed cat or in preventing recurrent episodes of obstruction or of hematuria and dysuria without urethral obstruction. To summarize current knowledge, the discussion will be divided into three parts: management of cats with urethral obstruction, management of cats without urethral obstruction, and prevention of recurrent episodes of FUS.

Feline Urethral Obstruction

The management of cats with urethral obstruction depends on the severity of clinical signs. These signs vary with the degree and duration of the obstruction. If the cat is not yet azotemic, relief of obstruction may be sufficient therapy. In an azotemic but nonuremic cat, relief of obstruction is essential, and fluid therapy is probably beneficial. In a uremic cat, both relief of obstruction and fluid therapy are essential. The value of fluid therapy, in addition to relief of obstruction, in cats with postrenal uremia was shown in experiments in which 10 of 13 cats treated only by relief of obstruction died, whereas eight of eight cats treated with fluid therapy as well as relief of obstruction survived.[83] Whether fluid therapy or relief of obstruction should be attempted first depends on the condition of the cat. If the cat is depressed and weak, we usually start fluid therapy first and may use cystocentesis to temporarily relieve bladder distention. If the cat is still alert, we try to relieve obstruction first.

Relief of obstruction is imperative and is most often accomplished by retrograde flushing of the urethra through a lubricated urethral catheter with a sterile solution such as saline or Ringer's solution. Another reverse flushing solution which has been recommended is Walpole's, buffered acetic acid.[5,93,94] Its beneficial effect has been attributed to the increased solubility of struvite crystals in acid solutions. Potential adverse effects are related to the acidity (pH 4.5) and potential absorption across the damaged urethral mucosa.[87] Controlled studies of efficacy and adverse effects are not available.

Many instruments are available for urethral catheterization. Since the urethra of an obstructed male cat is already damaged as the result of the pressure of the obstructing material, the pressure of the retained urine, and the pressure exerted during the cat's attempts to urinate, gentle technique is necessary to avoid further urethral trauma. Polyethylene catheters such as tom cat catheters or intravenous catheters are probably less traumatic than metal instruments such as a blunt lacrimal cannula or a silver abscess needle. However, the care of the operator is more important than the instrument in avoidance of urethral trauma.

Sufficient sedation should be used to facilitate catheterization. The degree of sedation required will depend on the cat's condition and temperament. All anesthetics should be administered cautiously because of the potential presence of postrenal azotemia. Intravenous short acting barbiturates, inhalant anesthetics, or low doses of ketamine can be used. Since ketamine is excreted by the kidneys, prolonged recovery may occur if the obstruction is not relieved or if renal function does not rapidly improve after relief of obstruction. Local anesthetic agents in reverse flushing solutions are not recommended because they may induce systemic toxicity if absorbed in sufficient quantity; absorption may be enhanced by uroepithelial damage and toxicity may be worsened by postrenal uremia.[90,97] A review of considerations for anesthesia of cats with urethral obstruction has recently been published.[98]

Once the necessary materials have been gathered and the cat has been restrained, the penis should be cleansed with warm water or dilute betadine scrub. The hair adjacent to the penis should be liberally wetted to decrease the chances for its contaminating the urethral catheter. The penis should be displaced dorsally until the long axis of the urethra is parallel to the vertebral column in order to eliminate the natural curvature of the male feline urethra. As aseptically as possible, a catheter coated with sterilized lubricant should be advanced to the site of obstruction. The location of the obstruction should be recorded. The sterile solution chosen should be flushed into the urethral lumen and allowed to reflux out the urethral orifice in the hope of dislodging the obstruction and flushing it out the urethra or into the bladder without greatly increasing intraurethral pressure. As possible, the catheter should be slowly advanced to the bladder. If the obstruction is not dislodged by backflushing, the tip of the penis is grasped with the thumb and index finger to prevent backleakage of fluid. Injection of fluid may then force obstructing material into the urinary bladder.

If the obstruction is not dislodged by initial retrograde flushing of the urethra, the bladder should be emptied by cystocentesis with a small gauge needle (22-gauge), a three-way valve, and a syringe. Manipulation of the bladder should be as gentle as possible, since its wall is distended and injured by the increased intravesicular pressure and it is vulnerable to rupture. Once bladder pressure has been relieved, flushing the obstruction out of the urethra via the urethral catheter is often successful.

If the above techniques do not relieve the obstruction, emergency surgery may be necessary. A cystostomy with placement of a Foley catheter in the bladder or percutaneous prepubic urinary drainage[99] will provide a means of urine elimination without repeated cystocentesis, in order to provide time to reverse uremia and hyperkalemia, stabilize the patient, and allow diagnostic testing to further localize and identify the cause of such a severe obstruction.

After the obstruction is relieved, a flexible #3.5 French rubber feeding tube type catheter should be inserted into the bladder, collecting a urine sample for urinalysis if one has not already been obtained by cystocentesis. A quantity of urine is saved for quantitative bacterial culture, if indicated by finding pyuria and/or bacteriuria on the urinalysis. Flexible catheters are preferred because of their longer length. Ten-cm polypropylene catheters often do not reach the bladder lumen.[100] Flexible rubber catheters also produce less bladder and urethral trauma.[100] The catheter should be inserted just to the bladder by determining the point at which urine is first obtained by aspiration. Inserting the catheter too deeply can result in trauma to the bladder. If large quantities of crystalline material or blood is evident in the urine, the bladder is repeatedly flushed with a sterile isotonic solution until the returning flushing solution is clear.

Whether the catheter is removed or sutured in place is based on the characteristics of each case. Leaving the catheter in place prevents immediate reobstruction and facilitates monitoring of urine output, but it also leads to bacterial urinary tract infection and urethral irritation.[101–103] Placing the cat on a broad-spectrum bactericidal antibiotic (ampicillin) while the catheter is in place reduces the incidence of UTI, but infection with antibiotic-resistant bacteria develops in some cats.[101] If the urethral catheter is left in place, a closed drainage system should be established by connecting the urethral catheter to a recently emptied sterile fluid bottle or bag with extension tubing. An Elizabethan collar is required to prevent the cat from removing the urethral catheter or disconnecting the drainage system.

At present, the best recommendation seems to be to leave the catheter in place only if one of the following four conditions is present: (1) the obstruction was relieved only with difficulty; (2) the urine stream is weak and small after relief of obstruction; (3) the cat is uremic (depressed, dehydrated, vomiting); or (4) detrusor dysfunction is present secondary to overdistention. In uremic cats rapid reobstruction should be prevented and urine output monitored. Unless clinical signs of bacterial infection develop, prophylactic antimicrobial therapy is not used, to avoid infection with resistant organisms. The catheter is left in place until the uremic signs abate, usually within 24 hours. To avoid catheter-induced complications, the catheter is left in place for as short a time as possible.[103] A urine sample is collected for urinalysis and culture when the catheter is removed. If bacterial infection is present, antibiotics are given for 7 to 10 days. A urine culture should be performed again 3 to 5 days after the antibiotic regimen is completed in order to ensure that the infection was eliminated. In evaluating the results of a culture of urine obtained when the urinary catheter is removed, less than 10^5 organisms per milliliter is considered significant.[103]

Obstructed cats are often hypothermic. Reestablishment of euthermia by application of blankets or a heating pad is recommended. Intravenous fluids can be warmed to body temperature prior to use. The cat should not be kept directly on a cold examining table during treatment. Warming should be continued until the cat's temperature reaches the low normal range and the cat's activity increases.

Uremic cats are usually also hyperkalemic and acidemic.[104] For survival of these cats, intravenous fluid therapy is required in addition to relief of obstruction.[84,85] The major goals of fluid therapy are to reduce hyperkalemia and azotemia, to improve acid-base balance, and to correct dehydration. Alkalinizing electrolyte solutions such as lactated Ringer's or Multisol have been shown to reverse acidemia and hyperkalemia in experimentally induced urethral obstruction, even though these fluids do contain a small amount of potassium.[84,85] Solutions containing dextrose and insulin have been recommended,[105–107] as well as combinations of saline and dextrose,[1,104,108] but no evidence exists that such therapy is more beneficial than alkalinizing electrolyte solutions alone.[84,85,109,110] Adding sodium bicarbonate to the treatment regimen will more rapidly reverse the acidemia of obstructed cats,[104] but no increase in survival over cats treated with electrolyte solutions containing the equivalent of 53 mEq/L $NaHCO_3$ has been shown.[84,85]

The amount of fluids to administer is based on the severity of dehydration, uremic signs, and hyperkalemia. Approximately 5 percent body weight should be given if the signs are mild, 8 percent if moderate, and 12 percent if severe (1 pound equals approximately 500 ml, and 1 kg equals 1,000 ml). This amount should be administered over approximately 1 to 2 hours. These are only general guidelines. Actual volume replacement must be individualized for each cat based on vital signs, changes in hydration status, mental attitude, and urine output. Hyperkalemia, acidemia, and uremia will not be rapidly reversed if the rate of fluid administration is too slow. Pulmonary edema may result from too rapid fluid replacement. No evidence of pulmonary edema developed when experimentally obstructed cats were given a balanced electrolyte solution at a rate of 50 to 60 ml/kg/h.[84,85]

In general, after the initial amount of fluid is given, the cat's mental attitude is improved, urine output is sustained, and severe hyperkalemia is reversed (as shown by biochemical measurement, the cat's improved attitude, and reversal of electrocardiographic abnormalities). When the cat's condition has thus improved, the rate of fluid administration can be reduced. Sufficient volume should be given over 24 hours to balance insensible water losses (estimated at 20 ml/kg/d) and to replace urine losses. If urine output is not measured, sufficient fluids should be given to provide maintenance needs (estimated at 60 ml/kg/d) and to correct any dehydration detected by physical examination. Food and water can be offered as soon as vomiting stops, which is usually within the first 24 hours.

Fluid therapy should be continued until the azotemia is resolved or minimal. Subcutaneous fluids can be substituted for intravenous fluids once the uremic signs abate and serum potassium is normal (usually within 4 to 24 hours). A postobstructive diuresis sometimes develops, making continued fluid therapy necessary. The cause of this diuresis is unknown, but both impaired renal tubular function and the necessity to excrete solutes retained during obstruction have been postulated. The actual percentage of cats that are affected by a diuretic phase during recovery from obstruction is unknown. Polyuria did occur in some experimental cats after relief of experimental obstruction.[85] In instances of postobstructive diuresis, the daily amount of fluids to be given can be determined by providing for insensible water losses and replacement of urine losses or by providing maintenance needs plus an amount sufficient to correct detectable dehydration.

Fluid therapy in cats with partial or total anorexia may lead to hypokalemia a few days after obstruction is relieved. Recurrent or worsening weakness and lethargy may be the only clinical signs. Hypokalemia was a problem within 24 hours in clinical cases treated with potassium-free fluids and sodium bicarbonate[104] but was not a problem in experimental cats treated with isotonic, balanced electrolyte solutions.[84,85] If hypokalemia is suspected, it should be confirmed by measurement of serum potassium concentration. If present, potassium supplementation can be given orally if the cat is not vomiting, or 20 mEq KCl can be added to each liter of balanced electrolyte solution. If hypokalemia is severe (less than 3.0 mEq/L), additional potassium supplementation may be needed. Recommended amounts have been tabulated.[111]

Experimentally obstructed cats were catabolic after relief of obstruction.[85] Weight loss occurred despite normal hydration, gradual return of food intake, and gradual normalization of laboratory data. Feeding cats highly palatable foods or force feeding after vomiting ceases might help to alleviate this catabolic state.

Prior to use of any drug in cats with urethral obstruction, the necessity, side effects, dose, and frequency of administration of each drug should be reviewed in light of the requirement for renal metabolism or excretion.[97] Urinary acidifiers should not be given to uremic or azotemic cats, because they may aggravate existing metabolic acidemia. Nephrotoxic drugs, such as aminoglycoside antibiotics, should be avoided unless required for treating bacterial infection known to be sensitive only to these antimicrobials. In general, cats with FUS do not have bacterial UTI at initial evaluation. Although hypocalcemia may be present, treatment with calcium is contraindicated. Treatment with calcium in the presence of hyperphosphatemia may result in dystrophic calcification, which could cause permanent renal damage. Treatment with calcium is unnecessary, since sufficient ionized calcium is usually present to prevent adverse clinical signs. Correction of hyperphosphatemia by restoring renal function results in return of eucalcemia.

The use of antiinflammatory drugs is controversial. Some investigators have advocated glucocorticoids to minimize urethral inflammation[69,112]; however, glucocorticoids may aggravate uremia by inducing gluconeogenesis and protein catabolism.[113] Glucocorticoids might increase the likelihood of catheter-associated UTI because of their immunosuppressive properties. A prospective study of the benefits versus risks of antiinflammatory drugs in obstructed cats is indicated. Some veterinarians believe that dimethyl sulfoxide (DMSO) is beneficial when instilled into the bladder after relief of urethral obstruction.[114] This compound also should be tested by a controlled study to determine benefits and risks.

Feline Urologic Syndrome Without Obstruction

Although antibiotic therapy has been recommended for cats with FUS without obstruction, the rationale is questionable, since urine cultures are negative. A prospective study of the efficacy of chloramphenicol versus placebo in 20 cats showed no difference in response.[77] Most cats were normal within 5 days, regardless of therapy.

A prospective study of subcutaneous fluids (100 ml lactated Ringer's) or a smooth muscle relaxant (probantheline bromide, 7.5 mg per os) versus 24 hours of hospitalization alone also indicated no benefits.[77] Again, most cats were normal within 5 days.

Based on the above limited studies[77] and the clinical impressions of others,[4] FUS without obstruction seems to be a self-limiting condition in the majority of cats. If the signs do not abate within 5 to 7 days, a diagnostic plan to rule out other causes of hematuria and dysuria should be instituted, including urine culture and survey and contrast radiography. Future studies to determine efficacious therapy for FUS cats without obstruction will have to be placebo-controlled because of the high rate of spontaneous resolution of clinical signs, and the term FUS will have to be well defined to a specific subpopulation of cats with hematuria and dysuria. Further drugs that warrant controlled study are antiinflammatory agents such as glucocorticoids[69,112] and megestrol acetate.[96] Potential risks and benefits of such agents have recently been discussed.[115] Diabetes mellitus has been described with long-term use of megestrol acetate. Diuretics such as furosemide have also been recommended to increase water turnover.[116] Again, no controlled studies are available.

Another group of drugs which should be studied are smooth or skeletal muscle relaxants for relief of dysuria. Probantheline bromide did not seem to improve duration of dysuria in one study.[77] In part, this may have been due to the 5-day time of evaluation in which most cats had total resolution of signs, and a beneficial earlier effect of the drug may have been masked. Since striated muscle surrounds much of the male cat urethra,[69,79,117] skeletal muscle relaxants should also be evaluated.

Considerable confusion exists in the treatment of this group of cats because of the use of the term FUS interchangeably with urolithiasis by some authors.[1] Thus, treatment recommendations shown effective for struvite uroliths are being advocated for all cats with hematuria and dysuria.[1] Such recommendations have not been tested prospectively in clinical cases without true uroliths and cannot at this time be considered efficacious.

Urinary products that contain methylene blue or phenazopyridine should not be used in cats because of their potential for causing methemoglobinemia and Heinz body anemia.[118–120]

Prevention of Recurrence of FUS

One of the most frustrating aspects of FUS is the high rate of recurrence of clinical signs.[11,77,121] Rate of recurrence in one study was 39 percent over 18 months in cats without urethral obstruction.[77] In cats with urethral obstruction, 22 percent died within 6 months.[11] In a study of cats with urethral obstruction, only 40 percent were alive without recurrence of obstruction at 6 months.[121] Cats experiencing their first episode of obstruction at less than 4 years of age appeared to have a higher incidence of recurrence (68 percent versus 32 percent).[121] Various recommendations have been made to reduce this recurrence rate, including long-term use of urinary acidifiers, low-Mg diets, and increasing water intake and urine output. None of these recommendations have been evaluated prospectively in clinical cases to date.

Only one acidifier has been evaluated in clinical cases of urethral obstruction. Ethylenediamine dihydrochloride (chlorethamine), when given for 21 days after obstruction, did not prevent future obstruction.[121] Whether obstruction would have been as likely if the acidifier had been continued was not answered by this study. Ethylenediamine hydrochloride has also been found to be only a weak urinary acidifier in cats.[121,122] DL-methionine slowed but did not prevent the development of urethral obstruction in cats fed an experimental calculogenic diet.[123] However, feeding an artificial diet which induces such a high rate of obstruction may overwhelm any potentially beneficial effect acidifiers may have. In normal cats, ammonium chloride (15 grains/day) was the only acidifier shown to prevent the postprandial alkaline tide.[124] However, higher doses of DL-methionine (1,000 to 1,500 mg/day) have also been reported to prevent postprandial alkaline urine production.[125] Inclusion of 1.5 percent ammonium chloride in food fed ad libitum to cats (approximately 668 mg/day)[126] was shown to maintain a lower urine pH (5.9 $\pm$ 0.3) than the same diet without ammonium chloride (pH 7.0 $\pm$ 0.5).[66] The administration of 500 to 1,500 mg of methionine or of 1,000 mg of ammonium chloride at feeding was also shown to cause a consistently lower urine pH than the same diet without acidifiers.[126] The reduction in urine pH with methionine was dose dependent. No adverse effects were found with methionine, but ammonium chloride caused adverse effects in four of five cats, consisting of diarrhea, partial anorexia, and vomiting. The vomiting and anorexia resolved after a few days, but the diarrhea remained throughout treatment in two of five cats.[126]

The majority of FUS cats with and without obstruction have acidic urine.[118,125] Whether maintenance of a more acidic urine with ammonium chloride would be beneficial in clinical cases of FUS is unknown. One report of four cats with recurrent urethral obstruction indicated prevention of recurrence with ammonium chloride but not with a magnesium-restricted diet.[128] Ammonium chloride apparently is of benefit in preventing struvite urolithiasis in cats fed an experimental calculogenic diet.[129] However, fatal toxicity of an ammonium chloride/DL-methionine combination (Uroeze-FUS) in kittens receiving the amount in food recommended for adult cats has recently been reported.[130] Toxicity studies of the high doses of acidifiers being recommended have apparently not been conducted.

Dietary recommendations have also been made for cats with FUS, based on reducing mineral intake and increasing water intake. Although a calculogenic diet has been formulated experimentally, no commercially available cat food has been shown to be calculogenic. Nor has any low-magnesium cat food been shown to prevent recurrence of FUS. Increasing water intake and thus urine output has been recommended for cats with FUS. Feeding moist cat foods, mostening dry cat foods, salting the food, or giving diuretics have been done to increase water turnover. Although one case-controlled study found a higher incidence of an initial episode of urethral obstruction in cats eating greater than 50 percent dry food,[37] the risk of recurrence of obstruction was not associated with percentage of dry food intake.[11,121] Addition of 4 percent NaCl to a calculogenic diet did not prevent calculi formation.[131] However, such an artificial diet which induces obstruction in the majority of normal cats may overwhelm any potentially beneficial effect of therapy, and negative results cannot be extrapolated to natural cases. One experimental study of six cats prone to hematuria showed decreased numbers of RBCs in urine, increased urine volume being associated with feeding canned or high salt dry foods.[61] One brief clinical report with few case details indicated prevention of recurrence of urethral obstruction by adding water to a low-magnesium diet.[5] Another clinical study that was not well controlled suggested a decreased risk of recurrence of FUS using addition of salt and water to the cats' food for life.[112] DL-methionine was also administered to affected cats for at least a month. Another poorly controlled study[132] is often cited as proving efficacy of a prescription diet (C/D), when in fact the study also employed commercial canned cat food, urinary acidifiers, and antimicrobial agents. A prospective, controlled study of the efficacy of low magnesium diets and/or of increasing water consumption is sorely needed.

Efficacy of crystallization inhibitors such as tripolyphosphate and of chelators of calcium and magnesium (CureCal) is unknown, but limited work has not demonstrated any efficacy.[133] The manufacturers' claim of efficacy is based solely on a limited number of uncontrolled empicical observations.[125] Addition of 15 percent alanine to calculogenic diets prevented the formation of magnesium phosphate uroliths in cats.[123] A high concentration of alanine in urine is postulated to increase the solubility of magnesium phosphate and to impair the aggregation of the proteinaceous matrix. No studies of the efficacy of alanine in preventing recurrence of urethral obstruction in clinical cases of FUS have been reported.

Various surgical techniques have been developed to prevent recurrence of urethral obstruction. These have been recently reviewed.[134] The current technique of choice is perineal urethrostomy.[134] Complications are possible, as with any surgical technique.[134] The incidence of complications and the efficacy of the technique in preventing reobstruction have not been determined by a prospective clinical trial. One uncontrolled series of reported cases indicated that reobstruction occurred in 2 of 10 cats,[132] which has led other authors to state a reobstruction rate of 20 percent.[1] This conclusion cannot be applied to perineal urethrostomies in general because of the few cases involved. Another study found an incidence of postoperative strictures of 9 percent,[135] while a third found no postoperative strictures and no reoccurrence of urethral obstruction.[89] To avoid the possibility that the obstruction occurs at a site cranial to perineal urethrostomy and thus that the surgery would be ineffective, one group recommends performance of urethrography routinely prior to surgery.[92] Surgery does not prevent recurrence of hematuria or dysuria without obstruction. In one study, recurrent dysuria was a problem in 10 of 35 cats which had a perineal urethrostomy.[89]

Surgical removal of urachal remnants has been reported to reduce the recurrence rate of lower urinary tract signs in both male and female cats and to reduce the rate of urethral reobstruction in males.[74] As discussed under etiology, this study needs to be extended, since the mechanism by which such a procedure should be so beneficial is difficult to understand.

Thus, at the present time there is no known method of preventing hematuria and dysuria in cats in which no predisposing cause for these problems can be identified.

CONSEQUENCES

FUS without Obstruction

Long-term consequences of repeated episodes of hematuria and dysuria without obstruction and without identifiable cause in cats (FUS without obstruction, by our definition) have not been described. Whether male cats with this history have a greater chance of later obstruction is not known. A prospective or retrospective study of the clinical course of this population of cats over a long period of time is indicated. Since each individual episode seems to be self-limiting without treatment, the clinician must be careful that treatment used does not cause any adverse effects.

FUS with Obstruction

The consequences of urethral obstruction can be divided into those related to the obstruction itself and those related to treatment of the obstruction.

The life-threatening consequences of urethral obstruction are related to the development of postrenal uremia and hyperkalemia as described under pathophysiology. In experimental ureteral obstruction, permanent renal dysfunction did not occur unless obstruction was maintained for longer than 96 hours.[83] Urethral obstruction for 96 hours or longer results in severe uremia, hyperkalemia, and death in cats.[85] Therefore, permanent renal lesions would be considered unlikely in most cats presented for urethral obstruction that are not this ill. However, one study of renal tissues from cats obtained more than 7 days after an episode of obstruction found a high incidence of renal lesions (five of eight cats), compared to the incidence in 300 cats of similar age.[63,136] Unfortunately, the incidence of renal lesions in cats in the same colony but without a history of urethral obstruction was not determined.[63]

A potential consequence of urethral obstruction is damage to the bladder detrusor muscle by prolonged bladder overdistension. Loss of the tight junctions between muscle fibers prevents the spread of motor nerve impulses that are required for normal bladder contraction. When such damage occurs, the cat cannot voluntarily empty its bladder after removal of obstruction, but the bladder can be expressed manually with a good urine stream.[137] For therapy, the bladder is kept empty so that the tight junctions can reform. This can be done by manually expressing the bladder frequently or by use of an indwelling urinary catheter. Bethanechol (2.5 mg) can be given a few days after frequent emptying is initiated.[138] Response to bethanechol should occur within a few hours of administration. If there is no response, either a higher dose must be used, observing for side effects, or the drug should be discontinued. The urethra must be patent during administration of parasympathomimetic drugs, or rupture of the bladder could theoretically occur. Time required for return of bladder function varies with degree of injury.

Another cause of micturition difficulty after relief of obstruction is increased outflow resistance. With this problem, the urine stream is weak even when digital compression of the bladder is forceful. Causes of such outflow resistance include reoccurrence of intraluminal obstruction, extraluminal obstruction, or urethral spasm.[137] Physical obstructions should be ruled out by passing a catheter or performing contrast radiography. If urethral spasm is present, drug therapy theoretically may be of benefit, but it has not been evaluated in cats. Extrapolating from other species, drugs to consider would include phenoxybenzamine to block urethral alpha adrenergic receptors and/or diazepam to relieve skeletal muscle spasm. Dosage recommendations and potential side effects have been recently reviewed.[135] For phenoxybenzamine, an initial dosage of 2.5 mg/day is recommended. If necessary, dosage can be increased by 2.5 mg every 3 to 5 days, to a maximum of 10 mg. Side effects are related to alpha adrenergic blockade. The drug should not be used in cats with cardiovascular disease. The recommended dosage of diazepam is 2.5 to 5.0 mg, but side effects such as sedation or unusual behavior are possible. It must be emphasized that any of these drugs should be used only if indicated and cautiously because of the extremely limited knowledge of dosages and side effects in cats.

Consequences of therapy include complications associated with removal of obstructing material and with urethral surgery. Use of urinary catheters during reverse flushing of the urethra can result in urethral injury ranging from mucosal erosions to complete tearing. Care must be taken in manipulation to minimize urethral trauma. Inflammation induced by catheterization may itself result in hematuria and dysuria. Use of indwelling urinary catheters can result in urinary tract infection and urethral and bladder inflammation. Urinary tract infection can occur in spite of prophylactic antibiotics, and infection in cats receiving antibiotics will be with more highly antibiotic-resistant organisms.[101] Indwelling urinary catheters in an open system left in place for 5 days is followed by a high rate of urethral obstruction (2 of 10 cats) and inflammatory urethral lesions that persisted up to 90 days in some cats.[102] Despite these problems, indwelling catheters are necessary in uremic cats when urine output must be monitored, in cats in which obstruction was difficult to remove and whose urine stream after relief of obstruction is small, and in cats with detrusor muscle dysfunction who cannot be frequently expressed manually. Our recommendations are that closed drainage systems be used and that antibiotics be given only if signs of infection are present. Otherwise we recommend a urine culture when the catheter is removed and treatment directed specifically to any organism detected.

Surgical complications of perineal urethrostomy have been studied retrospectively.[134,139] Urethral stricture is one major complication which predisposes the cat to obstruction and requires corrective surgery. Reported incidence of this complication has varied from 0 to 20 percent.[89,132,135] Other complications of perineal urethrostomy include predisposition to bacterial UTI.[89,102,139,140] Incidence of UTI was highest when indwelling urinary catheters were used in conjunction with surgery.[102] Urinary tract infection after perineal urethrostomy was usually present without causing clinical signs.[89] The long-term consequences of such infections are unknown. Perineal urethrostomy has been associated with decreased urethral pressure in normal cats[140,141] and in 7 of 18 cats that had surgery performed because of urethral obstruction.[140] This may result in urinary incontinence.[141]

REFERENCES

1. Lewis LD, Morris ML: Feline Urologic Syndrome: Causes and clinical management. Vet Med/Small Anim Clin 79:323, 1984
2. Fabricant CG: The feline urologic syndrome induced by infection with a cell-associated herpesvirus. Vet Clin North Am 14:493, 1984
3. Osborne CA, Johnston GR, Polzin DJ, et al: Feline urologic syndrome: A heterogeneous phenomenon? J Am Anim Hosp Assoc 20:17, 1984
4. Osborne CA, Johnston GR, Polzin DJ, et al: Redefinition of the feline urologic syndrome. Vet Clin North Am 14:409, 1984
5. Jackson OF: The treatment and subsequent prevention of struvite urolithiasis in cats. J Small Anim Pract 12:555, 1971
6. Jackson OF, Colles CM: Experimental matrix plug production in male cat urine following a natural case of urolithiasis due to matrix plug. J Small Anim Pract 15:701, 1974
7. Gaskell CJ: Urolithiasis in the dog and the cat. Vet Rec 102:546, 1978
8. Carbone G: Phosphocrystalluria and urethral obstruction in the cat. Am Vet Med Assoc 147:1195, 1965
9. Fennell C: Some demographic characteristics of the domestic cat population in

Great Britain with particular reference to feeding habits and the incidence of the Feline Urologic Syndrome. J Small Anim Pract 16:775, 1975
10. Tomey SL, Follis TB: Incidence rates of feline urological syndrome (FUS) in the United States. Feline Pract 8:39, 1978
11. Walker AD, Weaver AD, Anderson RS: An epidemiological survey of the feline urological syndrome. J Small Anim Pract 18:283, 1977
12. Joint BSAVA/PFMA FUS Committee: Feline Urolithiasis: interim report. Vet Rec 96:298, 1975
13. Frost RC: Cystic calculi in the cat. Vet Rec 70:765, 1958
14. Willeberg P: Epidemiology of naturally occuring feline urologic syndrome. Vet Clin North Am 14:455, 1984
15. Bernard MA: Feline Urological Syndrome: A study of seasonal incidence, frequency of repeat visits and comparison of treatment. Can Vet J 19:284, 1978
16. Willeberg P: A case-control study of some fundamental determinants in the epidemiology of the Feline Urological Syndrome. Nord Vet Med 27:1, 1975
17. Willeberg P, Priester WA: Feline Urological Syndrome: Associations with some time, space, and individual patient factors. Am J Vet Res 37:975, 1976
18. Holzworth J: Some important disorders of cats. Cornell Vet 53:157, 1963
19. Jackson OF: A springtime rise in the incidence of urolithiasis. Vet Rec 93:337, 1973
20. Aronson L: Discussion on microbial studies of feline urolithiasis. J Am Vet Med Assoc 158:980, 1971
21. Dorn CR, Saueressig S, Schmidt DA: Factors affecting use of urolithiasis-cystitis-urethritis in cats. Am J Vet Res 34:433, 1973
22. Foster SJ: The "urolithiasis" syndrome in male cats; a statistical analysis of the problems, with clinical observations. J Small Anim Pract 8:207, 1967
23. Barsanti JA, Finco DR, Shotts EB, et al: Feline urologic syndrome: further investigation into etiology. J Am Anim Hosp Assoc 18:391, 1982
24. Schechter RD: The significance of bacteria in feline cystitis and urolithiasis. J Am Vet Med Assoc 156:1567, 1970
25. Rich LJ, Kirk RW: The relationship of struvite crystals to urethral obstruction in cats. Am Vet Med Assoc 154:153, 1969
26. Gaskell RM, Gaskell CJ, Page W, et al: Studies on a possible viral aetiology for the feline urological syndrome. Vet Rec 105:243, 1979
27. Lees GE, Simpson RB, Green RA: Results of analyses and bacterial cultures of urine specimens obtained from clinically normal cats by three methods. Am Vet Med Assoc 184:449, 1984
28. Martens JG, McConnell S, Swanson CL: The role of infectious agents in naturally occurring feline urologic syndrome. Vet Clin North Am 14:503, 1984
29. Rich LJ, Fabricant CG: Urethral obstruction in male cats. Can J Comp Med 33:164, 1969
30. Rich LJ, Fabricant CG: Experimental production of urolithiasis in male cats. J Am Vet Med Assoc 158:974, 1971
31. Jackson OF: Feline urolithiasis report. Vet Rec 96:390, 1975
32. Shroyer EL, Shalaby MR: Isolation of feline syncytia-forming virus from oropharyngeal swab samples and buffy coat cells. Am J Vet Res 39:555, 1978
33. Seefeldt SL: The feline urological syndrome. Dissertation Abstracts Int 39B:110, 1978
34. Fabricant CG, Gillespie JH: Identification and characterization of a second feline herpesvirus. Infect Immun 9:460, 1974

35. Fabricant CG: Herpesvirus induced feline urolithiasis—A review. Comp Immunol Microbiol Infect Dis 1:121, 1979
36. Fabricant CG: Herpesvirus-induced urolithiasis in Specific-Pathogen-Free male cats. Am J Vet Res 38:1837, 1977
37. Reif JS, Bovee K, Gaskell CJ, et al: Feline urethral obstruction: a case control study. J Am Vet Med Assoc 170:1320, 1977
38. Fabricant CG, Krook L, Gillespie JH: Virus-induced cholesterol crystals. Science 181:566, 1973
39. Fabricant CG, Lein DH: Feline urolithiasis neither induced nor exacerbated by feeding a dry diet. J Am Anim Hosp Assoc 20:213, 1984
40. Osbaldiston GW, Taussig RA: Clinical report on 46 cases of feline urological syndrome. Vet Med/Small Anim Clin 65:461, 1970
41. Bloom F: The urine of the dog and cat. Gamma Pub., New York, 1960
42. Finco DR, Barsanti JA, Crowell WA: The Urinary System. p. 363. In Pratt PP (ed): Feline Medicine. Am Vet Pubns, Santa Barbara, CA, 1983
43. Osborne CA, Finco DR, Low D: Canine and Feline Urology. WB Saunders Co, Philadelphia, 1972
44. Fabricant CG, Gillespie JH, Krook L: Intracellular and extracellular mineral crystal formation induced by viral infection of cell cultures. Infect Immun 3:416, 1971
45. Fabricant CG: Serological responses to the cell associated herpesvirus and the manx calicivirus of SPF male cats with herpesvirus-induced urolithiasis. Cornell Vet 71:59, 1981
46. Barker J, Povey RC: The feline urolithiasis syndrome: a review and an inquiry into the alleged role of dry cat foods in its aetiology. J Small Anim Pract 14:445, 1973
47. Bressett JD, Kallfelz FA, Lubar J, et al: Relation of ration type and mineral content to the incidence of feline urologic syndrome. Proc Cornell Nutrition Conf for Feed Manufacturers. 1979, p. 108
48. Duch DS, Hamar DW, Chow FC, et al: Study on urine polyelectrolytes of cats with natural and exaperimental urolithiasis. Biochem Med 19:236, 1978
49. Lewis LD, Chow FHC, Taton GF, et al: Effect of various dietary mineral concentration on the occurrence of feline urolithiasis. J Am Vet Med Assoc 172:559, 1978
50. Rich LJ, Dysart I, Chow FC, et al: Urethral obstruction in male cats: experimental production by addition of magnesium and phosphate to diet. Feline Pract 4:44, 1974
51. Osborne CA, Clinton CW, Brunkow HC, et al: Epidemiology of naturally occurring feline uroliths and urethral plugs. Vet Clin North Am 14:481, 1984
52. Kallfelz FA, Bressett JD, Wallace RJ: Urethral obstruction in random source and SPF male cats induced by high levels of dietary magnesium or magnesium and phosphorus. Feline Pract 10:25, 1980
53. Finco DR, Barsanti JA, Crowell WA: Feline urethral obstruction: characterization of induced disease and comparison with naturally occurring feline urologic syndrome. (In press, 1984)
54. Feldman BM, Kennedy BM, Schelstraete M: Dietary minerals and the feline urologic syndrome. Feline Pract 7:39, 1977
55. Chow FC, Hamar DW, Dysart I, et al: Feline urolithiasis/cat foods: concentration of calcium, magnesium, phosphate and chloride in various cat foods and their relationship to feline urolithiasis. Feline Pract 5:15, 1975
56. Graser DH, Hamar DW, Lewis LD: The consistency of dietary minerals in com-

mercial cat foods and their relationship to feline urolithiasis. Feline Pract 11:41, 1981
57. Finco DR, Barsanti JA: Diet-induced feline urethral obstruction. Vet Clin North Am 14:529, 1984
58. Jackson OF: The dry cat food controversy: Urolithiasis in laboratory and domestic cats. Vet Rec 91:292, 1972
59. Jackson OF: PhD Thesis, University of London, 1971, referenced by Barker J, Povey RC. J Small Anim Pract 14:445, 1973
60. Thrall BE, Miller LG: Water turnover in cats fed dry rations. Feline Pract 6:10, 1976
61. Holme DW: Research into the feline urological syndrome. Proceedings on the Kal Kan Symposium. Vernon, CA, 1977
62. Jackson OF, Tovey JD: Water balance studies in domestic cats. Feline Pract 7:30, 1977
63. Lawler DF, Evans RH: Urinary tract disease in cats: water balance studies, urolith and crystal analyses, and necropsy findings. Vet Clin North Am 14:537, 1984
64. Rich LJ, Kirk RW: Feline urethral obstruction: mineral aspects. Am J Vet Res 29:2149, 1968
65. Lewis LD, Morris ML: Diet as a causative factor of feline urolithiasis. Vet Clin North Am 14:513, 1984
66. Taton GF, Hamar DW, Lewis LD: Evaluation of ammonium chloride as a urinary acidifier in the cat. J Am Vet Med Assoc 184:433, 1984
67. Willeberg P: Epidemiology of the feline urological syndrome. Adv Vet Sci Comp Med 25:311, 1981
68. Dickinson CD, Scott PP: Failure to produce urinary calculi in kittens by the addition of mineral salts, derived from bone-meal, to the diet. Vet Rec 68:858, 1956
69. McCully RM, Lieberman LL: Histopathology in a case of feline urolithiasis. Can Vet J 2:52, 1961
70. Sutor DJ, Wooley SE, Jackson OF: Crystalline material from the feline bladder. Res Vet Sci 11:298, 1970
71. Herron MA: The effect of prepubertal castration on the penile urethra of the cat. J Am Vet Med Assoc 160:208, 1972
72. Meier FW: Urethral obstruction and stenosis in the male cat. J Am Vet Med Assoc 137:67, 1960
73. Willeberg P: Interaction effects of epidemiologic factors in the feline urological syndrome. Nord Vet Med 28:193, 1976
74. Hansen JS: Urachal remnant in the cat: occurrence and relationship to the feline urological syndrome. Vet Med/Small Anim Clin 728:1735, 1977
75. Johnston GR, Feeney DA, Osborne CA: Urethrography and cystography in cats. Part II. Abnormal radiographic anatomy and complications. Compend Cont Ed 4:931, 1982
76. Klausner JS, Johnston GR, Osborne CA: Diverticula of the urinary bladder. p. 1093. In Kirk RW (ed): Current Veterinary Therapy. Vol 8. WB Saunders, Philadelphia, 1983
77. Barsanti JA, Finco DR, Shotts EB, et al: Feline urologic syndrome: Further investigation into therapy. J Am Anim Hosp Assoc 18:387, 1982
78. Johnston GR, Feeney DA: Localization of feline urethral obstruction. Vet Clin North Am 14:555, 1984
79. Cullen WC, Fletcher TF, Bradley WF: Morphometry of the male feline urethra. J Urol 129:186, 1983

80. Barsanti JA, Crowell W, Losonsky J, et al: Complications of bladder distention during retrograde urethrography. Am J Vet Res 42:819, 1981
81. Mehrotra RML: An experimental study of the vesical circulation during distention and in cystitis. J Pathol Bacteriol 66:79, 1953
82. Finco DR, Barsanti JA: Mechanism of urinary excretion of creatinine by the cat. Am J Vet Res 43:2207, 1982
83. Klahr S: Pathophysiology of obstructive uropathy. Kidney Int 23:414, 1983
84. Finco DR: Induced feline urethral obstruction: response of hyperkalemia to relief of obstruction and administration of parenteral electrolyte solution. J Am Anim Hosp Assoc 12:198, 1976
85. Finco DR, Cornelius LM: Characterization and treatment of water, electrolyte, and acid-base imbalances of induced urethral obstruction in the cat. Am J Vet Res 38:823, 1977
86. Parks J: Electrocardiographic abnormalities from serum electrolyte imbalance due to feline urethral obstruction. J Am Anim Hosp Assoc 11:102, 1975
87. Loeb WF, Knipling GD: Glucosuria and pseudoglucosuria in cats with urethral obstruction. Mod Vet Pract 52:40, 1971
88. Osborne CA, Lees GE: Feline cystitis, urethritis, urethral obstruction syndrome. Mod Vet Pract 59:173, 1978
89. Gregory CR, Vasseur PB: Long-term examination of cats with perineal urethrostomy. Vet Surg 12:210, 1983
90. Osborne CA, Lees GE, Polzin DJ, et al: Immediate relief of feline urethral obstruction. Vet Clin North Am 14:585, 1984
91. Osborne CA, Polzin DJ, Johnston GR: Diagnosis of the feline urologic syndrome. Vet Clin North Am 14:575, 1984
92. Johnston GR, Feeney DA: Localization of feline urethral obstruction. Vet Clin North Am 14:555, 1984
93. Zontine WJ, Andrews LK: Fatal air embolism as a complication of pneumocystography in two cats. J Am Vet Radiol Soc 19:8, 1978
94. Thayer GW, Carrig CB, Evans AT: Fatal venous air embolism associated the pneumocystography in a cat. J Am Vet Med Assoc 176:643, 1980
95. Jackson OF: The treatment of struvite urethral obstruction in cats using Walpole's acetate buffer solution pH 4.5. Feline Pract 6:52, 1980
96. Gaskell, CJ, Denny HR, Jackson OF, et al: Clinical management of the feline urological syndrome. J Small Anim Pract 19:301, 1978
97. Riviere JE: Adverse drug reactions in cats with feline urethral obstruction. Vet Clin North Am 14:703, 1984
98. Raffe MR, Caywood DD: Use of anesthetic agents in cats with obstructive uropathy. Vet Clin North Am 14:691, 1984
99. Botte RJ: Percutaneous prepubic urinary drainage in normal cats. Vet Surg 12:202, 1983
100. Lees GE, Osborne CA, Stevens JB, et al: Adverse effects caused by polypropylene and polyvinyl feline urinary catheters. Am J Vet Res 41:1836, 1980
101. Lees GE, Osborne CA, Stevens JB, et al: Adverse effects of open indwelling urethral catheterization in clinically normal male cats. Am J Vet Res 42:825, 1981
102. Smith CW, Schiller AG, Smith AR, et al: Effect of indwelling urinary catheters in male cats. J Am Anim Hosp Assoc 17:427, 1981
103. Lees GE, Osborne CA: Use and misuse of indwelling urinary catheters in cats. Vet Clin North Am 14:599, 1984
104. Burrows CF, Bovee KC: Characterization and treatment of acid-base and renal defects due to urethral obstruction in cats. J Am Vet Med Assoc 172:801, 1978

105. Schaer M: The use of regular insulin in the treatment of hyperkalemia in cats with urethral obstruction. J Am Anim Hosp Assoc 11:106, 1975
106. Schaer M: Polemical forum. J Am Anim Hosp Assoc 12:673, 1976
107. Schaer M: Letter to the editor. J Am Vet Med Assoc 173:147, 1978
108. Post K: Feline urological syndrome. Can Vet J 20:109, 1979
109. Finco D: Polemical forum. J Am Anim Hosp Assoc 12:675, 1976
110. Bovee K, Burrows CF: Letter to the editor. J Am Vet Med Assoc 173:148, 1978
111. Barsanti JA, Finco DR: Management of post-renal uremia. Vet Clin North Am 14:609, 1984
112. Bernard MA: Feline urologic syndrome: a study of seasonal incidence, frequency of repeat visits and comparison of treatments. Can Vet J 19:284, 1978
113. Osborne CA, Lees GE: Therapy of disorders of the upper and lower urinary tract. Mod Vet Pract 59:349, 1978
114. Koller LC: Clinical application of DMSO by veterinarians in Oregon and Washington. Vet Med/Small Anim Clin 71:591, 1976
115. Osborne CA, Polzin DJ, Klausner JS, et al: Medical management of male and female cats with nonobstructive lower urinary tract disease. Vet Clin North Am 14:617, 1984
116. Dingel RM: Diuretics in FUS treatment. Feline Pract 5:4, 1975
117. Meier FW: Urethral obstruction and stenosis. J Am Vet Med Assoc 147:67, 1960
118. Osborne CA, Lees GE: Feline cystitis, urethritis, urethral obstruction syndrome. Part IV. Mod Vet Pract 59:669, 1978
119. Harvey JW, Kornick HP: Phenazopyridine toxicosis in the cat. J Am Vet Med Assoc 169:327, 1976
120. Schechter RD, Schalm OW, Kaneko JJ: Heinz body hemolytic anemia associated with use of urinary antiseptics containing methylene blue in the cat. J Am Vet Med Assoc 162:37, 1973
121. Bovee KC, Reif JS, Maguire TG, et al: Recurrence of feline urethral obstruction. J Am Vet Med Assoc 174:93, 1979
122. Finco DR: Efficacy of ethylenediamine dihydrochloride in dogs and cats. Am J Vet Res 42:670, 1981
123. Chow FHC, Dysart I, Hamar DW: Effect of dietary additives in experimentally produce feline urolithiasis. Feline Pract 6:51, 1976
124. Chow FHC, Taton GF, Lewis LD, et al: Effect of dietary ammonium chloride, DL-methionine, sodium phosphate and ascorbic acid on urinary pH and electrolyte concentrations of male cats. Feline Pract 8:29, 1978
125. Polzin DJ, Osborne CA: Medical prophylaxis of feline lower urinary tract disorders. Vet Clin North Am 14:661, 1984
126. Lloyd WE, Sullivan DJ: Effects of orally administered ammonium chloride and methionine on feline urinary acidity. Vet Med/Small Anim Clin 79:773, 1984
127. Taussig RA: Cystitis in the female cat: therapy and prophylaxis. Feline Pract 3:52, 1975
128. Durham RM, Broom EL: A therapeutic preventive for feline urologic syndrome. Vet Med/Small Anim Clin 78:375, 1983
129. Taton GF, Hamar DW, Lewis LD: Urinary acidification in the prevention and treatment of feline struvite urolithiasis. J Am Vet Med Assoc 184:437, 1984
130. Brown JE, Fox LM: Ammonium chloride/methionine toxicity in kittens. Feline Pract 14:16, 1984
131. Hamar D, Chow FCH, Dysart MI, et al: Effect of sodium chloride in prevention of experimentally produced phosphate uroliths in male cats. J Am Anim Hosp Assoc 12:514, 1976

132. Engle GC: A clinical report on 250 cases of feline urological syndrome. Feline Pract 7:24, 1977
133. Rich LJ: Urthral Obstruction and Urolithiasis in Cats. p. 703. In Kirk RW (ed): Current Veterinary Therapy IV. WB Saunders, Philadelphia, 1971
134. Caywood DD, Raffe MR: Perspectives on surgical management of feline urethral obstruction. Vet Clin North Am 14:677, 1984
135. Tomchick TL, Green RW: Feline Urologic Syndrome, Surgical Prophylaxis. p. 1201. In Kirk RW (ed): Current Veterinary Therapy VII. WB Saunders, Philadelphia, 1980
136. Hamilton JM: Nephritis in the cat. J Small Anim Pract 7:445, 1966
137. Lees GE, Moreau PM: Management of hypotonic and atonic urinary bladders in cats. Vet Clin North Am 14:641, 1984
138. Moreau PM: Neurogenic disorders of micturition in the dog and cat. Compend Cont Ed Pract Vet 4:12, 1982
139. Smith CW, Schiller AG: Perineal urethrostomy in the cat: a retrospective study of compliactions. J Am Anim Hosp Assoc 14:225, 1978
140. Gregory CR, Vasseur PB: Electromyographic and urethral pressure profilometry: Long-term assessment of urethral function after perineal urethrostomy in cats. Am J Vet Res 45:1318, 1984
141. Gregory CR: Electromyographic and urethral pressure profilometry. Vet Clin North Am 14:567, 1984

4 Urologic Surgery—An Update

Elizabeth A. Stone

An update on urologic surgery involves the reassessment of past surgical recommendations and a better understanding of current techniques and procedures. The surgical treatment of some diseases is now being challenged. For example, although surgery will probably remain the primary treatment for urolithiasis, dissolution of calculi using dietary management has been reported in selected cases.[1] A review of long-term postoperative results and complications allows us to critically evaluate our treatment choices. A better understanding of surgical anatomy has simplified certain procedures such as urethrotomy and urethrostomy. This chapter will focus on selected areas of newer knowledge and on conditions with controversial surgical management choices.

SURGICAL REMOVAL OF UROLITHS

The disease syndrome of urolithiasis is discussed in Chapter 1. Medical treatment of urolithiasis with a combination of calculolytic diet, antimicrobial agents, and acetohydroxamine has been reported to cause dissolution of experimentally induced struvite uroliths within 6 weeks.[1] Clinical investigations also suggest that dissolution is possible in the canine patient. Surgical removal of uroliths is still indicated in many instances,[1] including the following:

1. Uroliths in immature dogs: Calculolytic diets have not been evaluated in puppies. Prolonged low protein diets may retard growth, and the effects of low magnesium in a growing animal are unknown.
2. Urinary tract obstruction: Uroliths causing obstruction of the renal

pelvis, ureter, or urethra should be removed to prevent and/or treat life-threatening postrenal uremia and to prevent further compromise of the kidney. Nonsurgical removal of urethral calculi by catheterization and hydropropulsion should be attempted before resorting to surgical removal.

3. Presence of urinary tract anomalies: Some anomalies of the urinary tract, such as a diverticulum of the urinary bladder, a patent urachus, and/or strictures of the urethra, may increase the susceptibility of the urinary tract to infections. Surgical correction may reduce the chances of recurrent urinary tract infection and calculi formation.

4. Unknown urolith composition: The most accurate method for determining urolith composition is by quantitative analysis of the urolith. The presence of struvite uroliths is suggested by the presence of radiopaque uroliths in alkaline urine infected with urease-producing bacteria. Medical dissolution therapy can be instituted based on this estimation. Uncertainty of mineral composition and/or failure of medical therapy necessitates surgical removal and analysis of the urolith.

5. Owner preference: Owner compliance is a major factor in the successful dissolution of calculi. Some owners will not feed their dogs calculolytic diets, and some dogs will not eat the diet. The costs of surgery and medical management may be similar, especially if multiple radiographs are required to monitor the progress of dissolution.

6. Uroliths in cats: Since the long-term effects of calculolytic diets and acetohydroxamine in cats are unknown, surgical removal is the treatment of choice.[1]

SURGICAL REMOVAL OF RENAL CALCULI

The decision to surgically remove nephroliths is based on the above considerations and the knowledge that renal function will continue to decline as long as nephroliths are present. Calculi act as a nidus for infection and may make antimicrobial therapy ineffective. Once the nephrolith is removed, there is a potential for compensatory hypertrophy even in a diseased kidney. The goals of the nephrolithotomy procedure are to relieve urinary obstruction, to assist in the eradication of urinary infection, and to minimize damage to renal parenchyma.[3]

Two procedures for removing renoliths are currently being used in small animal surgery. The bisection nephrolithotomy is routinely used in veterinary surgery to remove a single nephrolith within a normal sized renal pelvis or to remove multiple calculi within the diverticula.[4] A bisecting midline nephrotomy incision through the renal parenchyma was reported to temporarily decrease the glomerular filtration rate by 30 percent in dogs which previously had had a unilateral nephrectomy.[5]

To remove nephroliths by the pyelolithotomy procedure, an incision is made into the relatively avascular dorsolateral renal pelvis.[6] It does not require occlusion of blood flow to the kidney via a tourniquet. The pyelolithotomy procedure causes less parenchymal damage than does a bisection nephrotomy, but its use is restricted to instances when there is a single large calculus within a dilated renal pelvis.

Bilateral renoliths can be removed in one or two operations. Ideally, one kidney should be operated on, the animal and kidney should be allowed to recover, and then a second operation should be performed. The expense of two operations may discourage owners from pursuing any treatment. Therefore, if the animal is not azotemic, we assume there is sufficient reserve renal function and operate on both kidneys during the same surgery. If the animal is azotemic, only one kidney is operated on. After recovery from the first nephrotomy, the renal function is reassessed, and a decision regarding the second nephrotomy is made. Differential quantitative radionuclide scans are being used in human patients to assess individual kidney function before and after nephrotomy.[7] Radionuclide scans are being evaluated in dogs and should help with decisions regarding unilateral versus bilateral nephrotomy.

The decision to do a nephrectomy rather than a nephrotomy is made when there is a nonfunctional, infected kidney on one side and a functional kidney on the other side. A recent study in rats showed that the presence of a poorly functioning kidney induced compensatory renal hyperplasia in the opposite kidney. The amount of hyperplasia was significantly greater than that which occurred after removal of the damaged kidney.[8] This information suggests that a noninfected kidney with marginal renal function should not be removed.

URETHROTOMY AND URETHROSTOMY IN THE DOG

A *urethrotomy*, a temporary incision into the urethra, is performed for the temporary relief of urethral obstruction or for the removal of urethral calculi.

Urethrotomy incisions have been described in the prescrotal and the perineal regions in dogs. The most common site for uroliths to lodge is just caudal to the os penis. They can usually be retrieved through a prescrotal urethrotomy with alternate flushing between the end of the urethra and the urethrotomy site. The prescrotal urethra is more superficial and less vascular than the perineal urethra. A perineal urethrotomy is performed when calculi are lodged in the perineal or pelvic urethra. The calculi are retrieved through the urethrotomy site or flushed into the urinary bladder. A perineal urethrotomy can often be avoided by alternate flushing of the urethra between the urethral opening and a cystotomy. If calculi are lodged in the perineal or pelvic urethra, it may be possible to flush them back into the urinary bladder using a urethral catheter placed through a prescrotal urethrotomy or through the distal end of the intact urethra. Alternatively, the calculi can be flushed with a catheter placed into the proximal urethra via a cystotomy incision.

Some authors recommend a perineal urethrotomy following urethral surgery in a male dog so that a Foley catheter can be passed through the perineal urethrotomy into the bladder for temporary urinary drainage.[9] In most cases, however, a cystostomy catheter will allow temporary urine drainage without an additional incision into the urethra.

A *urethrostomy* is a permanent opening in the urethra which permits passage of larger uroliths from the urethra and prevents them from lodging in the more distal urethra. A urethrostomy is often indicated for dogs that are recurrent stone formers because of persistent urinary tract infection, metabolic abnormalities, unknown factors, or the inability of the owner to follow prevention recommendations. A urethrostomy may also be performed to bypass urethral obstruction from a more distal stricture. A urethrostomy at any site will make the dog infertile.

The preferred site for a permanent urethrostomy is at the level of the scrotal urethra. The procedure necessitates castration. The scrotal urethra is wider than the prescrotal urethra and more superficial than the perineal urethra. Care is taken to place the scrotal urethrostomy incision at the point where the urethra lies in a dorsal-ventral (or vertical) plane. Calculi can then pass directly out of the urethra without having to traverse the urethra as it curves into a cranial-caudal (or horizontal) plane.

A permanent opening can be made in the perineal urethra. However, a perineal urethrostomy is less cosmetically acceptable and is associated with more bleeding and urine scalding than a scrotal urethrostomy. In general, the technique of perineal urethrostomy in dogs is used only when there is irreparable damage to the perineal urethra.

TECHNIQUE FOR PRESCROTAL URETHROTOMY

A troublesome complication of urethrotomies and urethrostomies is hemorrhage. It can be minimized by careful attention to the anatomy of the urethra and penis. A cross section of the penis and urethra at the level of the prescrotal urethra shows that the urethra is surrounded by the corpus spongiosum. The paired bodies of the corpora cavernosa lie lateral to the urethra. An exact ventral midline urethral incision will pass through the corpus spongiosum but will avoid either corpus cavernosum. An incision into the corpus cavernosum causes considerable hemorrhage since it is a very vascular structure.

The skin incision for a prescrotal urethrotomy extends from just caudal to the prepuce to just cranial to the scrotum (Fig. 4-1A, insert). If the incision extends onto the scrotum, the dog is more likely to excoriate the site. There is also the risk that the testes will prolapse into the incision if the skin incision extends too far caudally.

Subcutaneous tissue is dissected to the level of the retractor penis muscle (Fig. 4-1A). The grayish corpus spongiosum and the white fibrous covered corpora cavernosa should be identified. If the corpora cavernosa is the most visible midline structure, it may be necessary to rotate the penis between the thumb and forefinger to bring the retractor penile muscle and corpus spongiosum to the midline.

The retractor penile muscle is retracted laterally. A longitudinal incision

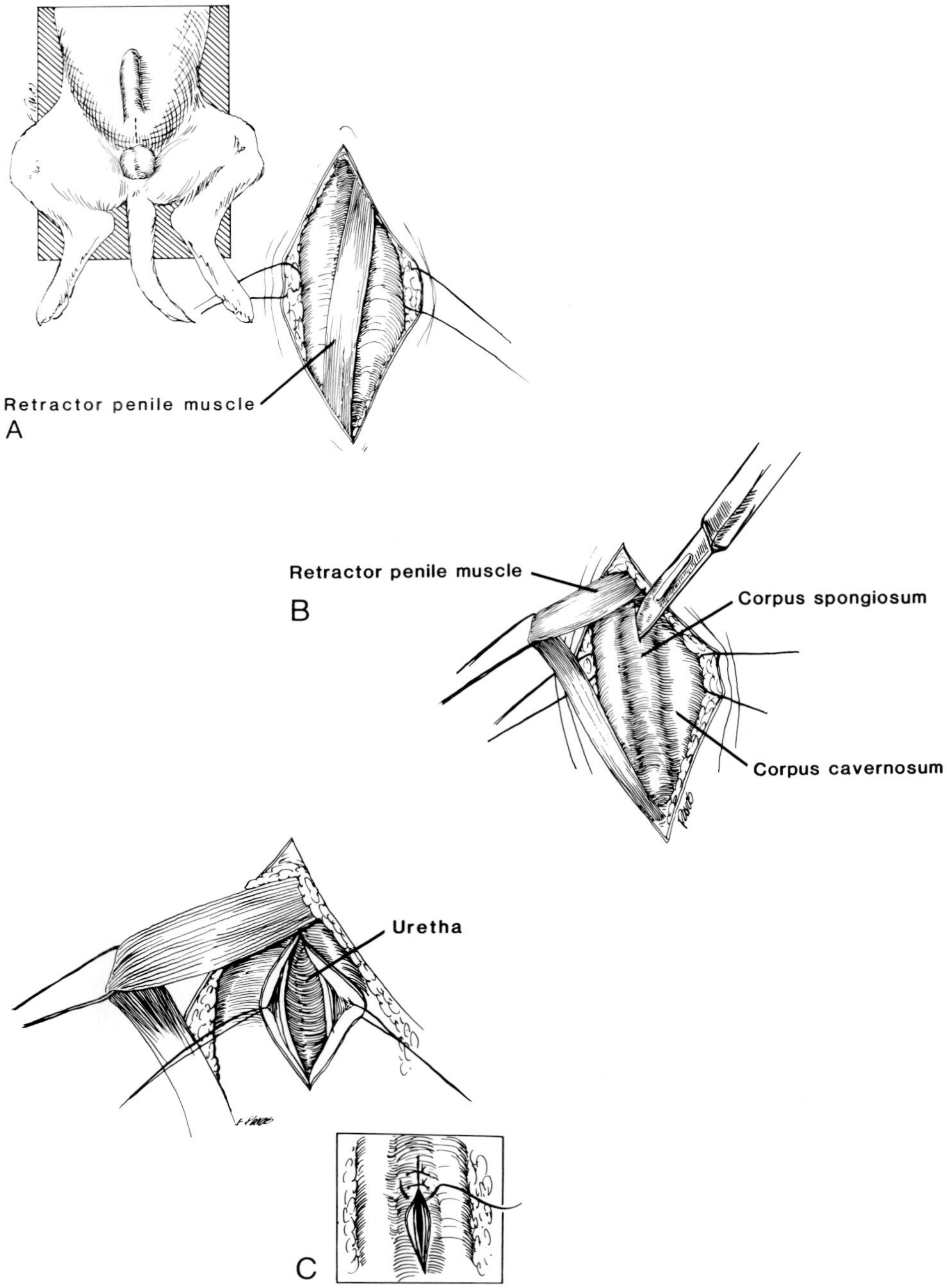

Fig. 4-1. Prescrotal urethrotomy. (A) The skin incision extends from just caudal to the prepuce to just cranial to the scrotum (insert). Subcutaneous tissue is dissected to the level of the retractor penile muscle. (B) The retractor penile muscle is retracted laterally. A longitudinal incision is made in the corpus spongiosum muscle and the urethra. The corpus cavernosum on either side of the urethra is avoided. (C) The urethral mucosa is shiny and white. Retention sutures can be placed in the corpus spongiosum to aid in the identification of the uretha. The urethrotomy can be closed with 4–0 or 5–0 synthetic absorbable suture material in a simple interrupted pattern (insert).

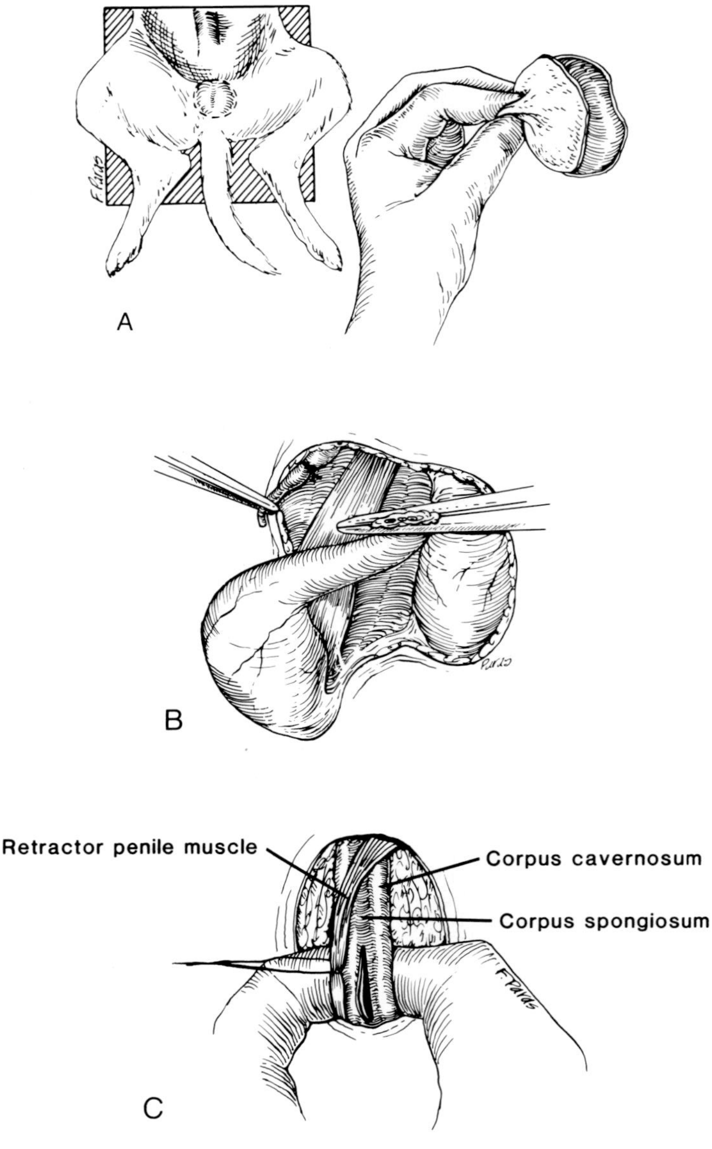

Fig. 4-2. Scrotal urethrostomy. (A) The skin is incised around the scrotum at the junction of the scrotal and inguinal skin. (B) If the dog is intact, a routine castration is done after the scrotal skin has been removed. (C) The subcutaneous tissue is dissected from the retractor penile muscle which is retracted laterally. An incision is made in the corpus spongiosum and urethra. (*Figure continues.*)

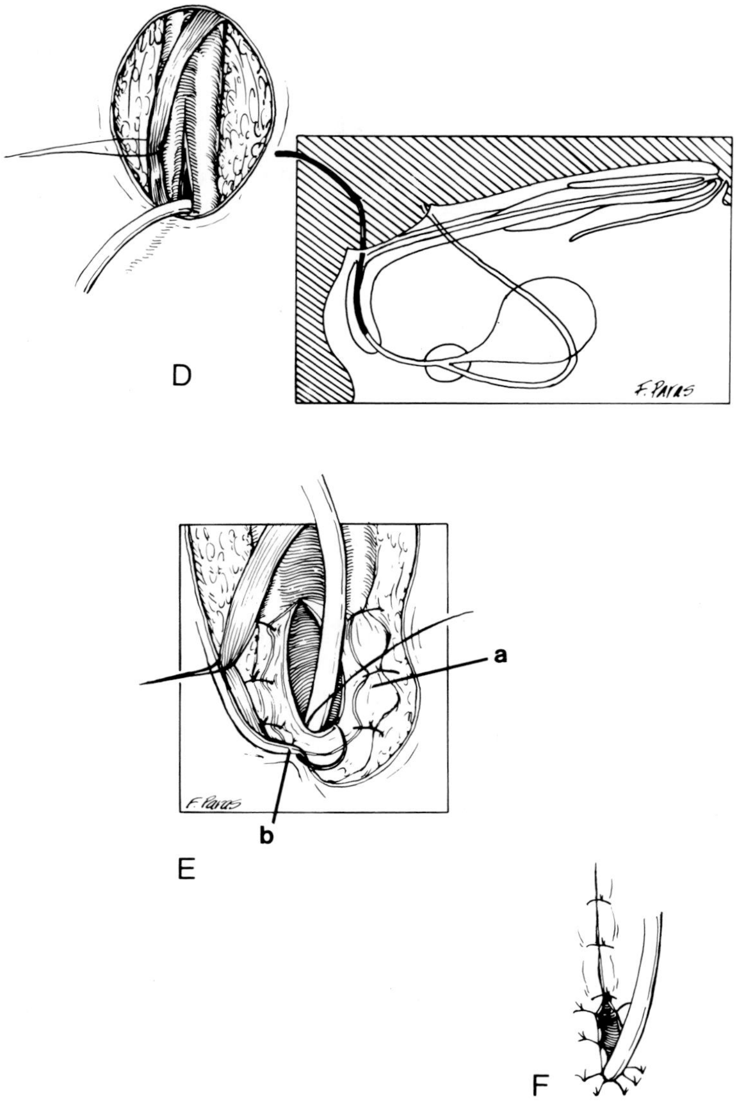

Fig. 4-2. (*continued*). (D) The urethral incision extends caudally to the point where the urethra turns dorsally. (E) The fascia of the corpora cavernosa is sutured to the subcutaneous fascia beneath the skin edges with absorbable suture material (a). The urethral mucosa is sutured to the skin with 4–0 nonabsorbable monofilament suture material (b). (F) The four most caudal sutures are placed first. The urethra-to-skin sutures are continued cranially for 2 cm. The remaining skin incision is apposed.

is made into the corpus spongiosum and urethra (Fig. 4-1B). The urethral mucosa lining is shiny and white and contrasts with the surrounding corpus spongiosum (Fig. 4-1C).

The uroliths are removed and saved for mineral analysis. A catheter is passed into the proximal urethra to check for additional uroliths. The catheter can be passed distally to dislodge calculi within the os penis urethra. If the catheter is to remain in the urethra for monitoring urine output, it is secured to the skin and connected to a closed urinary collection system.

Following removal of the urethral catheter, the urethrotomy can be left open to heal by second intention or it can be sutured with 4-0 or 5-0 synthetic absorbable suture material in a simple interrupted pattern (Fig. 4-1C). A recent study comparing the two techniques showed that there was more hemorrhage following surgery in the nonsutured group. Fine suture material (5-0 synthetic absorbable) was used to suture the urethra in a simple interrupted pattern. Suturing the urethra required more time, gentle tissue handling, and proper instruments and suture material. Stricture of the urethra did not occur with either technique.[8] Thus, the decision on whether or not to close the urethrotomy depends on the surgeon's preference and available materials.

TECHNIQUE FOR SCROTAL URETHROSTOMY

The skin is incised around the scrotum at the junction of the scrotal and inguinal skin (Fig. 4-2A). If the incision extends too far laterally, there will be excessive tension on the urethra-to-skin closure. The scrotal skin is removed. An intact dog is castrated through the scrotal incision (Fig. 4-2B). The subcutaneous tissue is dissected down to the level of the retractor penile muscle. The retractor penile muscle is retracted laterally. As with the prescrotal urethrotomy, it is important to stabilize the penis so that the urethral incision is made directly on the ventral midline through the corpus spongiosum and urethra (Fig. 4-2C). The urethral incision extends caudally to the point where the urethra turns dorsally. A catheter can be passed to identify this area (Fig. 4-2D).

The fascia of the corpora cavernosa is sutured to the subcutaneous fascia tissue beneath the skin edges with absorbable suture material (Fig. 4-2E). This step helps to relieve tension on the urethra-to-skin suture line. The urethral mucosa is sutured to the skin with 4-0 nonabsorbable monofilament synthetic suture material (Fig. 4-2E). The four most caudal sutures are placed first to align the urethral opening with the skin. The urethra-to-skin sutures are continued cranially for about 2 cm. The remaining skin incision is apposed.

SURGICAL MANAGEMENT OF PROSTATIC DISEASE

The diagnosis and medical management of prostatic disease have been discussed in Chapter 2. There is general agreement that benign prostatic disease should be treated with castration. Prostatic neoplasia may possibly be cured with surgical excision (prostatectomy) before metastasis has occurred. Unfortunately, early diagnosis is rare. Palliative therapy may include castration, estrogen therapy, and a cystostomy to divert urine from an obstructed urethra.

The surgical therapy for prostatic abscesses is quite controversial at the present time. Castration is usually performed along with either prostatic drainage or prostatectomy.

The drainage technique for prostatic abscesses in the dog involves the placement of drains through the prostatic parenchyma and out through the body wall. Some authors report the use of two to four one-half inch drains passed ventrally to dorsally through the gland, with additional drains in the periprostatic area.[10] With Johnston's technique, a single drain is used. The abscess is first opened lateral to the urethra with a closed hemostat and the purulent material is removed with suction. There is minimal dissection of the periprostatic fat. Loculation within the prostate is bluntly broken down with the surgeon's finger. A quarter-inch drain is passed into the abscess cavity, over the urethra and through the abscessed prostate gland on the opposite side. The ends of the drain are exteriorized through the body wall about 1 inch lateral to each side of the prepuce. The drain is left loose so that it will not constrict the urethra.[11]

Drains remain in place for 3 weeks. Antibiotics are administered for 3 weeks, based on culture and sensitivity testing of the abscess contents.

The prostatectomy technique has been described by Rawlings.[12] A urethral catheter is placed to help identify the urethra. A pubic splitting or pubic flap may be necessary for exposure of the caudal extent of the prostate. The branches of the urogenital artery and vein and the hypogastric and pelvic nerves are identified, if possible, and protected. The vas deferens is divided and ligated. The dissection of the prostate begins on the ventral midline and is continued to the urethra. The urethra is transected cranial and caudal to the prostate. The prostate is removed, and the urethra is anastomosed with 4–0 or 5–0 prolene. (I would prefer synthetic absorbable suture material such as polydioxanone or polyglactin 910). A cystostomy catheter is placed and left in place for 6 to 7 days. The urethral catheter is removed 1 day after surgery. Antibiotics are continued for at least 4 weeks.

There are advantages and disadvantages to each procedure. The prostatectomy is a more difficult and lengthy surgery and may require ostectomy and wiring of the pubis. Urinary incontinence is the most serious postoperative complication. Six of seven dogs were incontinent following prostatectomy in one report.[2]

Complications reported with drainage include reabscessation (5 of 12 dogs) and chronic recurrent urinary tract infections (8 of 12 dogs).[2]

Complications common to both procedures include postoperative shock, oliguria, and renal failure.

The confusion over treatment recommendations is partially related to the varied presentations and etiologies of the prostatic diseases and to the lack of uniformity in classification, treatment regimes, and follow-up times by the various investigators. At the present time the following guidelines are recommended:

Drainage techniques should be restricted to dogs with prostatic abscesses and should not be used for sterile or infected cysts. The wall of a cyst is thickened and lined with a smooth membrane. One surgeon suggests that many of the reports of unsuccessful treatment of prostatic abscesses by drainage refer to the treatment of infected prostatic cysts.[11] If a cyst comes down to a stalk, it can be completely removed. Partial removal may lead to leakage of cyst contents into the abdominal cavity and possible peritoneal irritation and adhesions. Broad-based cysts should be marsupialized, thereby avoiding damage to the bladder neck and urethra during attempted excision. The stoma should be at least 3 cm in length and should remain open for at least 2 months. Usually the stoma closes on its own. If drainage persists, it may be necessary to surgically remove the small stalk from the prostate to the stoma and close the opening in the skin.[11]

Prostatectomy is performed if there has been recurrence following proper drainage of an abscessed prostate. If the client is willing to accept the possibility of urinary incontinence and does not want to risk recurrent urinary tract and prostatic infections, prostatectomy can be used as the initial treatment for an abscessed prostate.

Client communication is extremely important in conjunction with the treatment of prostatic abscesses. Since either treatment can have significant complications, the owner must be able to make an informed decision regarding treatment recommendations. The dog should be thoroughly evaluated for urinary tract infection and urinary incontinence before surgery. The choice between drainage techniques and prostatectomy will depend on owner input, skill of the surgeon, and surgeon preference. Follow-up information should be carefully documented, and the dog should be examined periodically for complications.

TEMPORARY URINE DIVERSION

Temporary urinary diversion is indicated for urinary tract obstruction and for urine accumulation in the abdomen secondary to urinary tract trauma.

Peritoneal Catheter

A uremic animal is a poor anesthetic and surgical risk. When urine is leaking into the abdomen from a damaged distal ureter or ruptured bladder, the urine should be drained, if possible, and the animal rehydrated and diuresed. The urine can be removed simultaneously with a peritoneal catheter placed into the abdomen and a urethral catheter. A physiologic or osmotic diuresis will sufficiently dilute the fluid that is leaking into the abdomen. Peritoneal lavage is not necessary.

A local anesthetic can be used to place the peritoneal catheter in a depressed or calm dog. In the more excitable dog, a narcotic analgesic such as

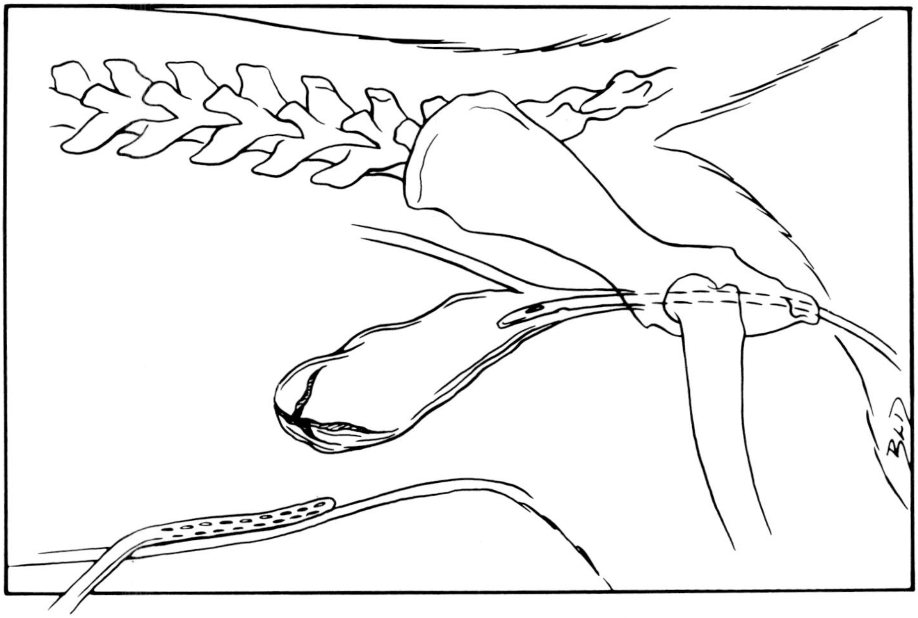

Fig. 4-3. Temporary urine diversion. For removal of urine following a urinary bladder tear, a peritoneal catheter is placed into the abdomen and a urethral catheter is inserted into the urinary bladder to the level of the trigone.

oxymorphone (0.1 to 0.2 mg/kg IV) is used. The narcotic effect is reversed with naloxone (0.02 mg/kg IV) after the catheter is placed. Aseptic technique is essential to prevent contamination of the abdominal cavity. A sterile rubber feeding tube with multiple holes cut in it or a manufactured peritoneal catheter (Abbot Laboratories, Chicago, IL) can be used. The manufactured peritoneal catheter comes with a stylet and can be inserted directly through the linea alba. For insertion of the rubber feeding tube, a small incision is made through the skin and into the linea alba. The catheter is directed caudally. It is connected to sterile tubing, such as an intravenous administration set, and then to a collection bottle or bag. If the urinary bladder retains urine, a urethral catheter can also be placed (Fig. 4-3A). The urethral catheter is also connected to a closed sterile drainage system.

Parenteral fluid therapy is administered to correct the water and electrolyte abnormalities. Urine output is monitored and recorded. Broad-spectrum antibiotics are administered to help combat possible gram-negative organisms in the urine. Once the animal is stable and no longer uremic, the definitive surgery to correct the urinary bladder rupture or ureteral tear can be performed.

Cystostomy Catheter

A cystostomy catheter is used to temporarily divert urine in the following situations: (1) urethral obstruction in a uremic animal which cannot be easily removed, (2) urethral trauma with periurethral leakage of urine, (3) after urethral anastomosis or prostatectomy (Fig. 4-4).

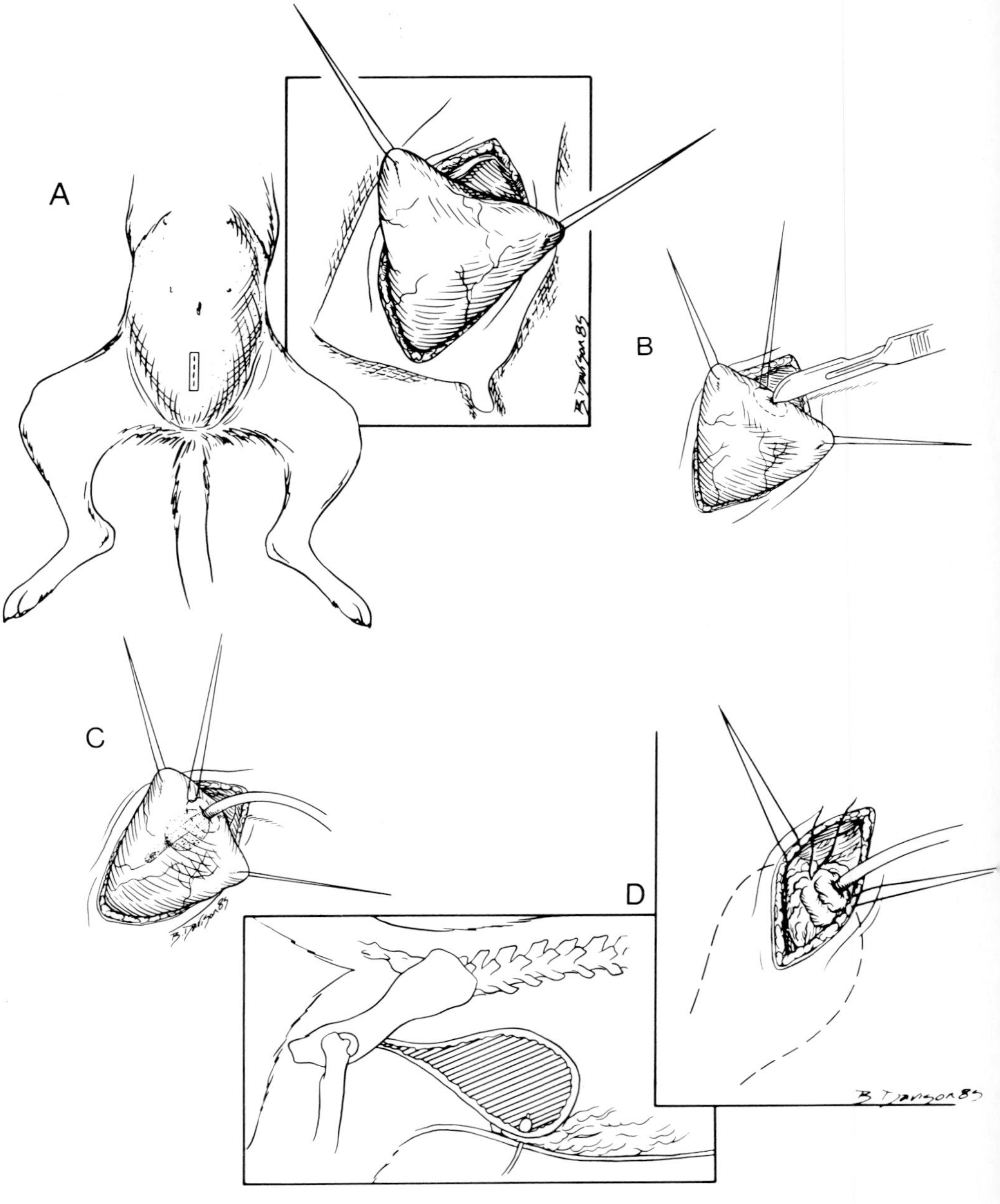

Fig. 4-4. Cystostomy catheter. (A) In a female dog or a male or female cat a 1 to 2 cm skin incision is made in the caudal one-third of the distance between the umbilicus and pubis. The urinary bladder is exteriorized and held with two retention sutures. (B) A purse-string suture is placed through the serosa and muscle layers of the cranial ventral bladder wall. A stab incision is made into the bladder. (C) The Foley catheter is inserted into the bladder and inflated. (D) The purse-string is tied. Omentum can be incorporated into the purse-string as it is tied. The retention sutures are passed through the linea alba or abdominal fascia and tied. After the linea alba and skin incisions are closed, the Foley catheter drains urine from the bladder into a closed drainage system.

The catheter is placed in the cranial-ventral region of the urinary bladder. If there is already an abdominal incision, the catheter is exited lateral to the midline. When the catheter is placed as the first procedure, a 1 to 2 cm skin incision is made in the caudal third of the distance between the pubis and the umbilicus. In cats and female dogs, it is made on the midline (Fig. 4-4A). In male dogs, it is made lateral to the prepuce. The incision is then continued through the body wall.

The bladder is exteriorized and held in position with two retention sutures (Fig. 4-4A). A purse-string using absorbable suture is placed through the serosa and muscle layers of the cranial ventral bladder wall. A stab incision is made into the urinary bladder within the purse-string (Fig. 4-4B). A size 8 French gauge or smaller Foley catheter is inserted into the bladder and inflated wth sterile saline (Fig. 4-4C). Omentum can be incorporated into the purse-string as it is tied around the Foley catheter. The retention sutures are passed through the linea alba or abdominal fascia and tied (Fig. 4-4D). The linea alba and skin incisions are closed. The Foley catheter is secured to the skin with two sutures tied around the catheter and passed through the skin and tied. Alternatively, a tape "butterfly" can be placed on the catheter and the tape sutured to the skin.

The catheter is connected to a closed drainage system. It can be deflated and removed percutaneously after 3 or more days.

REFERENCES

1. Osborne CA, Klausner JS, Abdullahi, S, Krawiec DR: Medical dissolution and prevention of canine struvite uroliths. p. 1066. In Kirk RW (ed): Current Veterinary Therapy VIII, WB Saunders, Philadelphia, 1983
2. Hardie EM, Barsanti JA, Rawlings CA: Complications of prostatic surgery. J Am Anim Hosp Assoc 20:50, 1984
3. Belis JA, Morabito RA, Kandzari SJ, et al: Anatrophic nephrolithotomy: Preservation of renal function demonstrated by differential quantitative radionuclide renal scans. J Urol 125:761, 1981
4. Stone EA: Surgical therapy for urolithiasis. Vet Clin North Am Small Anim Pract 14:77, 1984
5. Gahring DR, Crowe DT, Powers TE, et al: Comparative renal function studies of nephrotomy closure with and without sutures in dogs. J Am Vet Med Assoc 171:537, 1977
6. Greenwood KM, Rawlings, CA: Removal of canine renal calculi by pyelolithotomy. Vet Surg 10:12, 1981
7. Kawamura J, Itoh H, Okada Y, et al: Preoperative and postoperative cortical function of the kidney with staghorn calculi assessed by ^{99m}Technetium-dimercapto-succinic acid renal scintigraphy. J Urol 130:430, 1983
8. Castle WM, McDougal WS: Contralateral renal hyperplasia and increased renal function after relief of chronic unilateral ureteral obstruction. J Urol 132:1016, 1984
9. Weber WJ, Boothe HW, Brassard JA, et al: Comparison of the healing of prescrotal urethral incisions in the dog: Sutured versus nonsutured. Am J Vet Res 46:1309, 1985

10. Zolton GM, Greiner TP: Prostatic abscesses—A surgical approach. J Am Anim Hosp Assoc 172:806, 1978
11. Johnston DJ: Prostate. p. 1635. In Slatter DJ (ed): Textbook of Small Animal Surgery, WB Saunders, Philadelphia, 1985
12. Rawlings CA: Prostatectomy for prostatic abscesses. Proceedings for Small Animal Urogenital Session, American College of Veterinary Surgeons Surgical Forum, 1984, p. 74

5 Urinary Tract Infections

Timothy A. Allen

Urinary tract infection (UTI) constitutes one of the most common infectious bacterial diseases in veterinary practice. The severity of these infections range from asymptomatic bacteriuria to overwhelming bilateral kidney infections resulting in chronic renal failure. UTI due to nonbacterial microorganisms (e.g., mycoplasmas, chlamydias, viruses, and fungi) is rare.

It it helpful to define several terms. UTI is present when bacteria invade tissues of the urinary tract and multiply. Cystitis refers to infection limited to the urinary bladder. Pyelonephritis refers to immediate or delayed kidney damage resulting from bacterial invasion. Upper and lower urinary tract infection refer to pyelonephritis and cystitis, respectively. Acute pyelonephritis is characterized by relatively specific histopathologic features such as acute interstitial inflammation and tubular necrosis. The description of chronic pyelonephritis is more difficult. Chronic pyelonephritis produces less specific histologic changes such as interstitial inflammation and fibrosis and tubular dilation and atrophy. A number of physical, immunologic, and chemical injuries can produce these changes and are collectively called tubulointerstitial renal disorders. The presence of inflammation, fibrosis, and deformity of the renal pelvis distinguishes chronic pyelonephritis from the other tubulointerstitial diseases.[1] The diagnosis of chronic pyelonephritis does not require the presence of active bacterial infection.

There are no useful statistics on the prevalence of urinary tract infection in dogs and cats, since only limited surveys of small populations of animals have been performed.[2,3] Difficulties in localizing the site of UTI[4] make comparisons of the frequency of cystitis versus pyelonephritis virtually impossible.

INTRINSIC HOST MECHANISMS

Urine in the kidneys, ureters, and bladder is normally sterile. A number of systemic and local defense mechanisms play a role in maintaining sterility.[5] Perhaps the most efficient natural defense mechanism is normal micturition. The mechanical washout that occurs with complete and frequent voiding inhibits bacterial colonization by dislodging microorganisms that reach the bladder, ureters, or renal pelvis.

A number of anatomical defense mechanisms protect the urinary tract. Although there is a normal bacterial flora in the distal and mid-urethra, a functional high pressure zone in the mid-urethra prevents migration of bacteria proximal to this zone. Spontaneous contractions of the urethra also prevent retrograde movement of bacteria. Bactericidal prostatic secretions provide protection from ascending UTI in the male. The functional valve formed by the oblique course of the ureters through fibers of the detrusor muscle and unidirectional peristaltic waves in the ureters provides a protective function by preventing the ascent of contaminated urine from the bladder to the upper urinary tract.

The mucosa of the urinary bladder possesses inherent antibacterial properties and is involved in the production of local immunoglobulins. These inherent mucosal properties are complex and difficult to document. Secretory IgA plays an important role in the immunological response to UTI. IgG is present in large quantities in the urine; however, it is probably not functionally important since its action is dependent on phagocytosis, which is inhibited in urine.

Urine from normal animals inhibits bacterial multiplication. Factors responsible for this inhibition include the presence of high concentrations of urea, ammonia, and weak organic acids, and high osmolality. In addition, low urine pH will inhibit the growth of certain bacteria.

A recent study in women suggests that the normal flora of the distal urethral, cervical, and vaginal surfaces may play an important protective role in preventing uropathogens from adhering to the surface of uroepithelial cells.[6]

HOST PREDISPOSING FACTORS

Several host factors are important in predisposing the urinary tract to infection.[5] Urinary tract infections are associated with a variety of obstructive lesions of the upper and lower urinary tract (e.g., neoplasia or uroliths). Obstruction of the urinary bladder interferes with several of the normal defense mechanisms of the bladder. The greater residual urine volume increases the number of bacteria remaining in the bladder after voiding.[7] When the bladder is distended, the surface area of the bladder relative to the total volume of the bladder is decreased, thereby diminishing mucosal bactericidal factors. Obstruction also reduces blood flow and thus the delivery of leukocytes and other blood-borne defense factors to the bladder mucosa. Vesicourachal diverticula are of clinical significance because they appear to be a predisposing factor to recurrent urinary tract infection. Retention of urine and bacteria within the diverticulum may reduce bacterial clearance from the urinary tract.[8]

Any catheterization or instrumentation (e.g., vaginoscopic examination) of the genitourinary tract has the potential for causing UTI. UTI has been induced in normal bitches following a single catheterization.[9] The risk of infection is probably increased in the presence of a diseased or obstructed urinary tract. If multiple catheterizations are performed or if an indwelling catheter is utilized, the risk of UTI increases.

Ihrke et al have reported that 39 percent of dogs receiving long-term corticosteroid therapy for chronic skin diseases had urinary tract infections.[10] Females and castrated males had a greater frequency of bacteriuria. Pyuria is not a reliable predictor of urinary tract infection in dogs receiving chronic steroid therapy. Corticosteroid dose, daily versus alternate-day therapy, and duration of therapy did not correlate with the presence or absence of urinary tract infection in the dogs studied.

The relationship between urinary tract infection, vesicoureteral reflux, and pyelonephritis in humans is complex.[11] Some investigators feel that vesicoureteral reflux is an important event in the pathogenesis of pyelonephritis, while others state that reflux causes renal damage even in the absence of bacterial infection.[12,13]

Primary vesicoureteral reflux has been demonstrated by voiding cystourethrography in approximately 50 percent of dogs less than 6 months of age but in less than 10 percent of adult dogs.[14] The age-dependent difference in the incidence of vesicoureteral reflux appears to be a function of changes in the ratio of ureteral length to diameter that occur with normal growth.[15] Secondary vesicoureteral reflux has been associated with urinary tract infection, obstructive uropathy, neuropathic bladders, congenital ureteral defects, and iatrogenic causes.[16] It also has been reported that manual expression of the urinary bladder in normal dogs can cause vesicoureteral reflux.[17]

Radiographic studies that are used to demonstrate vesicoureteral reflux include voiding urethrography, maximum distention retrograde cystourethrography, and compression cystourethrography. Either voiding or retrograde cystourethrography are the preferred techniques and are described in Chapter 10.

Experimental studies, in laboratory rodents, using models of hematogenous pyelonephritis have revealed an increased susceptibility of the renal medulla to bacterial infection.[18,19] Increased vulnerability of the medulla has not been demonstrated in all models of pyelonephritis.[20] In some species, cortical and medullary lesions occur simultaneously, and in other species, cortical lesions occur first.[21] Nonetheless, various investigators have attributed the possible increased bacterial susceptibility of the renal medulla to a variety of mechanisms. These include decreased leukocyte migration and phagocytosis[22,23] and altered antigen-antibody reactions[24] in the hypertonic environment in the medulla.[24] Cell wall deficient bacterial variants, so called L-forms or protoplasts, can also survive in the hypertonic medulla.

IMMUNOPATHOGENESIS

Immunologic reactions may play an important role in the pathogenesis of pyelonephritis. First, it is possible that bacterial infection may stimulate an autoimmune response directed against renal tissue.[25] Secondly, the normal immunologic response may increase the damage to renal tissue, as well as serve a protective action by eliminating bacteria from the kidney.

An autoimmune mechanism has been suggested because renal scarring may progress in the absence of continued bacterial proliferation.[26] It has been proposed that renal infection can stimulate an autoimmune reaction against host renal antigens.[27] Preliminary immunoautoradiographic studies have revealed protein-containing subunits of *Escherichia coli* that cross react with anti-Tamm-Horsfall protein antibody.[28] Other studies suggest that autoimmune responses to Tamm-Horsfall protein may occur with vesicoureteral reflux.[29] An immunologic response to this normal urine protein may be the mechanism of the suggested autoimmune pathogenesis of pyelonephritis.[28,30] This mechanism would be consistent with the observation that pyelonephritis can occur in just one kidney. Investigators have failed to demonstrate locally synthesized immunoglobulins in the kidneys of humans or experimental animals with pyelonephritis.[31]

Despite conflicting experiments, it appears in general that the local antibody response eliminates bacteria and is, therefore, protective against both hematogenous and ascending infection.[32,33]

Investigators have suggested that the inflammatory response is responsible for a major part of the renal scarring that occurs in pyelonephritis. It has been demonstrated that complement depletion,[34] granulocyte depletion,[35] and rapid eradication of bacterial infection with antimicrobial agents[36] prevent inflammation and subsequent loss of renal tissue. The specific mechanism by which the inflammatory response damages the kidney appears to be phagocytosis.[37] Bacterial activation of complement leads to chemotaxis of granulocytes, release of lysozyme from granulocytes, and opsonization and phagocytosis of bacteria. One of the key events in phagocytosis is the release of superoxide from the granulocyte cell wall. This oxygen radical kills phagocytosed bacteria and produces further chemotaxis of additional granulocytes to the site of infection. The release of superoxide into the surrounding environment is toxic to renal tubular epithelial cells. It has not been determined whether the toxic species is the superoxide or one of the substances produced in its presence.[37]

ETIOLOGIC AGENTS

Pathogens of the canine and feline urinary tract include both gram-positive and gram-negative bacteria. Usually infections are due to a single strain of bacteria; rarely, mixed or polymicrobic infections occur.[3] Although specific incidence data vary slightly from hospital to hospital, *E. coli, Staphylococcus, Proteus, Klebsiella,* and *Streptococcus* are the most frequent isolates from canine urine, and *E. coli* and *Staphylococcus* are the most common isolates from feline urine. In both the dog and the cat, *E. Coli* is the single most common isolate. No unique group of clinical signs is associated with a particular species of bacteria.

In the dog, it is generally accepted that most urinary tract infections occur via an ascending route. A substantial number of bacteria that cause ascending pyelonephritis in human patients and experimental models originate from the gastrointestinal tract.[38,39] Although strict anaerobes predominate in the feces, they seldom cause UTI. It is presumed that the oxygen tension in the urine prevents their growth and multiplication.

Many bacteria that cause urinary tract infection possess the ability to attach to uroepithelial cells.[40,41] In many instances, the means of attachment are fimbriae, which are rigid, filamentous, proteinaceous appendages found on most gram-negative bacteria. Some investigators believe that fimbriae that adhere to glycolipids of the uroepithelial cells are responsible for the pathogenicity of certain strains of coli-forms.[42] The ability of bacteria to adhere to the uroepithelium prevents bacteria from being mechanically removed from the urinary system during micturition.[43] By resisting mechanical washout, bacteria multiply and invade urinary tract tissue. Experiments have shown that immunization with purified fimbriae prevents adherence and subsequent pyelonephritis, even when bacteria are inoculated directly into the kidney.[44]

Factors other than bacterial adhesion are probably important in the ability of certain strains to be pathogenic.[45] These include the capsule K antigens that may increase tissue invasiveness and interfere with opsonization and phagocytosis[46] and the O antigens contained in bacterial endotoxin.[47] Endotoxins have profound effects on smooth muscle and, therefore, decrease or stop ureteral peristalsis. The functional ureteral obstruction produced by endotoxin allows ascent and intrarenal reflux of bacteria at normal hydrostatic pressure.[48] Intrarenal reflux of bacteria, if untreated, will lead to acute and chronic pyelonephritis.[49]

The role of mycoplasms in UTI is not clear. These agents may be primary pathogens or may be opportunists that produce UTI in concert with bacteria. A recent report associated mycoplasma with canine UTI.[50] Mycoplasma were isolated from specimens obtained by cystocentesis and cultured on blood agar or a special medium supportive of mycoplasma growth (PPLO agar). The majority of isolates speciated were found to be *Mycoplasma canis*. Clinical signs associated with mycoplasma infection included pollakiuria, hematuria, stranguria, polyuria, polydipsia, urinary incontinence, and fever. Some dogs with positive mycoplasma cultures had no signs indicative of UTI. Although negative mycoplasma cultures were reported following treatment with tylosine, tetracycline, and cephalexin, it was not clear from this report whether elimination of mycoplasma resulted in clinical improvement.

Urinary tract candidiasis is rare in dogs and cats.[51] *Candida* species are normal inhabitants of the canine and feline gastrointestinal tract. It is presumed that candidiasis UTI can occur by means of either the hematogenous or ascending routes. Infection is frequently associated with altered intrinsic host defense mechanisms. Conditions associated with an increased risk include diabetes mellitus, indwelling urinary catheters, or long-term antimicrobial or glucocorticoid therapy.

Candiduria may or may not be associated with clinical signs. If signs are present, they are indistinguishable from signs associated with bacterial UTI. The significance of asymptomatic candiduria is unclear. The problem may resolve spontaneously when host defense mechanisms become normal, or clinical signs may develop as host defense deteriorates.

The diagnosis of candiduria depends on demonstrating the organism either in serial urine sediment examinations or cultures. Since yeasts are potential contaminants, it is important to verify candiduria in more than one urine specimen before recommending treatment. Sabouraud's dextrose agar and blood agar without cycloheximide are suitable media for isolation of *Candida* species.

Treatment of candiduria should be based on the specific clinical situation. If predisposing factors (e.g., indwelling urinary catheters) are present they should be eliminated. Since the optimal pH for growth of *Candida* is 5.0 to 6.5, alkalinization of the urine with sodium bicarbonate is beneficial. If warranted, more aggressive therapy with ketoconazole is possible.

LABORATORY FINDINGS

The value of the specimen submitted for urinalysis is influenced by the method of collection. Gross examination of urine (e.g., odor, turbidity, and cloudiness) often provides initial evidence of urinary tract infection. An alkaline urine pH may indicate infection with a urea-splitting organism such as *Proteus*. The urine sediment can be influenced by the method of collection. Voided urine samples can be contaminated with bacteria and white blood cells from the distal urethra, vagina, or prepuce.

Most bacterial infections of the urinary tract are accompanied by pyuria; however, the correlation of pyuria with bacterial infection is only approximate. Bacteriuria may be present without pyuria, and pyuria is not always accompanied by bacteriuria. Noninfectious causes of pyuria include inflammation and sterile or chemical cystitis due to cyclophosphamide.

A Gram-stained smear of a drop of uncentrifuged urine is a good rapid technique for the initial evaluation of bacteriuria. The presence of one or more bacteria per oil immersion field suggests significant bacteriuria, and the results of the Gram stain can be used to guide initial antimicrobial therapy.

Rapid dipstick techniques based on bacteria-induced chemical reactions are not recommended as screening tests for UTI in dogs and cats. The nitrite, glucose consumption, catalase, and leukocyte esterase tests are subject to both false-positive and false-negative results.

SIGNIFICANT BACTERIURIA AND QUANTITATIVE URINE CULTURES

Urine obtained directly from the urinary bladder is normally sterile; however, urine that passes through the distal urethra and genital tract may become contaminated by the endogenous bacterial flora present in these locations. Consequently, the presence of bacteria in voided or catheterized specimens does not always indicate UTI.

Significant bacteriuria and quantitative urine culture are concepts used to aid in the differentiation between contaminants and pathogens associated with UTI. Qualitative urine culture merely indicates the isolation and identification of the bacteria present in the specimen. Quantitative urine culture involves not only the isolation and identification of bacteria but also the enumeration of the number of bacteria per unit volume of urine. The technique provides criteria for differentiating a pathogen from a contaminant. The numerical criteria established for the interpretation of quantitative urine cultures are valid only if the urine sample has been properly collected and handled prior to culture. Voided midstream or catheterized urine samples from normal dogs usually contain fewer than 10,000 colony-forming units (CFU) per milliliter.[52] Specimens containing more than 100,000 CFU/ml have significant bacteriuria indicative of UTI. Cystocentesis samples avoid contamination in the distal urethra, vagina, and prepuce, and consequently, any growth is probably significant. Cystocentesis samples are preferred for both qualitative and quantitative cultures.

A study by Lees and coworkers suggests there are important differences between cats and dogs regarding culture results obtained by catheterization.[53] In dogs, contaminating bacteria are more commonly present in catheterized samples obtained from females,[54] but in the cat, contaminating bacteria are more common in males. Furthermore, in cats most specimens obtained by catheterization do not contain bacteria, and therefore, on quantitative culture fewer than 1,000 CFU/ml of urine are found in normal cats. Urethral catheterization is not routinely recommended in the cat because of the possibility of iatrogenic trauma or catheter-induced infection and because sedation or anesthesia is usually required.

HANDLING OF URINE SPECIMENS FOR BACTERIOLOGIC CULTURE

If the urine specimen cannot be plated within 30 minutes of collection, the urine specimen should be cooled to 4°C (refrigerated) as soon as possible follwing collection. Since bacteria in urine may double their numbers every 45 minutes at room temperature, immediate refrigeration is necessary in order to prevent false positives due to contamination of the specimen. False-negative results (i.e., failure to isolate pathogens) may occur if the urine is refrigerated for more than 12 to 24 hours, depending on the bacterial species present, or if the specimen is allowed to freeze. Bacterial culture of the urine specimen must be performed within 6 hours of the time of collection. If this is not possible, a bacterial support medium (Urine Culture Kit, Becton-Dickinson, Rutherford, NJ) should be used.[55] An alternative approach would be to inoculate culture plates as soon as the specimen is collected, incubate them overnight at 37°C, and submit the plates to an outside bacteriologic laboratory for species identification and antimicrobial sensitivity determination the next day. Blood agar and MacConkey agar culture plates are suitable culture media for primary isolation. A measured volume (0.01 or 0.1 ml) of well-mixed urine should be inoculated onto each plate using a calibrated loop. The urine should be streaked for individual colony isolation.

DIFFERENTIATION OF UPPER AND LOWER URINARY TRACT INFECTION

The main indication for differentiating upper from lower urinary tract infections is to prevent renal damage by identifying the animals that require long-term antimicrobial therapy and careful bacteriologic follow-up.[56] Common laboratory procedures can sometimes be helpful in localizing urinary tract infection. The presence of azotemia and leukocytosis are not specific for pyelonephritis; however, their presence suggests an upper urinary tract infection. The presence of cylinduria is of localizing value; however, the absence of casts does not exclude pyelonephritis.

Radiography is sometimes useful in localization of the site of infection. The presence of radiographic changes provides only circumstantial evidence that the lesion and the urinary tract infection are related. The spectrum of radiologic findings associated with urinary bladder infection range from none to focal or diffuse lesions demonstrated by contrast cystography. Diffuse or focal thickening of the bladder wall is consistent with but not diagnostic of bacterial cystitis. Radiographic changes associated with bacterial pyelonephritis have not been systematically investigated in the dog and cat. Nonhomogeneous opacification of the nephrogram stage of the excretory urogram can occur with chronic pyelonephritis. Symmetrical dilation of the renal pelvis with either no filling or asymmetrical filling of the diverticula suggests acute pyelonephritis. Radiographic lesions recognized in dogs with experimental pyelonephritis include a slight increase or decrease in kidney size, and ureteral and pelvic dilation within 10 days following inoculation. Kidney size decreased progressively following experimental pyelonephritis.[57]

Traditionally, the presence of pyelonephritis has been based on the presence of pain at the costovertebral angle, fever, and leukocytosis. However, these clinical criteria are neither sensitive or specific for pyelonephritis. A number of specialized differentiation techniques are used in humans with urinary tract infection.[56] Although the applicability of these techniques to animals with urinary tract infection has not been documented, familiarity with these techniques is useful to the veterinary clinician.

Histologic examination and bacteriologic culture of biopsy specimens also have limitations in localizing the site of infection to the kidney. Unless the infection is generalized, percutaneous or keyhole biopsy techniques may miss the area of involvement. Furthermore, specimens obtained by needle biopsy generally do not include the pelvis; thus, the differentiation of pyelonephritis from other tubulointerstitial diseases may be impossible. Open biopsy does not obviate these limitations.

Culture of urine obtained by ureteral catheterization (Stamey test) is considered the definitive technique for localizing urinary tract infection to the kidneys in humans. The urinary bladder is irrigated with copious volumes of water by means of a cystoscope to reduce the number of bacteria that may be introduced into the ureters with passage of the catheters. Ureteral catheters are passed up both ureters and urine specimens are obtained for quantitative culture. A variation of the Stamey test that warrants evaluation in veterinary medicine is the percutaneous aspiration of urine from the renal pelvis using ultrasonic or fluoroscopic guidance.[58]

Another test for differentiating upper from lower urinary tract infection is the bladder washout (Fairley) test. In this technique an indwelling Foley catheter is inserted, and a control urine specimen is obtained for Gram staining and culture. A solution containing normal saline, an enzyme preparation, and an antimicrobial selected based on the Gram stain is instilled into the bladder and allowed to remain for 45 minutes in order to detach organisms from the bladder wall and inhibit their multiplication. The bladder is drained and rinsed with 1 to 2 liters of sterile normal saline. The final 50 ml portion of the saline rinse remains in the bladder for a few minutes and is cultured in order to obtain the zero time sample. Furosemide is given intravenously, and specimens are obtained for culture at 10, 20, 30, and 60 minutes.

The bladder washout technique does not require specialized equipment; however, it did not appear to be reliable when applied to dogs with experimentally induced urinary tract infection.[4] It is possible that the experimental infection created by these investigators damaged the bladder wall more severely than spontaneous infection, and thus the bladder could not be washed out.

Another test for localizing UTI is the antibody-coated bacterial (ACB) test. The theoretical basis for the ACB test is that organisms that have invaded tissues will stimulate the production of specific antibodies which adhere to the bacteria. Thus, bacteria associated with pyelonephritis will bind fluorescent antibodies directed against immunoglobulins, but bacteria from an infected bladder will not. Although the theoretical principle is sound, there are practical problems with reliability and interpretation.

The definition of what constitutes a positive test has been debated. The original reports considered a positive reaction to be greater than 25 percent of the bacteria fluorescing in the centrifuged urine sediment. A recent study has suggested that just 1 percent fluorescent organisms is a more appropriate cutoff point. It has also been recommended that the conditions (e.g., hydration and time between voiding) under which the urine is obtained be standardized.

Both false-positive and false-negative antibody-coated bacterial tests have been reported. A potential explanation for a false-negative test is that the ACB test has been performed before an immunologic response to the invading organism has occurred. Another possible explanation for a false-negative ACB test is that the formed antibody is unable to adhere to the pathogenic organism. Such urinary pathogens as *Pseudomonas aeruginosa* develop mucoid coats that may interfere with adherence of antibody. Technical problems can also cause false-negative results; for example, if a urine sample is not tested immediately, bacterial multiplication may dilute the antibody sufficiently to cause a negative interpretation. False-positive results are possible because the antibody used in the test is nonspecific. Situations where patients with infection confined to the lower urinary tract have false-positive ACB reactions include patients with proteinuria, patients who have had a kidney infection with an antigenically similar organism in the last few months, and women with recurrent bladder infections. Women also will have false-positive results if the urine sample is contaminated with antibody-coated bacteria from the vaginal vestibule, and men with prostatic infections will have false-positive ACB tests due to antibody-coated bacteria from the prostate. If the bladder mucosa is disrupted or eroded due to cystic calculi, hemorrhagic cystitis or bladder neoplasia antibody may escape into the urine and nonspecifically coat the bacteria, producing a false-positive test. The ACB test was evaluated in 12 female dogs with urinary tract infection established by means of bacteriologic culture of bladder urine obtained by antepubic cystocentesis.[59] The authors concluded that the ACB test was not useful in localizing bacterial infection within the urinary tract.

Measurement of a variety of urinary enzymes has been advocated as a means of differentiating upper from lower urinary tract infection. The hypothesis is that, with pyelonephritis, renal cell damage results in the elaboration of enzymes that are specific to the upper urinary tract. Lactic dehydrogenase (LDH) has several isoenzymatic forms that are specific for certain sites of origin. Isoenzyme fractions are present in the renal medulla but not in the serum or bladder. Thus, if they are found in the urine, pyelonephritis should be suspected. The test involves measurement of total LDH activity and subsequent electrophoresis to determine the isoenzyme fractions. Since this enzyme is labile, the specimen must be kept cool after collection. *N*-acetyl glucosaminidase is another enzyme that has been reported to be of value in localizing urinary tract infection. The principal advantage of *N*-acetyl glucosaminidase is that it is stable and relatively easy to measure.[60]

Studies in children with UTIs have strongly associated p-fimbriated *E. coli* with acute pyelonephritis. Therefore, it has been suggested that detection of p-fimbriated strains might be a useful indicator of the site of UTI. Recently, Latham and Stamm[61] studied a small group of adult women and found that the presence of p-fimbriae was not a useful localization test.

The administration of a single dose of an antimicrobial is an empirical method for differentiating upper from lower urinary tract infections. In an uncomplicated lower urinary tract infection it is anticipated that the comparatively high antimicrobial concentrations achieved in the urine will eliminate the infection after just a single dose. In upper urinary tract infection the deep medullary location and poor delivery of the antimicrobial to the infected tissues will not resolve the infection after a single dose.

TREATMENT

The treatment of urinary tract infection has been reviewed.[62] There are no controlled clinical studies of therapy of UTI in the dog and cat that establish the superiority of one antimicrobial agent over another or define the optimum duration of therapy. Consequently, therapy must be individualized based on culture and sensitivity testing and specific clinical and laboratory findings.

The standard method for determining antimicrobial sensitivity is the disk-diffusion (Kirby-Bauer) method. This method is based on anticipated serum concentrations of antimicrobials rather than urine concentrations. Since antimicrobials excreted in an active form in the urine can attain concentrations 10 to 100 times their serum concentrations, organisms that appear resistant may, in fact, be sensitive to the concentrations present in the urine.[63] The determination of minimum inhibitory concentrations (MIC) is a better method of predicting in vivo response to therapy.[64] If the ratio of the MIC of an antimicrobial to the expected urinary concentration of that antimicrobial is approximately 1:4, clinical improvement can be anticipated. Unfortunately, the MIC method is more expensive and less readily available than the disk-diffusion method.

Based on retrospective analysis of sensitivity patterns and the urine concentrations of various antimicrobials, recommendations have been established for empirical therapy or urinary tract infections.[62] Virtually all gram-negative organisms isolated during the period of study at a veterinary teaching hospital were sensitive to the penicillins.[65] Ampicillin at a dose of 66 mg/kg daily in three divided doses is, therefore, recommended in treating a gram-positive organism. With gram-negative organisms, response to therapy is predicted approximately 80 percent of the time with the following drugs and doses. A trimethoprim-sulfa combination at a dose of 30 mg/kg daily in 2 divided doses is recommended for *E. coli*.[62] Ampicillin at the above dose is suggested for *Proteus* species.[63] *Pseudomonas aeruginosa* will respond to tetracycline at a dose of 60 mg/kg daily in 3 divided doses.[66] Community acquired *Klebsiella pneumoniae* infections can be treated with oral cephalexin at a daily dose of 60 mg/kg divided twice per day.[67]

Unfortunately, it cannot be assumed that urine concentrations of an antimicrobial reflect concentrations achieved in pyelonephritis-damaged renal parenchma.[68] Some authors have advised that serum concentrations are a better predictor of renal parenchyma concentrations than urine concentrations.[69] It would be helpful in selecting an antimicrobial to differentiate pyelonephritis from lower urinary tract infection. Unfortunately, there is no reliable, practical technique for localizing the site of urinary tract infections.[4] If pyelonephritis is suspected based on clinical findings (i.e., fever, leukocytosis, and pain at the costovertebral angle), prompt therapy is indicated since septicemia is a potential sequela to pyelonephritis.[70] If by the third or fourth day of therapy clinical and laboratory improvement has not occurred, a change in antimicrobial agents is warranted. The decision to switch antimicrobials should not be made too hastily. In pyelonephritis the long-term prognosis with regard to preservation of renal function does not depend on the severity of clinical signs, but rather it depends on the presence of underlying abnormalities that alter urine flow, normal host resistance, and the rapid elimination of the bacterial infection.[71]

In a case of presumed pyelonephritis, the duration of therapy should be a minimum of 3 to 4 weeks, and appropriate bacteriologic follow-up is essential. If cystitis is suspected, antimicrobial therapy should be continued for at least 1 week. Ideally, a follow-up culture and sensitivity should be done 2 and 6 weeks after the cessation of antimicrobial therapy.

Potentially nephrotoxic drugs should be avoided whenever possible; however, if in vitro susceptibility testing indicates there are no safer alternatives, the patient should be carefully monitored for signs of nephrotoxicity. If renal insufficiency is present prior to the start of therapy and the only sensitive antimicrobial is nephrotoxic, the dose or dosage interval will require modification.[72]

Catheterization and instrumentation should be kept to an absolute minimum in patients with UTI in order to reduce the risk of introducing infection to an already compromised urinary tract. In order to facilitate cystocentesis at the time of bacteriologic follow-up, furosemide can be administered if the urinary bladder cannot be palpated.

ADJUNCTIVE THERAPY

Manipulation of urine pH by alkalinizing or acidifying agents can be a useful adjunct to antimicrobial therapy. The activity of the aminoglycosides (kanamycin, gentamicin, tobramycin, amikacin, netilmicin) is greatly enhanced in an alkaline pH. Erythromycin also has increased activity against common enteric bacilli at highly alkaline urine pH. By comparison, an acid urine pH improves the antibacterial activity of certain tetracyclines, and carbenicillin and is mandatory for the antimicrobial effect of methenamine mandelate or hippurate. Oral sodium bicarbonate is used for alkalinization and ammonium chloride for acidification of urine. The dose of these drugs should be adjusted based on daily monitoring of the urine pH.

Induction of polyuria by salting the diet has several beneficial effects in the treatment of UTI. Polyuria dilutes the number of microorganisms and thus may produce clinical improvement. Polyuria will also increase the number of voidings and consequently increase mechanical washout of bacteria from the urinary tract. Induced polyuria will reduce the urine concentration of the antimicrobial selected for therapy; however, the concentrations achieved will still usually exceed minimum inhibitory concentrations. The advantages of induced polyuria outweigh the disadvantage of reduced antimicrobial concentrations.

SUPPRESSION OF URINARY INFECTION WITH LOW-DOSE INTERMITTENT ANTIMICROBIAL THERAPY

When an animal suffers recurrences of urinary tract infection more than three times per year despite the appropriate use of a sensitive antimicrobial and if underlying complicating factors such as cystic calculi and bladder diverticuli have been ruled out, long-term management with antimicrobial agents may be necessary to prevent or reduce the frequency of further recurrences. The use of trimethoprim-sulfa, nitrofurantoin, or cephalexin at about one-third of the total recommended daily dose in dogs with recurrent gram-negative or mixed infections has reduced the incidence of recurrence about tenfold.[73] Similarly, ampicillin has been used to reduce the recurrence of gram-positive infections. The reduced dosage is given once daily at bedtime. It is very important to prevent urination after the dose has been administered. By administering the dose following the last voiding at night, the urine concentration of the antimicrobial will be high enough to kill susceptible bacteria during this period. Subtherapeutic concentrations of antimicrobials have also been shown to prevent adherence to the uroepithelium of some bacteria by inhibiting the development of fimbriae. Since urination during the night will reduce the concentration of the antimicrobial to ineffective levels, this regimen will be less effective in dogs that have pollakiuria or continuous opportunity to void. Patients receiving this regimen should have monthly bacteriologic rechecks. If trimethoprim-sulfa is the antimicrobial used, a Schirmer tear test should be performed monthly to assess tear production. There are legitimate concerns about the development of resistance, toxicity, and superinfection with the long-term use of any antimicrobial. However, there is no evidence of any of these problems with this suppression regimen.

SEPSIS ASSOCIATED WITH URINARY TRACT INFECTION

In humans, more than one-half of gram-negative septicemias originate from the genitourinary tract.[74] The majority of these cases of sepsis are associated with diagnostic or therapeutic manipulations. The uroepithelium of both the prostatic portion of the urethra and the renal pelvis is vulnerable to traumatic injury and subsequent loss of its ability to serve as a barrier to microbial invasion. The ample venous supply of the prostate allows access of bacteria to the systemic circulation following damage to the uroepithelial barrier.

Since one of the aminoglycosides is generally considered the antimicrobial of choice in the treatment of sepsis, extreme caution should be exercised in treating septic patients with reduced renal function. The risk of aminoglycoside-induced nephrotoxicity is increased by the tendency of patients in septic shock to develop oliguric acute renal failure.

CATHETER-ASSOCIATED URINARY TRACT INFECTION

The indwelling urinary catheter is an essential part of quality small animal patient care. Urinary catheters are used in the following situations: in the relief of mechanical or functional obstruction of the lower urinary tract, in the pre- and postoperative management of lower urinary tract trauma, in the nursing

Table 5-1. Measures to Improve Indwelling Catheter Care

Aseptic method of insertion
Sterile technique during catheter care
Avoidance of breaking the closed collection system
Proper positioning of the drainage bag below the patient's bladder
Handwashing between patients

care of animals with neurologic disease, and as a means of accurately measuring urine output in patients at risk for acute renal failure. Unfortunately, if used improperly or poorly maintained, the indwelling urinary catheter can result in a serious urinary tract infection. Indwelling urinary catheters are the most important predisposing factor in fatal gram-negative sepsis in hospitalized human patients, and the acquisition of urinary tract infection during indwelling catheterization is associated with a threefold increase in mortality among hospitalized patients.[75]

The best means of reducing the hazards associated with indwelling urinary catheters is to avoid their use when unnecessary and to promptly remove the catheters when no longer needed. The frequency of catheter-induced urinary tract infection depends on the technique of catheterization, the length of time the catheter remains in the urinary tract, and the immunological status of the patient. Single (in and out) catheterization of healthy adult female dogs is associated with a 20 percent risk of catheter-induced urinary tract infection.[9] If an indwelling catheter is required, measures should be taken to minimize the risk of infection (Table 5–1).

The use of closed urine drainage systems has reduced the incidence of catheter-induced UTI in human patients.[76] A closed urine drainage system protects the lumen of the catheter from the contaminated environment. In normal male cats, 3 days of open urine drainage resulted in UTI in 8 of the 12 cats evaluated.[77] Attempts to reduce the incidence of infection by irrigating the bladder with acetic acid or polymyxin B–neomycin solutions have not been successful. In fact, irrigation of the bladder may eventually result in colonization of the urine with yeasts.

In a properly managed closed urinary drainage system, the major pathway of infection is the migration of bacteria extraluminally in the periurethral space. Consequently, measures to reduce bacterial colonization of the periurethral space have been evaluated. Antimicrobial lubricants (e.g., povidone-iodine gel) used at the time of insertion reduce initial infection rates but are probably of minimal long-term benefit.[78] The daily application of an antimicrobial ointment to the urethral meatus does not appear to be beneficial in human patients. Proper maintenance of the urine collection system is very important. Disconnections of catheter junctions are associated with a high rate of infection.[75] Urine samples should be obtained via the ports present on most drainage tubes, thereby eliminating the need to disconnect the drainage tube. A major problem is reflux of urine from the bag into the bladder, so it is essential that the drainage bag be kept below the level of the bladder at all times.

Several reports claim that the addition of antiseptics to the drainage system decreases the rate of infection in catheterized patients.[79,80] The agents claimed to be effective include: povidone-iodine, 3 percent hydrogen peroxide, chlorhexidine, and formalin. The efficacy of these agents has been disputed in other studies.[81]

Systemic antimicrobial therapy eradicates catheter-associated infections only temporarily, and excessive use of antimicrobials leads to the emergence of resistant strains.[82] Therefore, this form of control is not recommended.

Methenamine does not decrease the frequency of urinary tract infection in human patients with indwelling catheters.[83] The antimicrobial action of methenamine depends on its hydrolysis in an acid environment to formaldehyde. The generation of formaldehyde from methenamine is a time-dependent reaction that requires a minimun of 60 to 90 minutes to achieve a bacteriostatic concentration. Thus, an indwelling urinary catheter that continually drains the bladder of urine will not allow an appropriate setting for the effective use of methenamine.

REFERENCES

1. Heptinstall RH: The enigma of chronic pyelonephritis. J Infect Dis 120:104, 1969
2. Finco DR, Barsanti JA: Bacterial pyelonephritis. Vet Clin North Am [Small Anim Pract] 9:645, 1979
3. Wooley RE, Blue JL: Bacterial isolations from canine and feline urine. Mod Vet Pract 57:535, 1976
4. Finco DR, Shotts EB, Crowell WA: Evaluation of methods for localization of urinary tract infection in the female dog. Am J Vet Res 40:707, 1979
5. Sobel JD, Kaye D: Host factors in the pathogenesis of urinary tract infections. Am J Med 76:122, 1984
6. Chan CYR, Bruce AW, Reid G: Adherence of cervical, vaginal and distal urethral normal microbial flora to human epithelial cells and the inhibition of adherence of gram-negative uropathogens by competitive exclusion. J Urol 131:596, 1984
7. Cox CE, Hinman F: Experiments with induced bacteriuria, vesical emptying and bacterial growth on the mechanism of bladder defense to infection. J Urol 86:739, 1961
8. Wilson JW, Klausner JS, Stevens JB, Osborne CA: Canine vesicourachal diverticula. Vet Surg 8:63, 1979
9. Biertuempfel PH, Ling GV, Ling GA: Urinary tract infection resulting from catheterization in healthy adult dogs. J Am Vet Med Assoc 178:989, 1981
10. Ihrke PJ, Norton AL, Ling GV, Stannard AA: Urinary tract infection associated with long-term corticosteroid administration in dogs with chronic skin diseases. J Am Vet Med Assoc 186:43, 1985
11. Salvatierra D, Tanagho EA: Reflux as a cause of end-stage kidney disease: Report of 32 cases. J Urol 117:441, 1977
12. Rolleston GL, Shannon FT, Utley WL: Follow-up of vesicoureteral reflux in the newborn. Kidney Int 8:S59, 1975
13. Smellie J, Edwards D, Hunter N, et al: Vesico-ureteric reflux and renal scarring. Kidney Int 8:565, 1975
14. Christie BA: Incidence etiology of vesicoureteral reflux in apparently normal dogs. Invest Urol 10:184, 1971

15. Hutch JA: Theory of maturation of the intravesicular ureter. J Urol 86:534, 1961
16. Christie BA: Vesicoureteral reflux in dogs. J Am Vet Med Assoc 162:772, 1973
17. Klausner JS, Feeney DA: Vesicoureteral reflux. p. 1041. In Kirk RW (ed): Current Veterinary Therapy VIII. WB Saunders, Philadelphia, 1983
18. Rocha H, Guze LB, Freedman LR, et al: Experimental pyelonephritis. III. The influence of localized injury in different parts of the kidney on susceptibility to bacillary infection. Yale J Biol Med 30:341, 1958
19. Freedman LR, Beeson PB: Experimental pyelonephritis. IV. Observations on infections resulting from direct inoculation of bacteria in different zones of the kidney. Yale J Biol Med 30:406, 1958
20. Miller TW, North JDK: Host response in urinary tract infections. Kidney Int 5:179, 1974
21. Cotran RS, Pennington JE: Urinary tract infection, pyelonephritis and reflux nephropathy. p. 1579. In Brenner BM, Rector FC (eds): The Kidney. 2nd ed. WB Saunders, Philadelphia, 1981
22. Andriole VT: Acceleration of the inflammatory response of the renal medulla by water diuresis. J Clin Invest 45:847, 1966
23. Chernew I, Braude AI: Depression of phagocytosis by solutes in concentrations found in the kidney and urine. Clin Invest 41:1945, 1962
24. Hubert EG, Montgomerie JZ, Kalmanson GM, et al: Effect of renal physiochemical milieu on serum bactericidal activity. Am J Med Sci 253:225, 1967
25. Losse H, Intorp HW, Lison AE, et al: Evidence of an autoimmune mechanism in pyelonephritis. Kidney Int 8(4):S44, 1975
26. Angell ME, Relman AS, Robins SL: Active chronic pyelonephritis without evidence of bacterial infection. N Engl J Med 278:1303, 1968
27. Kalmanson GM, Glassock RJ, Harwick HJ, et al: Cellular immunity in experimental pyelonephritis. Kidney Int 8(4):S35, 1975
28. Mayrer AR, Miniter P, Andriole VT: Immunopathogenesis of chronic pyelonephritis. Am J Med 75:59, 1983
29. Zager RA, Cotran RS, Hoyer JR: Pathologic localization of Tamm-Horsfall protein in interstitial deposits in renal disease. Lab Invest 38:52, 1978
30. Fasth A, Bengtsson U, Kaijser B, et al: Antibodies to Tamm-Horsfall protein associated with renal damage and urinary tract infection in adults. Kidney Int 20:500, 1981
31. McClusky RT, Colvin RG: Immunologic aspects of renal, tubular and interstitial disease. Annu Rev Med 29:191, 1978
32. Kaijser B, Larrson P, Olling S: Protection against ascending *E. coli* pyelonephritis in rats and significance of local immunity. Infect Immun 20:78, 1978
33. Smith JW, Kaijser B: The local immune response to *E. coli* O- and K-antigen in experimental pyelonephritis. J Clin Invest 58:276, 1976
34. Roberts JA, Roth JK, Domingue G, et al: Immunology of pyelonephritis in the primate model VI. Effect of complement depletion. J Urol 129:193, 1983
35. Roberts JA, Domingue GJ, Martin LN, Kim JCS and Rangan SRS: Immunology of pyelonephritis in the primate model II. Effect of immunosuppression. Invest Urol 19:148, 1981
36. Slotki IN, Asscher AW: Prevention of scarring in experimental pyelonephritis in the rat by early antibiotic therapy. Nephron 30:262, 1982
37. Roberts JA, Roth JK, Domingue G, et al: Immunology of pyelonephritis in the primate model V. Effect of superoxide dismutase. J Urol 128:1394, 1982
38. Beeson PB: Factors in the pathogenesis of pyelonephritis. Yale J Biol Med 28:81, 1955

39. Vivaldi E, Cotran RS, Zongwill DP, et al: Ascending infection as a mechanism in the pathogenesis of experimental nonobstructive pyelonephritis. Proc Soc Exp Biol Med 102:242, 1959
40. Aronson M, Medalia O, Schori L, et al: Prevention of colonization of the urinary tract of mice with *Escherichia coli* by blocking of bacterial adherence with methyl alpha-D-m-annopyranoside. Infect Dis 139:329, 1979
41. Svanbord-Eden CS, Hanson A, Jodal U, et al: Variable adherence to normal urinary tract epithelial cells of *E. coli* strains associated with various forms of UTI. Lancet 2:490, 1976
42. Kallenius G, Mollby R, Hultberg H, et al: Structure of carbohydrate part of receptor on human uroepithelial cells for pyelonephritogenic *Escherichia coli*. Lancet 2:604, 1981
43. Roberts JA, Kaack B, Kallenius G, et al: Receptors for pyelonephritogenic *Escherichia coli* in primates. J Urol 131:163, 1984
44. Roberts JA: Pathogenesis of pyelonephritis. J Urol 129:1102, 1983
45. Hanson LA: Host-parasite relationships in urinary tract infections. Infect Dis 127:726, 1973
46. Kaijser B, Hanson LA, Jodal V, et al: Frequency of *E. coli* K antigens in urinary tract infections in children. Lancet 1:663, 1977
47. Teague N, Boyarsky S: Further effects of coliform bacteria on ureteral peristalsis. J Urol 99:720, 1968
48. Roberts JA, Angel JR, Roth JK: The hydrodynamics of pyelorenal reflux. II. The effect of chronic obstructive changes on papillary shape. Invest Urol 18:296, 1981
49. Bourne HH, Condon NR, Hoyt TS, et al: Intrarenal reflux and renal damage. J Urol 113:400, 1975
50. Jang SS, Ling GV, Yamamoto R, Wolf AM: Mycoplasma as a cause of canine urinary tract infection. J Am Vet Med Assoc 185:45, 1984
51. Polzin DJ, Klausner JS: Treatment of urinary tract candidiasis. p. 1055. In Kirk RW (ed): Current Veterinary Therapy. 8th Ed. WB Saunders Co, Philadelphia, 1983
52. Carter JM, Klausner JS, Osborne CA: Comparison of collection techniques for quantitative urine culture in dogs. Am Vet Med Assoc 173:296, 1978
53. Lees GE, Simpson RB, Green RA: Results of analyses and bacterial cultures of urine specimens obtained from clinically normal cats by three methods. J Am Vet Med Assoc 184:449, 1984
54. Gomer KM, Ling GV: Results of urinalysis and bacterial culture of canine urine obtained by antepubic cystocentesis, catheterization, and the midstream voided methods. J Am Vet Med Assoc 179:891, 1981
55. Guenther KL, Washington JA: Evaluation of the B-D urine culture kit. J Clin Microbiol 14:628, 1981
56. Sheldon CA, Gonzalez R: Differentiation of upper and lower urinary tract infections: how and when? Med Clin North Am 68:321, 1984
57. Barber DL, Finco DR: Radiographic findings in induced bacterial pyelonephritis in dogs. J Am Vet Med Assoc 175:1183, 1979
58. Ling GV, Ackerman N, Lowenstine LJ, et al: Percutaneous nephropyelocentesis and nephropyelostomy in the dog: a description of the technique. Am J Vet Res 40:1605, 1979
59. Ling GV, Cullem M, Kennedy PC, et al: Relationship of upper and lower urinary tract infection and bacterial invasion of uroepithelium to antibody-coated bacteria test results in female dogs. Am J Vet Res 46:499, 1985
60. Vigano J, Assael BM, Villa AD, et al: N-acetyl-B-D-glucosaminidase (NAG) and

NAG isoenzymes in children with upper and lower urinary infection. Clin Chem Acta 130:297, 1983

61. Latham RH, Stamm WE: Role of fimbriated Escherichia coli in urinary tract infections in adult women: correlation with localization studies. J Infect Dis 149:835, 1984
62. Ling GV: Treatment of urinary tract infections with antimicrobial agents. p. 1051. In Kirk RW (ed): Current Veterinary Therapy VIII. 8th Ed. WB Saunders, Philadelphia, 1983
63. Ling GV, Hirsh DC: Antimicrobial susceptibility tests for urinary tract pathogens. p. 1048. In Kirk RW (ed): Current Veterinary Therapy VIII. Philadelphia, WB Saunders Co, 1983
64. Rohrich PJ, Ling Gv, Ruby AL, et al: In vitro susceptibilities of canine urinary bacteria to selected antimicrobial agents. J Am Vet Med Assoc 183:863, 1983
65. Ling GV, Gilmore CJ: Penicillin G or ampicillin for oral treatment of canine urinary tract infections. J Am Vet Med Assoc 171:358, 1977
66. Ling GV, Creighton SR, Ruby AL: Tetracycline for the oral treatment of canine urinary tract infection caused by *Pseudomonas aeruginosa*. J Am Vet Med Assoc 179:578, 1981
67. Ling GV, Ruby AL: Cephalexin for oral treatment of canine urinary tract infection caused by *Klebsiella pneumoniae*. J Am Vet Med Assoc 182:1346, 1983
68. Bergeron MG, Bastille A, Lessard C, et al: Significance of intrarenal concentrations of gentamicin for the outcome of experimental pyelonephritis in rats. J Infect Dis 146:91, 1982
69. Whelton A: Antibiotic pharmacokinetics and clinical application in renal insufficiency. Med Clin North Am 66:267, 1982
70. Tunn UW, Thieme H: Sepsis associated with urinary tract infection. Arch Intern Med 142:2035, 1982
71. Huland H, Busch R: Chronic pyelonephritis as a cause of end-stage renal disease. Urology 127:642, 1982
72. Riviere JE, Coppoc GL: Dosage of antimicrobial drugs in patients with renal insufficiency. J Am Vet Med Assoc 178:70, 1981
73. Ling GV: The use of antimicrobial agents in the management of urinary tract infections. Proc Kal Kan Symposium 1983, p. 101
74. Tunn UW, Thieme H: Sepsis associated with urinary tract infection. Arch Intern Med 142:2035, 1982
75. Platt R. Murdock B, Polk BF, Rosner B: Reduction of mortality associated with nosocomical urinary tract infection. Lancet, April 23. 893, 1983
76. Kunin CM, McCormack RC: Prevention of catheter-induced urinary tract infections by sterile closed drainage. New Engl J Med 274:1155, 1966
77. Lees GE, Osborne CA, Stevens JB, Ward GE: Adverse effects caused by polypropylene and polyvinyl feline urinary catheters. Am J Vet Res 41:1836, 1980
78. Harrison LH: Comparison of a microbicidal povidone-iodine gel and a placebo gel as catheter lubricants. J Urol 124, 347, 1980
79. Maizels M, Schaeffer AJ: Decreased incidence of bacteriuria associated with periodic instillations of hydrogen peroxide into the urethral catheter drainage bag. J Urol 123:841, 1980
80. Gillespie WA, Jones JE, Teasdale C, et al: Does the addition of disinfectant to urine drainage bags prevent infection in catheterized patients. Lancet 1:1037, 1983
81. Warren JW, Hoopes JM, Muncie HL, Anthony WC: Ineffectiveness of cephalexin

in treatment of cephalexin-resistant bacteriuria in patients with chronic indwelling urethral catheters. J Urol 129:71, 1983
82. Bjork DT, Pelletier LL, Tight RR: Urinary tract infections with antibiotic resistant organisms in catheterized nursing home patients. Infect Control 5:173, 1984
83. Warren JW, Muncie HL, Bergquist EJ, Hoopes JM: Sequelae and management of urinary infection in the patient requiring chronic catheterization. J Urol 125:1, 1981

6 Feline Renal Failure

Linda A. Ross

Renal failure is defined as the inability of the kidneys to perform their normal functions. Consequences of renal failure include loss of the ability to eliminate metabolic waste products, abnormal water and electrolyte metabolism, and abnormal endocrine function. Renal failure may be due to prerenal factors such as hypovolemia secondary to dehydration, shock, or heart failure; primary renal disease; or postrenal factors such as an obstruction or tear in the ureters, bladder, or urethra. This review is limited to a discussion of renal failure due to primary renal disease.

Disorders of the urinary system are common in cats. In one study, diseases of the urinary tract were diagnosed twice as often in cats as in dogs. This reflects in part the high incidence of feline lower urinary tract disease (81 percent of all feline urinary tract diseases). In contrast, diseases of the upper urinary tract (kidneys and ureters) and lower urinary tract (bladder and urethra) were diagnosed with approximately equal frequency in dogs. Diseases of the kidney also differed between the species. Amyloidosis and hydronephrosis were diagnosed much less frequently in cats than in dogs. Glomerular diseases had a similar but less pronounced disparity[1] (Table 6-1).

Despite the lower incidence of renal disease in cats as compared to dogs, renal failure still accounts for a significant incidence of feline morbidity and mortality. While acute obstructive uropathy is probably the most common cause of renal failure in cats, chronic renal failure of various etiologies also occurs. Unfortunately, much of the information about the pathogenesis, diagnosis, and treatment of renal failure in cats has been extrapolated from dogs or human beings. Differences between cats, dogs, and other species will be pointed out where appropriate in the following discussion.

Table 6-1. Frequency of Diagnosis of Selected Urinary Tract Diseases in the Dog and Cat[a]

	Dogs		Cats	
Disease	1970–74	1975–79	1970–74	1975–79
Renal calculi	13(8.4)	15(5.7)	2(1.9)	0
Ruptured kidney	3(1.9)	4(1.5)	0	2(1.7)
Infarcted kidneys	19(12.3)	42(15.9)	3(2.8)	8(6.7)
Amyloidosis	16(10.4)	20(7.6)	3(2.8)	1(6.7)
Hydronephrosis	14(9.1)	33(12.5)	3(2.8)	1(0.8)
Glomerular disease	174(112.6)	314(118.9)	60(56.4)	89(74.8)
Renal neoplasia	17(11)	44(16.7)	12(11.3)	12(10.1)

[a] Numbers without parentheses indicate actual number of times each diagnosis was made in dogs and cats at the University of California, Davis, for the 5-year period indicated. Numbers in parenthesis indicate the frequency of diagnosis of each disease per 1000 diagnoses of disease of the urinary tract.

(Modified from Low DG: Cats aren't small dogs. Carnation Research Digest 17:1, 1981.)

PATHOPHYSIOLOGY OF RENAL FAILURE

The response of the kidney to injury has been extensively studied in other species. It has been assumed that cat kidneys function similarly to dog kidneys. The cat, however, has a number of structural and functional differences from other species. The kidney of the cat contains more lipid than that of any other species. It has a subcapsular network of veins that drains the superficial renal cortex.[2] It has no transport maximum for glucose or phosphate reabsorption by the tubules. Glucose reabsorption is depressed by increasing levels of blood glucose in the cat, whereas in the dog and man it is enhanced. In cats, phosphate and glucose reabsorption appear to have a parallel rather than an inverse relationship.[2] Sodium, potassium, and chloride content of feline urine is quantitatively different from canine urine, probably due to dietary or fluid intake difference. Urine concentrating ability in the cat is greater than many other species. These differences suggest that the pathophysiologic consequences of renal failure in the cat may vary somewhat from other species. Since few studies of feline renal failure have been done, we are forced to use information obtained from studies in rats, dogs, and man.

Prerenal Azotemia

Renal insufficiency can result from decreased renal blood flow due to a variety of causes. Dehydration resulting in hypovolemia is probably the most common cause of prerenal azotemia. Blood loss and shock will also cause decreased renal blood flow, as will heart failure. In cats, congestive heart failure is most commonly associated with cardiomyopathy (dilatative or hypertrophic forms).

Extrarenal factors may cause mild azotemia. Blood urea nitrogen (BUN) is generated by the liver as a product of protein metabolism. Factors causing increased protein catabolism (such as massive muscle trauma, intestinal hemorrhage, or steroid administration) may cause azotemia, as can high dietary levels of protein. Blood urea nitrogen levels have been shown to rise slightly in dogs after feeding; occasionally the BUN concentration may exceed the upper limit of normal.[3] While this has not been studied in cats, it may well occur in this species—especially in light of their high dietary protein requirements.[4]

While renal function is diminished due to decreased renal perfusion of short duration, kidney structure remains normal. Correction of the cause of prerenal azotemia will promptly restore renal function to normal. However, prolonged hypoperfusion may result in renal ischemia and renal damage.

Primary Renal Failure

Renal failure may be caused by a number of diseases (see section entitled "Causes of renal disease and renal failure"). However, the resulting alterations in renal function are similar no matter what the inciting cause. The clinical and laboratory changes in acute and chronic renal failure have been discussed elsewhere.[5,6] Table 6-2 lists selected abnormalities which can be used to differentiate various forms of renal failure.

Acute Renal Failure. Acute renal failure may be defined as the sudden inability of the kidneys to regulate water and solute balance; this may occur with reduced, normal, or increased urine flow. Clinically, oliguria is urine flow of less than 20 ml/kg body weight per day, and anuria is urine flow less than 4 ml/kg per day.

The pathophysiology of oliguria in renal failure remains an engima. There are several theories, each of which has been shown to play a role in specific experimental models of acute renal failure.[7,8] How these factors interact in naturally occurring disease is not known.

Failure to produce adequate urine volume leads to water retention and expansion of the extracellular fluid compartment. This may result in heart failure and/or pulmonary edema, especially if coupled with a positive sodium balance. Hyperkalemia is the second major threat in oliguria. It results from inability of the kidney to excrete potassium, as well as potassium released by tissue catabolism.[7]

Metabolic acidosis occurs in renal failure due to inability of the diseased kidneys to excrete a hydrogen load.[7,8] Although acidosis per se does not usually cause problems, it tends to potentiate hyperkalemia.

Hyperphosphatemia occurs in patients with oliguria and may cause a reciprocal decrease in serum calcium concentration.[7] Hyperphosphatemia does not result in clinical problems unless the patient undergoes rapid therapeutic alkalinization. This may result in further lowering of the serum ionized calcium levels and subsequent hypocalcemic tetany or seizures.

Chronic Renal Failure. Chronic renal failure results in a wide variety of pathophysiologic changes. Metabolic acidosis occurs primarily as the result of inability of the kidney to produce sufficient ammonia to excrete hydrogen ions.[8,9] The acidosis is partially buffered by bone apatite; this, however, results in decreased bone growth in growing animals and children.[9]

There is a progressive decrease in the fractional reabsorption of sodium

Table 6-2. Selected Clinical and Laboratory Findings in Renal Failure

Findings	Prerenal	Acute Renal	Chronic Renal	Postrenal
	Type of Renal Failure Suggested			
Blood chemistry				
↑ BUN or creatinine	N[a]	N	N	N
↑ Potassium	—	○[a]	○	○
↑ Chloride or bicarbonate	—	○	○	○
↑ Phosphorus	—	○	○	○
Hematology				
Anemia: normocytic, normochronic	—	—	●[a]	—
Urinalysis				
sp gr > 1.040	N	○	○	○
sp gr 1.008–1.012	—	○	●	○
sp gr ≥ 1.008	—	—	○	—
Proteinuria	—	○	○	—
Hematuria	—	○	○	—
Granular casts	—	○	○	—
Broad casts	—	—	●	—
Other casts	—	○	○	—
Other tests				
Urine sodium < 10 mEq/L	●	—	○	—
Urine sodium > 25 mEq/L	—	●	○	—
Urine: plasma osmolarity > 1.1	●	—	○	—
Urine: plasma osmolarity < 1.1	—	●	○	—
Urine: plasma urea > 20:1	●	—	○	—
Urine: plasma urea < 3:1	—	●	○	—
Urine: plasma creatinine > 40:1	●	—	○	—
Urine: plasma creatinine < 15:1	—	●	○	—
Renal size				
Small	—	—	○	—
Normal to large	●	●	—	○
Miscellaneous				
Renal pain	—	●	—	—
Dysuria/inability to void	—	—	—	S[a]
History polydipsia/ polyuria	—	—	●	—
Osteodystrophy (radiographically)	—	—	●	—

[a] KEY: ○ = occurs in the syndrome.
● = important clue to the syndrome.
N = necessary for the diagnosis of the syndrome.
S = sufficient for diagnosis of the syndrome unless clearly caused by another disease.

(Modified from Coe FL: Clinical and laboratory assessment of the patient with renal disease. p. 1135. In Brenner BW, Rector FC (eds): The Kidney. 2nd Ed. WB Saunders, Philadelphia, 1981.)

and water. The mechanism for this is not fully understood, although the presence of a natriuretic hormone has been proposed. A compound causing natriuresis has been isolated but not characterized.[9] Tubular secretion of potassium is increased. In the late stages of renal failure, fecal excretion of potassium may also increase. The ability to excrete a water load is decreased.[5,9] The activity of Na,K-ATPase is inhibited with subsequent alterations in cellular ion flux and membrane potential.[9]

A normocytic, normochromic, nonregenerative anemia is common in cats with chronic renal failure. Three factors play a role in the pathogenesis of this anemia: (1) decreased levels of erythropoietin due to decreased renal mass, (2) serum inhibitors of erythropoiesis, (3) shortened red blood cell life span.[9–11]

Although platelet numbers are normal in animals with chronic renal failure, their function is abnormal, as shown by decreased platelet adhesiveness and aggregation in response to ADP and decreased release of platelet factor III. These changes are caused by elevated plasma levels of toxic metabolites such as guanidinosuccinic acid, phenols, and urea. In addition, elevated levels of PGI_2 (prostacycline, which inhibits platelet aggregation) are found.[9–11]

Secondary hyperparathyroidism is an inevitable consequence of chronic renal failure,[12] although the exact mechanism remains controversial.[13,14] There are numerous clinical consequences of hyperparathyroidism, and parathyroid hormone (PTH) has been proposed as a primary uremic toxin.[15] Hyperparathyroidism causes calcium depletion of the skeletal system. Soft tissue calcification may occur.[15] In people, pruritus, proximal myopathy, and neurologic dysfunction have been related to elevated levels of PTH.[5,15,16] Parathyroid hormone has been implicated in the phenomenon of relative insulin resistance at the cellular level. It may also play a role in the progression of renal failure. Uremic animals with increased PTH levels had progressive functional and structural deterioration of remaining renal tissue.[17,18]

Reproductive failure occurs in both sexes in patients with chronic renal failure. The pathogenesis is complex, involving both hypothalamic-pituitary dysfunction and direct uremic toxicity upon reproductive tissues. Luteinizing hormone (LH) levels are elevated due to increased secretion, as well as decreased metabolic clearance. Follicle-stimulating hormone (FSH) levels increase less frequently and to a lesser extent. Elevations in both these hormones probably also reflect end-organ resistance with subsequent effects on the pituitary-hypothalamic feedback mechanism. Levels of testosterone are decreased in males, and levels of estrogen and progesterone are decreased in females.[9,19]

Stomatitis and oral ulceration are frequent manifestations of chronic renal failure, as are vomiting and diarrhea. Serum gastrin levels are elevated in chronic renal failure because of decreased renal degradation; this may cause increased gastric acid secretion and uremic gastropathy.[20] In humans, uremia results in decreased gastric acid secretion in the face of hypergastrinemia.[21]

The effects of uremia on small bowel function are not well defined. The results of measurements of brush border enzymes have been conflicting. Iron and calcium absorption are both depressed. Increased gastrointestinal losses of albumin have been reported. Inflammatory changes in the colon may contribute to diarrhea. Pancreatic and liver involvement are reported in people with chronic renal failure but are uncommon in animals.[5,21]

Neurologic abnormalities are common in people with chronic renal failure but have been infrequently reported in animals. This is undoubtedly due to the ability to determine minor changes in intellectual ability in people. Recent data suggest that these alterations may be due to increased PTH levels. Increased PTH levels have been associated with EEG abnormalities and decreased motor nerve conduction velocity.[16]

Both humoral and cellular immunity may be depressed with chronic renal failure. Lymphopenia is common in both dogs and cats, and serum immunoglobulin concentrations may be low. Complement activation and granulocyte function may be impaired.[5]

Hypertension is common in both people[7] and dogs[6,22] with chronic renal failure. The incidence in cats has not been reported, but hypertension has been documented in clinical cases. Abnormalities in cardiac rate or rhythm may occur.[9] Pericarditis, pericardial effusion, and pulmonary edema are not uncommon in people with uremia but have been rarely reported in animals.[5] It is not clear whether the edema is due to increased lung vascular permeability from uremia or increased extracellular fluid volume due to renal dysfunction.[9]

Primary glomerular diseases result in loss of the normal size- and charge-selective properties of the glomerular basement membrane (GBM). Albumin does not normally cross the GBM because of its size and because as an anion it is repelled by the fixed negative electrostatic charge of the GBM. Alterations in pore size and membrane charge result in marked albuminuria and proteinuria,[5,6] the hallmark of glomerular disease.

Clinical signs associated with glomerular disease may be related to the proteinuria and subsequent hypoproteinemia rather than to renal insufficiency. These include weight loss, peripheral edema, ascites, or dyspnea due to pulmonary edema or hydrothorax. Severe glomerulonephritis will eventually result in destruction of sufficient numbers of nephrons to cause renal failure.

Nephrotic syndrome is a term that refers to a set of four clinical and laboratory parameters associated with glomerular disease: proteinuria, hypoproteinemia (due to hypoalbuminemia), hypercholesterolemia, and peripheral edema. It is not an etiologic or pathologic classification. The pathogenesis of the hypercholesterolemia is not clear but appears to be related to altered levels of lipoproteins. Peripheral edema results from hypoalbuminemia and the subsequent reduction in plasma oncotic pressure.

Postrenal Failure

Postrenal failure is caused by obstruction to urine flow distal to the kidneys. In cats, urethral obstruction due to struvite crystals and a mucoprotein substance (the feline urologic syndrome) is the most common cause of postrenal failure. This syndrome has been discussed elsewhere[2,23,24] and is reviewed in Chapter 3.

CAUSES OF FELINE RENAL DISEASE AND RENAL FAILURE

Congenital and Familial Renal Disease

A variety of congenital abnormalities of the kidney have been reported in cats, although they do not necessarily result in renal failure. These include unilateral renal agenesis, renal ectopia,[25] hydronephrosis,[26] polycystic disease,[2,27,28] and fused kidneys.[2] Renal amyloidosis has been reported in related Abyssinian cats, suggesting that it is a familial disease.[29,30] Congenital renal disease is discussed in Chapter 7.

Acquired Renal Disease

Glomerulopathies. ***Amyloidosis.*** Amyloidois in all species is now known to represent a group of diseases rather than a distinct disease entity. Amyloid does not represent one substance but may be composed of one of several proteins. Each of these proteins shares one vital characteristic; they are deposited in tissue in a beta-pleated sheet conformation. It is this conformation which results in the unique appearance and chemical properties of amyloid.[31,32]

In dogs, amyloid is usually deposited in the glomeruli. While glomerular deposition may occur in cats, amyloid is more frequently found in the medullary interstitium.[2,31,32] If glomerular deposition is marked, the cat may show clinical signs of the nephrotic syndrome.

Glomerulonephritis. Glomerulonephritis is an uncommon disease in cats, although it represents a significant percentage of feline renal disease.[33] In two studies of 493 cats, only one case of glomerulonephritis was found at necropsy.[34,35] Despite this data, glomerulonephritis can be a cause of significant morbidity and mortality, especially in certain groups of cats.

Glomerulonephritis may be classified according to the morphological changes it produces. However, this classification is not necessarily helpful in determining the pathogenesis because the glomerulus can react in only a limited number of ways to injury. The major pathologic changes in the glomerulus are proliferation of cells in the mesangial matrix (proliferative glomerulopathy) and thickening of the basement membrane (membranous glomerulopathy). Both changes may be seen in the same patient (membranoproliferative glomerulopathy).[8]

Membranous glomerulopathy can be further subdivided into two types. In the first, circulating antiglomerular basement membrane antibodies react with the glomerular basement membrane (GBM). Immunofluorescent staining of these glomeruli reveals that immunoglobulins and complement are deposited in a smooth, linear fashion along the basement membrane.[6,36–38] Anti-GBM glomerulonephritis has not been reported in the cat.[6]

In immune-complex glomerulonephritis, immune complexes formed by antibodies to various antigens are deposited in the glomerulus, most commonly on the epithelial side of the basement membrane. Electron microscopy or immunofluorescent stains show that the GBM has a "lumpy-bumpy" appearance, attributed to the irregular deposition of the immune complexes. In severe cases, thickening of the basement membrane with spike-like protrusions may be seen by light microscopy.[6,36–38]

The antigens involved in immune complex formation in cats with membranous glomerulonephritis are usually difficult to identify. Suggested sources include chronic viral respiratory infections, bacterial abscesses or infections, systemic lupus erythematosus (SLE), pancreatic disease, and feline infectious peritonitis (FIP).[38] Infection with the feline leukemia virus (FeLV) has been associated with increased incidence of glomerulonephritis.[39–41] Glomerulonephritis was the leading cause of death in one study of a large group of cats living in a virus-endemic household.[39] Another study found glomerulonephritis in approximately one-third of cats with lymphosarcoma or myeloproliferative diseases.[40] It was assumed that all of these cases were FeLV-associated, although tests for FeLV antigens were not reported.

Membranous glomerulopathy has twice been reported in sibling cats.[42,43] The cause for the immune complex deposition could not be identified, although FeLV infection, pancreatic disease, SLE, and FIP were ruled out. Environmental causes could not be ruled out, since the related cats lived in the same household in both reports. However, the close relationship of the cats sugests that a familial form of glomerulonephritis may exist.

Several miscellaneous cases of feline glomerulonephritis have been reported. Immune complex glomerulonephritis was reported in a cat with pyogranulomatous pericholangiohepatitis and depletion of T-lymphocyte-dependent areas in the lymph nodes and spleen.[44] Tests for FeLV infection were negative; tests for SLE were not reported. The etiology of the lesions in this case was not determined but was speculated to be immune-mediated or infectious.

A necrotizing glomerulopathy has been described in cats euthanatized with a combination of ketamine hydrochloride and sodium pentobarbitol.[45] Since no glomerular lesions were seen in cats given either drug alone, the authors speculated that an in vivo interaction of the two drugs resulted in peracute necrosis of the glomerular endothelium and mesangium.

Pyelonephritis. Pyelonephritis is the bacterial infection of the renal pelvis and parenchyma. It has been discussed clinically in the cat[46] and has been produced and characterized experimentally.[47–49] However, most of the clinical information about feline pyelonephritis has been extrapolated from the canine literature.

While lower urinary tract disease (the feline urologic syndrome) is common in cats, bacterial urinary tract infections are infrequent. The bacteria most commonly isolated are *E. coli, Proteus sp., Pseudomonas* sp.,[46] and *Staphylococcus aureus*. It has been suggested that the high osmolality of feline urine may be bacteriostatic, rendering cats as a species more resistant to urinary tract infection than dogs.[50,51] Cats would be expected to have a lower incidence of pyelonephritis than dogs since pyelonephritis is usually the result of an ascending urinary tract infection.

Interstitial Nephritis. The term *chronic interstitial nephritis* has been applied to a type of renal disease common in both dogs and cats. It is characterized by mononuclear cell infiltration and fibrosis of the renal interstitium. In advanced cases, glomerular sclerosis may also be seen. Originally, it was thought that the interstitial inflammatory changes represented the primary disease process. It is now known, however, that virtually any form of renal disease can cause similar pathologic changes. It is difficult to separate true "interstitial nephritis" from the terminal stages of any renal disease.[5]

Polyarteritis Nodosa. Polyarteritis nodosa is a rare cause of renal failure in cats.[52,53] It is a disease of unknown etiology characterized by fibrinoid necrosis and inflammation of small- and medium-sized arteries and arterioles. Multiple organs may be affected. Two of the reported cases had lesions confined to the kidneys[52]; two others had multisystem involvement.[52,53]

Feline Infectious Peritonitis. Feline infectious peritonitis (FIP) is a multisystem disease caused by infection with a coronavirus. The disease has two clinical manifestations. The first form is characterized by pleural or peritoneal effusion (effusive or "wet" FIP). The second form involves granulomatous inflammation of various organs, including the central nervous system, lymph nodes, and kidneys. Extensive lesions may result in renal insufficiency. Affected kidneys are typically enlarged and have an irregular, lumpy contour. A few cats may have glomerulonephritis with concurrent proteinuria.[54]

Neoplasia. Lymphosarcoma is by far the most common neoplasm affecting feline kidneys, and indeed, it is the most common feline neoplasm. It is generally associated with infection by the feline leukemia virus (FeLV). The feline leukemia virus is a retrovirus which can be transmitted horizontally, primariy through saliva. Most infected cats remain persistently viremic, although a latent form of infection exists in some cats. These cats have high circulating levels of neutralizing antibody which protect against viremia, but they have persistent infection of the bone marrow cells. Either category of cat may develop lymphosarcoma as a result of neoplastic transformation of lymphocytes by FeLV.[55]

Renal lymphosarcoma may be part of a generalized neoplastic process involving multiple organs, or the kidney may be the sole site of involvement. In one study, renal involvement produced the most common clinical signs in 20 percent of a group of cats with lymphosarcoma. A second study found renal involvement in 31 of 78 cases of feline lymphosarcoma.[2] Renal involvement is usually diffuse, interstitial, and bilateral resulting in large, irregular kidneys.[55] Signs of renal failure do not occur until the kidneys have undergone massive infiltration by neoplastic lymphocytes. Owners may seek veterinary attention because they have noticed "lumps" in their cat's abdomen (the enlarged kidneys) rather than signs of uremia.

Primary renal neoplasms are rare. One study reported 43 cases which consisted of 17 renal carcinomas, three transitional cell carcinomas, two squamous cell carcinomas, eight unclassified sarcomas, two leiomyosarcomas, nine nephroblastomas, and two adenomas.[56] Renal neoplasms do not necessarily result in renal failure unless both kidneys are involved or the contralateral kidney is diseased.

Hydronephrosis. Hydronephrosis is the result of obstruction to urine flow from the kidneys. Obstruction is usually mechanical and may occur anywhere in the urinary tract distal to the kidneys. Hydronephrosis may be unilateral or bilateral, depending on the location of the obstruction. Hydronephrosis in the cat may be due to congenital or acquired causes. Congenital causes include ureteral or urethral abnormalities such as stenosis, torsion, kinking, and atresia; ureteral constriction may also be caused by aberrant renal vessels.[26] The most common causes of acquired hydronephrosis are ureteral and urethral masses and calculi. A number of cases of hydronephrosis in cats have been reported in which there is no apparent cause.[2]

Hydronephrosis must be differentiated from a perirenal cyst. Perirenal cysts (perinephric pseudocyst, perirenal pseudocyst, renal capsular cyst, capsulogenic renal cyst, capsular hydronephrosis, retroperitoneal perirenal cyst) have been reported occasionally in male cats over 8 years of age. These cysts can reach large sizes but do not usually cause renal failure unless underlying renal disease exists. The fluid in the cysts is classified as a transudate and may be located either between the renal parenchyma and the renal capsule or enclosed in a separate sac attached to the kidney.[57]

Toxicities. A number of chemicals are nephrotoxic and can result in acute tubular necrosis. Those most commonly affecting cats are the heavy metals, especially lead, mercury, and arsenic; ethylene glycol (antifreeze); and the aminoglycoside antibiotics (gentamicin, kanamycin, neomycin, tobramycin).

DIAGNOSIS

One of the major difficulties in the diagnosis of renal disease and renal failure is that common clinical tests fail to detect mild or moderate decreases in renal function. These tests also do not localize abnormalities in function; that is, they do not determine whether renal insufficiency is prerenal, primary renal, or postrenal in origin. The clinician must interpret and correlate the history, physical findings, and laboratory tests in order to make the diagnosis of renal failure (Table 6-2).

History and Clinical Signs

A thorough history is essential when pursuing any clinical problem. Older cats are more likely to have chronic renal failure due to interstitial nephritis, whereas lymphosarcoma and glomerulonephritis are more common in younger cats. The signs of renal failure vary, are nonspecific, and may include anorexia, depression, lethargy, weight loss, vomiting, and diarrhea. Cats with acute renal failure will generally show more severe signs than those with chronic disease. If acute renal failure is suspected, the owner should be carefully questioned as to exposure to nephrotoxic agents (especially ethylene glycol). A history of polydipsia and polyuria may be elicited, although its absence does not rule out renal failure. Prior urinary tract disorders (such as repeated urethral obstructions) may increase the risk of renal disease.

Physical Examination

Physical examination may or may not provide clues to the presence of renal failure, depending on its cause and severity. The cat's general condition may be poor, with muscle wasting and a poor hair coat. Dehydration may be detected by decreased skin turgor, dry mucous membranes, and sunken eyeballs. Oral ulcerations or stomatitis may be present. The mucous membranes may be pale if the cat is anemic, and a systolic murmur may be present if the anemia is severe. The kidneys are easily palpated in most cats. It should be ascertained whether both kidneys are present; whether they are small, normal-sized, or enlarged; and whether their surface is regular. The urinary bladder should also be thoroughly palpated to determine whether a urethral obstruction is present. Some cats, particularly those with chronic renal failure, have no physical abnormalities.

Laboratory Assessment

A number of laboratory parameters should be evaluated by the clinician in making a diagnosis of renal failure and in attempting to differentiate acute from chronic disease. Several tests of renal function are available to the clinician. Different tests assess the integrity of different parts of the nephron and vary according to their sensitivity and specificity.

Glomerular Function. The glomerular filtration rate (GFR) is generally assessed clinically by the determination of BUN and serum creatinine concentrations. Both substances are freely filtered through the glomerular basement membrane. Much of the urea that is filtered is reabsorbed as it passes through the renal tubules; the amount reabsorbed is dependent on the rate of flow through the tubules. The BUN concentration is dependent on several nonrenal factors, as well as intrinsic renal function; the serum creatinine concentration is less dependent on such nonrenal factors. Since creatinine is an end product of muscle metabolism, extreme cachexia with muscle wasting may in rare instances result in decreased creatinine production and a low serum creatinine concentration. The dog has a weak proximal tubular secretory mechanism for creatinine,[23] which does not appear to be important clinically. In the cat, no such mechanism exists, and essentially all of the creatinine that is filtered by the glomerulus appears in the urine.[59] The serum creatinine concentration is considered to be a more accurate index of GFR than BUN because it is less dependent on nonrenal factors. The BUN concentration is still useful, however, because of its simplicity, reproducibility, and low cost.

Both BUN and serum creatinine concentrations are, at best, only crude reflections of GFR. With primary renal disease, neither value will rise above the normal range until approximately three-fourths of renal function is lost. Conversely, both values will rise under conditions which produce a decrease in GFR, despite normal renal function (pre- or postrenal azotemia). The BUN to serum creatinine ratio has been used to determine the pathogenesis of azotemia in humans. However, in the dog it does not differentiate between prerenal, renal, and postrenal causes.[60] It has not been studied in the cat. Both BUN and serum creatinine concentrations are highest when there is lack of urine output, either from anuric primary renal failure or from postrenal failure.

In some cases the diagnosis of renal disease may be unclear. Cats with marginally elevated BUN or serum creatinine concentrations, relatives of cats with suspected familial renal disease, or cats infected with the feline leukemia virus may fall into this category. In such instances, it may be desirable to obtain a more precise measurement of GFR. Such a measurement may be obtained by measuring the clearance of a substance. The term *clearance* refers to the amount of plasma which is completely cleared of a given substance per unit of time. In order to provide an accurate estimate of GFR, the substance measured must be freely filtered through the glomerulus and neither reabsorbed nor secreted by the renal tubules. Inulin and creatinine are two such substances which have been shown to accurately reflect GFR.[60] Inulin is rarely used in clinical situations because of technical difficulties in providing a constant intravenous infusion of this substance and difficulties in its chemical assay. Interestingly, creatinine clearance determinations slightly underestimate GFR as measured by inulin clearance in the cat, although there is good correlation between the two. It has been suggested that this discrepancy may be due to the methodology used in the laboratory determination of the serum creatinine concentration.[59] The discrepancy is not important clinically, since the creatinine clearance correlates well with GFR.

A creatinine clearance may be performed by measuring either endogenous or exogenous creatine. Exogenous clearances usually require a constant intravenous infusion of the substance whose clearance is being measured. A method utilizing one subcutaneous injection of creatinine has recently been shown to provide an accurate index of GFR in the dog.[61] This method has not been validated in the cat but would seem to be applicable to this species as well.

All clearance procedures have the inherent disadvantage of requiring the collection of a timed urine sample. In cats, catheterization of the urinary bladder to obtain an accurate urine collection may require general anesthesia. Anesthesia not only depresses GFR[60] but may be dangerous in a clinical patient. Catheterization also carries the risk of inducing a urinary tract infection. Manual expression of the bladder can be traumatic, and accurate urine collection is difficult. Creatinine clearances, therefore, are generally not performed in cats.

Another method for estimation of GFR is to determine the rate of excretion of a substance known to be excreted primarily by glomerular filtration. Sodium sulfanilate is one such substance whose excretion has been shown to correlate with GFR in the cat.[18] In this test, a 5 percent solution of sodium sulfanilate is injected intravenously at a dose of 0.2 ml/kg. Blood samples are collected at 30, 60, and 90 minutes and analyzed for sodium sulfanilate concentration. The plasma half-life is then calculated; half-life in the normal cat is 48 to 50 minutes.[18]

Tubular Function. Renal tubular function is usually determined by the ability of the animal to produce a concentrated or dilute urine. While osmolarity gives a more accurate reflection of urine concentrating ability than does specific gravity, the latter provides sufficient information to assess tubular function in most clinical situations.

Urine specific gravity should always be evaluated with respect to the hydration status of the cat, as well as other renal function tests. A normal cat may produce urine that is dilute, isosthenuric, or concentrated, depending upon its water balance at that point in time. However, it is unusual for a cat to have isosthenuric or dilute urine without the existence of some disease process. It has been stated that the ability to concentrate urine is lost when two-thirds of the nephrons are lost and that azotemia occurs after loss of three-fourths of renal mass.[5] This axiom is not always true. Animals with glomerulonephritis may have azotemia in conjunction with concentrated urine if the glomeruli are more severely affected than the tubules. Cats with renal insufficiency may become azotemic prior to losing urine concentrating ability.[18] This is probably related to their ability to normally produce very concentrated urine.

Normal urine concentrating ability has been defined as the production of urine of specific gravity greater than 1.025. However, this figure was taken from the human literature. Since people have a maximal urine concentrating ability of approximately 1.040 and cats have one of 1.080, a more accurate but still conservative figure for the cat would be 1.035.[62] Urine concentrating ability in kittens has not been studied but is assumed to be similar to puppies. The kidneys of puppies are able to concentrate urine to some degree but not to the same level as an adult dog.[63] The exact age at which normal urine concentrating ability develops is also not well documented but is suggested to be at 12 to 16 weeks of age. These factors are important when assessing renal function in kittens.

Excretion of phenolsulphonphthalein (PSP) dye has been described as a renal function test in dogs.[60,64,65] At the dose used, the test is a reflection of renal plasma flow. Evaluation of this test in cats showed poor correlation with renal plasma flow, indicating that it is not a reliable test of renal function.[18] Phenolsulphonphthalein may be excreted by other routes (possibly hepatic) in the cat.

Radiology. Radiographic studies may provide some information about the cause of renal failure; they are less important in the assessment of renal function, since the information they provide is qualitative rather than quantitative. Survey abdominal radiographs may be helpful in determining renal size, shape, and contour. Since the kidneys of cats are usually palpable, this information may be less important than it is in dogs. Intravenous urography can be helpful in determining differences in function between the two kidneys as shown by differences in radiographic density; it can illustrate the presence of hydronephrosis or changes in the renal pelvis suggestive of pyelonephritis; and it may show the presence of obstructive uropathy. One of the most important pieces of information that can be gained from contrast radiography is the diagnosis of a tear in the urinary collecting system (postrenal failure).

Histopathology. Renal biopsy and histopathologic study is the only definitive method to establish an etiologic diagnosis for renal failure. Both aspiration and needle biopsies are easily performed in the cat, due to the location and mobility of the kidneys. The left kidney is usually biopsied in the case of generalized renal disease, because it is slightly more accessible. The platelet count, prothrombin time, partial thromboplastin time, and plasma fibrinogen concentration should be determined prior to biopsy.

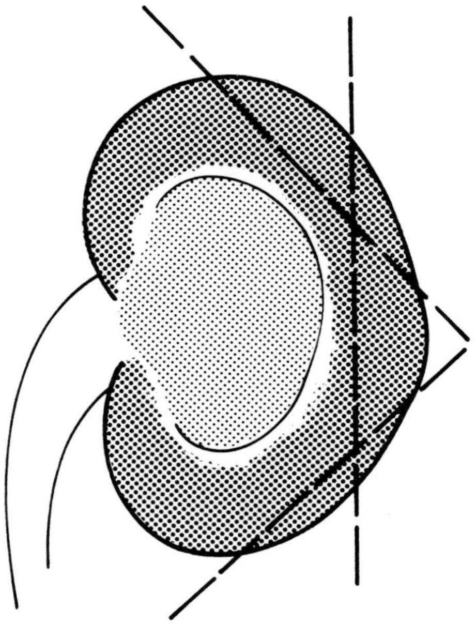

Fig. 6-1. Dotted lines indicate recommended paths for aspiration or needle biopsy of the kidney.

Aspiration biopsies may be performed in the conscious cat or under light sedation; use of a local anesthetic is optional. The area over the left kidney is clipped free of hair and surgically prepared. A 22-gauge, 2-inch spinal needle is attached to a 12 or 20 ml syringe. The kidney is held against the body wall and immobilized with one hand. The needle is inserted through the skin into the kidney. The needle should be positioned along the long axis of the kidney, on the abaxial surface from the renal vessels (Fig. 6-1). Suction is applied with the plunger of the syringe for a few seconds, released, and the needle withdrawn. The syringe is detached from the needle, filled with air, reattached, and the contents of the needle forced out.[2] Larger pieces of tissue may be fixed in formalin for histopathology or may be cultured; smaller pieces of tissue or fluid can be smeared on slides for cytologic evaluation. Aspiration biopsies are most useful in establishing a diagnosis of lymphosarcoma and less helpful when renal morphology must be evaluated.

Needle biopsies are performed in much the same way as aspiration biopsies. Several types of biopsy needles are available, including the Vim-Silverman and the Tru-Cut. The latter has the advantages of being relatively inexpensive and easy to use. General anesthesia with an ultra-short-acting barbiturate or halothane is recommended. The biopsy site is surgically prepared. A stab incision is made through the skin, and the biopsy needle is positioned against the kidney so that the thrust will follow the same line as that described for aspiration biopsies. The needle is thrust into the kidney, the biopsy is taken, and the needle and specimen are removed. The tissue obtained can be cultured or fixed for histopathologic study. Digital pressure is applied to the kidney at the point of penetration for 5 minutes to control hemorrhage. Up to three biopsy specimens can be taken from one kidney. The skin incision may be sutured if desired. The color of the mucous membranes, capillary refill time, and hematocrit should be monitored for 12 hours following the procedure. Microscopic or macroscopic hematuria has been reported during the 48-hour period after biopsy in up to 50 percent of dogs in one study[66] and up to 73 percent of cats in another.[67] However, the high incidence of hematuria in the second study may have been due to the method of collecting urine, since even the control cats had hematuria. The same study reported severe thrombosis, infarction, and fibrosis in the kidneys of 7 of 11 cats subjected to a single percutaneous needle renal biopsy. The lesions were more severe in kidneys in which the biopsy track passed through the corticomedullary junction. While these cats remained clinically normal for several months following the biopsy, such lesions could be detrimental in cats already suffering from renal insufficiency. Correct placement of the biopsy needle should minimize this complication.

THERAPY OF RENAL FAILURE

Therapy of renal failure will vary with the cause, duration of disease, and clinical status of the patient. Specific therapy should be directed at eliminating the cause of renal disease, if known. General therapeutic measures are intended to alleviate signs of uremia, improve renal function, and slow the progression of renal failure. Few studies have been conducted to determine the efficacy of such therapy in cats with renal failure; most of the following recommendations have been extrapolated from canine or human studies.

Specific Therapy

Amyloidosis. There is no form of therapy to date that has documented efficacy in the treatment of amyloidosis. Several drugs may have some benefit, but controlled studies are lacking.

Dimethyl sulfoxide (DMSO) has been shown to cause dissolution in vitro of amyloid fibrils formed from light chains. Results of in vivo studies and clinical trials in mice, hamsters, ducks, dogs, and humans had conflicting results,[31,68,69] and further studies are needed to determine its efficacy. Oral administration of DMSO may cause nausea and halitosis; this in turn may produce anorexia and decreased water consumption in animals. The use of intravenous DMSO in cats may cause hemolysis and hemoglobinuria.[31] Colchicine has also been used to treat amyloidosis in certain patients. It apparently prevents the formation of amyloid, rather than causing dissolution of existing deposits.[54] Clinical veterinary trials have not been performed. The use of both DMSO and colchicine must still be regarded as experimental.

Corticosteroid administration will accelerate amyloid deposition, and its use in cats with amyloidosis is to be discouraged.[32]

Glomerulonephritis. A number of therapeutic regimens for different types of glomerulonephritis are currently used in humans; however, no uniformly efficacious drugs have been described in veterinary medicine. Elimination of the antigen involved in immune complex formation would be the ideal therapy, but this is not possible in cats with FeLV infections. Immunosuppressive drugs used in humans to decrease antibody formation (corticosteroids, azathioprine, cyclophosphamide, chlorambucil) may be contraindicated in a cat already immunosuppressed by FeLV. The use of corticosteroids in an azotemic animal frequently causes a decline in the clinical condition, probably as a result of the catabolic effects of the drug. The decision to use immunosuppressive therapy in a cat with glomerulonephritis must be made on an individual basis. Spontaneous remissions have been reported in animals.[36]

Pyelonephritis. Pyelonephritis is treated with long-term antibiotic therapy, based on bacterial culture and sensitivity of urine or tissue from a renal biopsy. When possible, antibiotics that reach high concentrations in the renal parenchyma or urine should be used, and those that are nephrotoxic should be avoided. Antibiotic therapy should be continued for a minimum of 30 days. Urine cultures should be repeated at 30- to 60-day intervals after termination of antibiotic therapy, until three consecutive negative cultures are obtained. A positive culture during follow-up indicates the need for another 30- to 60-day course of antibiotics. Some cats have persistent reinfections despite appropriate therapy. Chronic low-dose antibiotic therapy may be effective in controlling the infection in these cats (ampicillin, trimethoprim-sulfa, or nitrofurantoin; one third of the total daily dose given at bedtime). Such low-dose therapy should be instituted after a course of antibiotics and a negative urine culture; it should not be used in an attempt to clear an active infection.

No specific therapy is known for interstitial nephritis, polyarteritis nodosa, or feline infectious peritonitis at this time.

Neoplasia. Cats with renal lymphosarcoma have been successfully treated with chemotherapy; specific protocols are described in detail elsewhere.[70,71] Other renal tumors must be treated by surgical excision, which usually involves nephrectomy. No effective forms of chemotherapy have been described for renal tumors other than lymphosarcoma.

Hydronephrosis. Hydronephrosis is best treated by removing the cause of the obstruction to urine flow. The degree of resolution of renal failure will depend upon its duration and whether the obstruction can be removed. Every effort should be made to salvage residual renal tissue, as some renal function may return with even marked hydronephrosis. Experimentally, canine kidneys resumed some function after total ureteral ligation for up to 4 weeks.[2] Nephrectomy may be indicated if no renal tissue remains in the hydronephrotic kidney, although function in the contralateral kidney must also be impaired if renal failure exists. Little improvement in the cat's clinical condition can be expected in such instances.

Perirenal cysts do not necessarily require treatment. Surgical drainage and resection of the cyst should be performed if the size of the cyst is causing discomfort.[57]

Toxicities. Heavy metal toxicities are treated by the administration of chelating agents. Lead toxicity is treated with calcium EDTA (ethylenediaminetetraacetate) at a dose of 25 mg/kg body weight four times daily subcutaneously for 5 days.[72] Oral penicillamine is an alternative chelating agent. It is administered at a dose of 100 mg/kg body weight daily for 7 to 14 days.[72]

Ethylene glycol toxicity can be prevented if treated within 8 hours of ingestion of the chemical. An emetic should be given and gastric lavage performed. Administration of ethanol will block the enzymes necessary to convert ethylene glycol to oxalic acid; sodium bicarbonate will reverse the acidosis. The recommended treatment schedule is 5 ml of 20 percent ethanol and 6 ml of 5 percent sodium bicarbonate per kg body weight intraperitoneally every 6 hours for five treatments and then every 8 hours for four treatments.[73] Ethanol can alternatively be given intravenously. If clinical signs of renal failure are present, treatment is the same as for acute renal failure of any cause, although mortality in such cases approaches 100 percent.

Treatment for aminoglycoside nephrotoxicity is based upon the severity of renal dysfunction and clinical signs. Administration of the antibiotic should be stopped as soon as signs of renal damage occur, since the drug continues to accumulate in renal proximal tubular cells for several days after administration is stopped.[74]

General Therapy

Acute Renal Failure. Cats with acute renal failure may have profound fluid and electrolyte abnormalities associated with polyuria or oliguria, vomiting and diarrhea, and lack of water consumption. Fluid therapy remains the cornerstone of treatment for these cats. The cat should be weighed prior to therapy and at least twice daily thereafter to monitor hydration status. Fluids should be administered intravenously through a catheter inserted under sterile conditions. A polyionic fluid such as lactated Ringer's is satisfactory in most cases. Cats with oliguric renal failure may be hyperkalemic; 0.9 percent saline is the fluid of choice for such patients. Sodium bicarbonate can be added to the saline if acidosis is severe (serum bicarbonate concentration less than 12 mEq/L).

The volume of fluid administered should be carefully calculated and monitored. Initially, the volume necessary to rehydrate the cat is given over a 6-hour period. This is determined by estimating the percent dehydration and using the formula:

$$\text{Fluid volume necessary for rehydration} = \text{Percent dehydration} \times \text{body weight (kg)} \times 1000 \text{ ml}$$

The amount of urine produced during rehydration should not be used as an indication of oliguria, since little urine will be produced until hydration is restored.

After the cat is rehydrated, the amount of fluid to be administered is calculated based upon the normal daily requirement (60 ml/kg body weight) and an estimate of daily losses from abnormalities such as vomiting and diarrhea. Urine production should be monitored closely, ideally by an indwelling catheter attached to a closed collection system. However, because it is difficult to catheterize conscious cats, estimation of the amount of urine voided and frequent palpation of the urinary bladder to assess urine volume may be substituted. Urine specific gravity will probably not be helpful in determining the efficacy of fluid therapy since cats in acute renal failure usually have dilute urine.

The amount of fluid administered on a daily basis should be gradually increased as long as urine volume increases proportionately and overhydration (as evidenced by weight gain, pulmonary edema, or peripheral edema) does not occur. Intravenous fluid therapy should be continued until renal function improves and the cat is eating and drinking. Overhydration is a serious complication which is better prevented than treated. If the cat is not oliguric, temporarily suspending fluid administration may alleviate the problem. Diuretics such as furosemide (at a dose of 2 mg/kg body weight) can be given to promote urine flow.

Oliguria or anuria is the most serious complication of acute renal failure. If urine production remains low after rehydration, various measures should be taken to promote diuresis. Furosemide should be administered at a dose of 2 mg/kg. This dose can be doubled and then tripled at hourly intervals if urine volume fails to increase.

Osmotic diuresis may be tried if diuretics are ineffective; 20 percent mannitol (0.5 g/kg body weight) or dextrose (25 to 65 ml/kg body weight) is administered intravenously at the rate of 2 ml/min for 10 to 15 minutes. Urine production will increase to 1 to 4 ml/min if osmotic diuresis is effective. The remainder of the osmotic solution is infused more slowly. Lactated Ringer's solution at a dose of 30 to 60 ml/kg body weight should be alternated with the osmotic solution to prevent dehydration. Osmotic diuresis can be administered as long as necessary to maintain urine flow.[75]

Vasodilators can be extremely effective in increasing urine production by decreasing glomerular afferent arteriolar constriction. Dopamine is diluted in 5 percent dextrose solution and administered at the rate of 2 to 5 μg/kg/min.[76] A prompt diuresis will be noted if the drug is going to be effective. Electrocardiographic monitoring is desirable since dopamine is arrhythmogenic, especially at higher dose rates. The infusion can be continued as long as necessary to maintain urine flow.

In the event that none of the above measures result in diuresis, peritoneal or hemodialysis will be necessary. These procedures are described elsewhere.[77–79]

Occasionally, a cat may present in the polyuric phase of acute renal failure. Parenteral fluid administration may not be required in these cats if they are drinking sufficient quantities of water. Serum electrolytes should be monitored at 48-hour intervals, as hyponatremia and hypokalemia can occur. Some cats will drink polyionic fluids such as lactated Ringer's solution, which is beneficial in maintaining normal serum electrolyte levels.

The duration of acute renal failure depends upon the type and degree of insult to the kidneys. Improvement in renal function is frequently not evident for 7 to 10 days. Intensive therapy and monitoring should not be discontinued before this time, on the assumption that irreversible renal damage has occurred.

Chronic Renal Failure. Therapy for chronic renal failure is based on alleviating the abnormalities in fluid, electrolyte, endocrine, and acid-base status. Although renal lesions cannot be eliminated, residual renal function can be maximized, and the progression of renal failure may be slowed. Cats with renal insufficiency have lived as long as 3 years with careful management.[80]

Water should always be available to cats with chronic renal failure. The polyuria of chronic renal failure will result in a compensatory increase in water intake. Some cats become very choosy about the source and freshness of their drinking water. Owners should be made aware of this and encouraged to modify the cat's water supply accordingly.

Stress may precipitate a uremic crisis by straining the compensatory mechanisms already in use by the kidneys and the body as a whole. Stressful events include high environmental temperatures, travel, change of residence, introduction of a new pet, and hospitalization. Treatment for cats with chronic renal failure should be administered on an outpatient basis when at all possible, and hospital stays should be kept to a minimum.

Dietary Therapy. The efficacy of dietary therapy in alleviating the signs of chronic renal failure in cats has not been proven. The following discussion is based on data from dogs and humans and on clinical experience.

Reduced levels of dietary protein have been recommended in patients with chronic renal failure. Many protein catabolites are felt to contribute to the signs of uremia. Urea nitrogen is not felt to be a significant uremic toxin; however, its concentration in the blood or serum is an indication of levels of other unmeasured substances. A reduction in BUN concentration is generally associated with an increase in well-being.

Recent studies[17,81–83] have associated restricted protein diets to stabilization of renal function or at least slowing of the progression of renal failure. The mechanism responsible for this effect remains obscure. In one study, rats were subjected to a five-sixths nephrectomy to induce renal failure. Rats fed normal or increased dietary levels of phosphate had mineralization, mononuclear cell infiltration, and fibrosis in residual renal tissue and showed deterioration of renal function with time. The rats fed a phosphate-restricted diet showed no such changes.[17] It was suggested that the hyperphosphatemia and secondary hyperparathyroidism associated with chronic renal failure might be responsible for these changes. Similar findings were observed in cats subjected to a three-fourths reduction of renal mass.[84] Since most of dietary phosphate is associated with protein, such a theory would be consistent with the beneficial effects of a low-protein diet.

The role of phosphate in the progression of renal failure is not yet clearly defined, however. More recent studies have produced conflicting data. Several trials have been conducted in dogs with experimental renal failure; none have shown histologic or function deterioration in dogs ingesting phosphate levels comparable to those in normal foods.[81,85–87] Severe phosphate restriction can have detrimental effects, including anorexia and rickets.[85]

A theory of glomerular hyperfiltration has also been proposed to explain the benefits of feeding a low-protein diet. Protein ingestion causes increases in both GFR and renal blood flow, changes which are probably mediated by a circulating hormone (possibly glucagon).[81,88] Single-nephron GFR (SNGFR) varies with the amount of protein ingested. In animals with experimental chronic renal failure, high protein diets cause SNGFR to rise above normal (hyperfiltration). It is hypothesized that this hyperfiltration causes glomerular damage and eventually glomerulosclerosis by an as yet unidentified mechanism.[88] Further studies are needed to prove or disprove this theory.

Regardless of the mechanism, reduced levels of dietary protein appear to be indicated in cats with chronic renal failure. The exact amount of protein to feed is still a matter of conjecture, since no clinical trials have been performed in cats. Normal cats have a higher protein requirement than dogs—29 percent of the diet for kittens versus 12 percent for puppies; 19 percent for adult cats versus 4 percent for adult dogs.[89] This requirement appears to be due to a higher requirement for certain essential amino acids but also to a lower efficiency of use.[90] It would seem logical that recommended levels for cats in chronic renal failure would be proportionately greater than dogs. A level of 3.3 to 3.8 g of protein per kg body weight per day has been suggested.[4,89] One commercial diet (Feline K/D) provides this level of protein. Homemade diets may also be formulated. It should be remembered that cats require taurine as an essential amino acid, and that it is found solely in animal sources of protein. The daily caloric requirement for normal cats is 70 to 80 kcal/kg body weight. Since no studies have been performed to determine the caloric requirements of uremic cats, the same amount of calories is recommended for these patients.

Cats have the ability to metabolize high levels of dietary fat and, in fact, prefer to eat and do better on high fat diets.[4,89] The level of dietary fat can range from 15 to 40 percent. This is advantageous when formulating a low-protein diet with sufficient calories to fulfill the cat's requirements. Cats must ingest both arachidonic and linoleic acids as essential fatty acids. Linoleic acid is found in fats from both animal and plant sources; arachidonic acid, however, is found only in animal sources.[4,89]

Vitamin requirements of cats in renal failure have not been determined. The obligatory polyuria of chronic renal failure may "wash out" the water-soluble vitamins (B and C), resulting in an increased requirement. Vitamin B and C supplements are recommended, especially since excess amounts do not appear to be harmful. Vitamin A must be ingested by cats since they are unable to convert β-carotene (from plant sources). Excessive vitamin A supplementation should be avoided, since hypervitaminosis A may increase parathormone secretion.[4,89]

Vitamin D levels in animals with chronic renal failure are subnormal. Vitamin D supplementation must be done cautiously and with close monitoring of serum calcium levels. If hyperphosphatemia is not controlled prior to supplementation, the increase in calcium absorption can lead to mineralization of various soft tissues, including the kidney. High levels of vitamin D may lead to frank hypercalcemia, which will cause further renal damage. A number of formulations of vitamin D with varying potencies and durations of action are commercially available. Discussion of these formulations and indications have been reviewed elsewhere.[91]

Anemia. Although the anemia of chronic renal failure is multifactorial, only a limited number of therapeutic measures are available. Cats with a hematocrit above 25 percent generally do not require therapy. Those with hematocrits in the range of 15 to 25 percent may benefit from administration of anabolic steroids. Administration of erythropoietin would be the therapy of choice, but this hormone is not commercially available. Various anabolic steroids are available, including nandrolone (Deca-Durabolin), oxymethalone, testosterone, and stanazolol (Winstrol-V). No studies have been done in cats to determine the relative efficacy of each of these drugs. Very anemic cats (hematocrit less than 15 percent) may require a blood transfusion.

Vomiting. Administration of histamine H_2-receptor antagonists may help to decrease the vomiting associated with hypergastrinemia and gastric hyperacidity.[20] Cimetidine (Tagamet) is administered at a dose of 4 mg/kg body weight every 6 hours orally, intramuscularly or intravenously. There appears to be a rebound effect on gastric acid secretion if the dose interval is too long or if the drug is withdrawn abruptly. Cimetidine can be obtained as an oral liquid which enables accurate dosing; it unfortunately has a bitter taste.

Ranitidine (Zantac) is another H_2-receptor antagonist which has the advantage of requiring only twice-daily dosage. A dose of 2.2 mg/kg body weight every 12 hours has been used in cats without side effects. Accurate dosage can be difficult, since the drug is supplied only as 150 mg tablets.

Hypertension. There are no clinical studies in cats or dogs to document whether antihypertensive therapy is beneficial in slowing the progression of renal failure, and indeed, there are few reports on methods of controlling hypertension. Antihypertensive measures have been extrapolated from those used in human medicine.

Dietary sodium restriction should be the initial form of therapy. Feline K/D (Hill's) is a sodium-restricted diet. Although the diseased kidney is able to excrete sodium normally, it is not able to make rapid adjustments to changes in sodium load. Rapid institution of a low-sodium diet could theoretically lead to volume depletion, as water is excreted with sodium. Changes in dietary intake of sodium should therefore be done gradually. Mild diuretics such as the thiazides may be tried; more potent drugs such as furosemide (Lasix) may be required. Furosemide administration may lead to dehydration and worsening of azotemia because of its profound diuretic effect.

If the above measures are not successful, sympatholytic drugs may be tried. Propanolol is the drug of choice in this category and should be given at a dose of 2.5 to 5 mg two to three times daily.

Vasodilators constitute the last group of antihypertensive drugs. Hydralazine (Apresoline) at a dose of 2.5 mg three times daily or prazosin (Minipress) at a dose of 0.25 mg twice daily can be used. Overdosage of these drugs may result in weakness or collapse.

Hyperphosphatemia. The control of hyperphosphatemia began to receive attention when it appeared to be a major contributing factor to the progression of renal failure.[17] Although this theory is now being questioned, lowering serum phosphate levels to alleviate secondary hyperparathyroidism may decrease some of the signs of uremia.

Dietary protein restriction is the most important factor in reducing serum phosphate levels. Oral phosphate-binding gels may be used in conjunction with a low-protein diet. These gels bind phosphorus from ingested food in the gut to prevent absorption; they do not remove phosphorus from the body. Phosphate-binding gels usually contain aluminum hydroxide, are produced under a variety of trade names (AlternaGEL, Basaljel, Amphojel), and are marketed as antacids. Magnesium-containing formulations should be avoided, since magnesium cannot be excreted normally during renal failure. Both liquid and tablet formulations are available. The tablets are a chewable formulation; this may explain why they seem to be somewhat less effective than the liquid. The large size of the tablet makes administration difficult, although they can be divided.

The dose of phosphate-binding gels is empiric; suggested initial dose is 30 to 90 mg/kg body weight daily. Since the gel binds only the phosphate in ingested food, it must be given at the same time that the cat is fed. The serum phosphate concentration should be monitored periodically and the dose of the gel adjusted to maintain the concentration at 4 to 6 mg/dl. Blood for serum phosphate analysis should be taken after a 12-hour fast, since the serum phosphate concentration normally rises postprandially. Hemolysis will also artificially elevate serum phosphate levels.

Unfortunately, many cats object to the taste of phosphate-binding gels and may refuse to eat if they associate administration of the gel with food. Administration of phosphate-binding gels should be attempted only after the cat is well adjusted to the low protein diet.

Acidosis. Sodium bicarbonate is administered orally to correct metabolic acidosis. It is impossible to predict the onset or degree of acidosis from clinical signs or degree of renal dysfunction. Serum bicarbonate levels should be determined by arterial or venous blood gas measurement or measurement of the total serum carbon dioxide concentration. Alkalinizing therapy should be instituted when serum bicarbonate levels fall below 16 mEq/L. Sodium bicarbonate supplementation is started at a dose of 15 grains/day. The serum bicarbonate concentration should be monitored periodically and bicarbonate administration adjusted to maintain a concentration of 20 to 24 mEq/L. Large quantities of sodium bicarbonate may aggravate hypertension by increasing the sodium load.

Uremia. Signs of uremia will appear when compensatory mechanisms are exhausted. Conservative medical management will fail to be effective at this point, and fluid therapy should be instituted (refer to discussion of therapy for acute renal failure). Fluid therapy may be successful in improving renal function if there was a significant prerenal component to the uremia. If renal function does not improve after 48 to 72 hours or if clinical signs persist, the cat may be in terminal renal failure. Euthanasia is indicated, since neither long-term dialysis or renal transplantation are feasible in cats at this time.

REFERENCES

1. Low DG: Cats aren't small dogs. Carnation Research Digest 17:1, 1981
2. Finco DR, Barsanti JA, Crowell WA: The Urinary System. p. 3102. In Pratt PW (ed): Feline Medicine. 1st Ed. American Veterinary Publications, Santa Barbara, CA, 1983
3. Finco DR: Clinical evaluation of renal function. p. 95. In Marthens EV (ed): Seventh Annual Kal Kan Symposium for the Treatment of Small Animal Diseases Proceedings. Kal Kan Food Inc, Vernon, CA, 1984
4. Osborne CA, Polzin DS, Abdullahi S, et al: Role of diet in management of feline chronic polyuric renal failure: Current status. J Am Anim Hosp Assoc 18:11, 1982
5. Osborne CA, Finco DR, Low DG: Pathophysiology of renal disease, renal failure, and uremia. p. 1733. In Ettinger SJ (ed): Textbook of Veterinary Internal Medicine. 2nd Ed. WB Saunders, Philadelphia, 1983
6. Cowgill LD: Diseases of the kidney. p. 1793. In Ettinger SJ (ed): Textbook of Veterinary Internal Medicine. 2nd Ed. WB Saunders, Philadephia, 1983
7. Levinsky NG, Alexander EA, Venkatachalam MA: Acute renal failure. p. 1181. In Brenner BM, Rector FC (eds): The Kidney. 2nd Ed. WB Saunders, Philadelphia, 1981
8. Leaf A, Cotran RS: Renal Pathophysiology. 2nd Ed. Oxford University Press, New York, 1980
9. Knochel JP, Seldin DW: The pathophysiology of uremia. p. 2137. In Brenner BM, Rector FC (eds): The Kidney. 2nd Ed. WB Saunders, Philadelphia, 1981
10. Anagnostou A, Fried W, Kurtzman NA: Hematologic consequences of renal failure. p. 2184. In Brenner BM, Rector FC (eds): The Kidney. 2nd Ed. WB Saunders, Philadelphia, 1981
11. Fried W: Hematologic abnormalities in chronic renal failure. Semin Nephrol 1:176, 1981
12. Coburn JW, Slatopolsky E: Vitamin D, parathyroid hormone, and renal osteodystrophy. p. 2213. In Brenner BM, Rector FC (eds): The Kidney. 2nd Ed. WB Saunders, Philadelphia, 1981
13. Slatopolsky E, Caglar S, Pennell JP, et al: On the pathogenesis of hyperparathyroidism in chronic experimental renal insufficiency in the dog. J Clin Invest 50:492, 1971
14. Massry SG, Coburn JW: Divalent ion metabolism and renal osteodystrophy. p. 304. In Massry SG, Sellers AL (eds): Clinical Aspects of Uremia and Dialysis. Charles C Thomas, Springfield, IL, 1976
15. Massry SG: Is parathyroid hormone a uremic toxin? Nephron 19:125, 1977
16. Arieff AI: Neurologic complications of uremia. p. 2306. In Brenner BM, Rector FC (eds): The Kidney. 2nd Ed. WB Saunders, Philadelphia, 1981
17. Ibels LS, Alfrey AC, Haut L, et al: Preservation of function in experimental renal disease by dietary restriction of phosphate. N Engl J Med 298:122, 1978
18. Ross LA, Finco DR: Relationship of selected clinical renal function tests to glomerular filtration rate and renal blood flow in cats. Am J Vet Res 42:1704, 1981

19. Emmanouel DS, Lindheimer MD, Katz AI: Endocrine abnormalities in chronic renal failure: Pathogenetic principles and clinical implications. Semin Nephrol 1:151, 1981
20. Thornhill JA: Control of vomiting in the uremic patient. p. 1022. In Kirk RW (ed): Current Veterinary Therapy VIII. WB Saunders, Philadelphia, 1983
21. Zelnick EB, Goyal RK: Gastrointestinal manifestations of chronic renal failure. Semin Nephrol 1:124, 1981
22. Cowgill LD, Kallet AJ: Recognition and management of hypertension in the dog. p. 1025. In Kirk RW (ed): Current Veterinary Therapy VIII. WB Saunders, Philadelphia, 1983
23. Greene RW, Scott RC: Diseases of the bladder and urethra. p. 1890. In Ettinger SJ (ed): Textbook of Veterinary Internal Medicine. 2nd Ed. WB Saunders, Philadelphia, 1983
24. Osborne CA (ed): Disorders of the feline lower urinary tract. Vet Clin North Am [Small Anim Pract] 14:407, 1984
25. Johnson CA: Renal ectopia in a cat: A case report and literature review. J Am Anim Hosp Assoc 15:599, 1979
26. North DC: Hydronephrosis and hydro-ureter in a kitten—A case report. J Small Anim Pract 19:237, 1978
27. Northington JW, Julians MM: Polycystic kidney disease in a cat. J Small Anim Prac 18:663, 1977
28. Crowell WA, Hubbell JJ, Riley JC: Polycystic renal disease in related cats. J. Am Vet Med Assoc 175:286, 1979
29. Chew DJ, DiBartola SP, Boyce JT, et al: Renal amyloidosis in related Abyssinian cats. J Am Vet Med Assoc 181:139, 1982
30. DiBartola SP, Stephen P: Familial nephropathy in the Doberman Pinscher dog and familial renal amyloidosis in the Abyssinian cat. p. 35. In Marthens EV (ed): Seventh Annual Kal Kan Symposium for the Treatment of Small Animal Diseases Proceedings. Kal Kan Foods Inc, Vernon, CA, 1983
31. DiBartola SP, Stephen P: The diagnosis and management of renal amyloidosis in the dog and cat. p. 87. In Marthens EV (ed): Kal Kan Symposium for the Treatment of Small Animal Diseases Proceedings. Kal Kan Foods Inc, Vernon, CA, 1983
32. Chew DJ, DiBartola SP: Feline renal amyloidosis. p. 976. In Kirk RW (ed): Current Veterinary Therapy VIII. WB Saunders, Philadelphia, 1983
33. Slauson DO, Lewis RM: Comparative pathology of glomerulonephritis in animals. Vet Pathol 16:135, 1979
34. Hamilton JM: Nephritis in the cat. J Small Anim Pract 7:445, 1966
35. Lucke VM: Renal disease in the domestic cat. J Pathol 95:67, 1968
36. Osborne CA, Hammer RF, Stevens JB, et al: Immunologic aspects of glomerular disease in the dog and cat. p. 15. In the Newer Knowledge About Dogs, 26th Gaines Veterinary Symposium. Gaines Dog Research Center, White Plains, NY, 1976
37. Osborne CA, Vernier RL: Glomerulonephritis in the dog and cat. A comparative review. J Am Anim Hosp Assoc 9:101, 1973
38. August JR, Leib MS: Primary renal diseases of the cat. Vet Clin North Am [Small Anim Pract] 14:1247, 1984
39. Francis DP, Essex M, Jakowski RM, et al: Increased risk for lymphoma and glomerulonephritis in a closed population of cats exposed to feline leukemia virus. Am J Epidemiol III:337, 1980
40. Glick AD, Horn RG, Holscher M: Characterization of feline glomerulonephritis associated with viral-induced hematopoietic neoplasms. Am J Pathol 92:321, 1978

41. Thornburg LP, Kinden D, Digilio K: Immune glomerulitis in a cat. Vet Pathol 16:604, 1979
42. Nash AS, Wright NG: Membranous nephropathy in sibling cats. Vet Rec 113:180, 1983
43. Crowell WA, Barsanti JA: Membranous glomerulopathy in two feline siblings. J Am Vet Med Assoc 182:1244, 1983
44. Johnson ME, DiBartola SP, Gelberg HB: Nephrotic syndrome and pericholangiohepatitis in a cat. J Am Anim Hosp Assoc 19:191, 1983
45. Wright NG, Minto AW, Nash AS: Necrotizing glomerulopathy in cats euthanased with ketamine hydrochloride and sodium pentobarbitone. Vet Rec 111:127, 1982
46. Scott RC: Feline urologic diseases. Vet Clin North Am 6:479, 1976
47. Kelly DF, Lucke VM, McCullagh KG: Experimental pyelonephritis in the cat. 1. Gross and histologic changes. J Comp Pathol 89:125, 1979
48. Kelly DF, Lucke VM, McCullagh KG: Experimental pyelonephritis in the cat. 2. Ultrastructural observations. J Comp Pathol 89:563, 1979
49. McCullagh KG, Bishop KA, Lucke VM, et al: Experimental pyelonephritis in the cat. 3. Collagen alterations in renal fibrosis. J Comp Pathol 93:9, 1983
50. Lees GE, Osborne CA, Stevens JB: Antibacterial properties of urine: Studies of feline urine specific gravity, osmolality, and pH. J Am Anim Hosp Assoc 15:135, 1979
51. Lees GE, Osborne CA: Feline urinary tract infections. p. 1058. In Kirk RW (ed): Current Veterinary Therapy VIII. WB Saunders, Philadelphia, 1983
52. Lucke VM: Renal polyarteritis nodosa in the cat. Vet Rec 1:622, 1968
53. Altera KP, Bonasch H: Periarteritis nodosa in a cat. J Am Vet Med Assoc 149:1307, 1966
54. Pederson NC: Feline coronavirus infections. p. 514. In Greene CE (ed): Clinical Microbiology and Infectious Diseases of the Dog and Cat. WB Saunders, Philadelphia, 1984
55. Cotter SM: Feline viral neoplasia. p. 490. In Greene CE (ed): Clinical Microbiology and Infectious Diseases of the Dog and Cat. WB Saunders, Philadelphia, 1984
56. Caywood DD, Osborne CA, Johnston GR: Neoplasms of the canine and feline urinary tract. p. 1203. In Kirk RW (ed): Current Veterinary Therapy VII. WB Saunders, Philadelphia, 1980
57. Brace JJ: Perirenal cysts (pseudocysts) in the cat. p. 980. In Kirk RW (ed): Current Veterinary Therapy VIII. WB Saunders, Philadelphia, 1983
58. Swanson RE, Hakim AA: Stop-flow analysis of creatinine excretion in the dog. Am J Physiol 203:980, 1962
59. Finco DR, Barsanti JA: Mechanisms of urinary excretion of creatinine by the cat. Am J Vet Res 43:2207, 1982
60. Finco DR: Kidney function. p. 338. In Kaneko JJ (ed): Clinical Biochemistry of Domestic Animals. Academic Press, New York, 1980
61. Finco DR, Coulter DB, Barsanti JA: Simple, accurate method for clinical estimation of glomerular filtration rate in the dog. Am J Vet Res 42:1874, 1981
62. Osborne CA, Polzin DJ: Azotemia: A review of what's old and what's new. Part II. Localization. Compend Cont Ed Prac Vet 5:561, 1983
63. Lage AL: Neonatal clinical nephrology. p. 1085. In Kirk RW (ed): Current Veterinary Therapy VII. WB Saunders, Philadelphia, 1980
64. Coles EH: Veterinary Clinical Pathology. WB Saunders, Philadelphia, 1980
65. Osborne CA, Low DG, Finco DR: Canine and Feline Urology. WB Saunders, Philadelphia, 1972

66. Osborne CA: Clinical evaluation of needle biopsy of the kidney and its complications in the dog and cat. J Am Vet Med Assoc 158:1213, 1971
67. Nash AS, Boyd JS, Minto AW, et al: Renal biopsy in the normal cat: An examination of the effects of a single needle biopsy. Res Vet Sci 34:347, 1983
68. Ravid M, Shapira J, Lang R, et al: Prolonged dimethylsulphoxide treatment in 13 patients with systemic amyloidosis. Ann Rheum Dis 41:587, 1982
69. van Rijswijk MH, Marrink J, Ockhuizen T, et al: Successful treatment with dimethylsulfoxide of human amyloidosis secondary to rheumatoid arthritis. p. 570. In Glenner GG, Costas PP, Freitas F (eds): Amyloid and Amyloidosis. Excerpta Medica, Amsterdam, 1980
70. Cotter SM: Treatment of lymphoma and leukemia with cyclophosphamide, vincristine, and prednisone: II. Treatment of Cats. J Am Anim Hosp Assoc 19:166, 1983
71. Theilen GH, Madewell BR: Leukemia-sarcoma disease complex. p. 208. In Theilen GH, Madewell BR (eds): Veterinary Cancer Medicine. Lea & Febiger, Philadelphia, 1979
72. Kowalczyk DF: Lead poisoning. p. 107. In Kirk RW (ed): Current Veterinary Therapy VIII. WB Saunders, Philadelphia, 1983
73. Oehme FW: Ethylene glycol (antifreeze) poisoning. p. 114. In Kirk RW (ed): Current Veterinary Therapy VIII. WB Saunders, Philadelphia, 1983
74. Spangler WL, Adelman RD, Conzelman GM, Jr, et al: Gentamicin nephrotoxicity in the dog: Sequential light and electron microscopy. Vet Pathol 17:206, 1980
75. Finco DR, Low DG: Intensive diuresis in polyuric renal failure. p. 1091. In Kirk RW (ed): Current Veterinary Therapy VII. WB Saunders, Philadelphia, 1980
76. Parker HR: Evaluation and management of acute renal failure in the emergency patient. p. 202. In Salter F, Knowles R, Whittich W (eds): Veterinary Critical Care. Lea & Febiger, Philadelphia, 1981
77. Thornhill JA: Continuous ambulatory peritoneal dialysis. p. 1028. In Kirk RW (ed): Current Veterinary Therapy VIII. WB Saunders, Philadelphia, 1983
78. Parker HR: Current status of peritoneal dialysis. p. 1106. In Kirk RW (ed): Current Veterinary Therapy VII. WB Saunders, Philadelphia, 1980
79. Cowgill LD: Current status of veterinary hemodialysis. p. 1111. In Kirk RW (ed): Current Veterinary Therapy VII. WB Saunders, Philadelphia, 1980
80. Barsanti JA, Gitter ML, Crowell WA: Long-term management of chronic renal failure in a cat. Feline Pract 11:10, 1981
81. Finco DR: Progression of renal failure. p. 139. Proc 2nd Annual Forum ACVIM, Washington, DC, 1984
82. Adler SG, Kopple JD: Factors influencing the progression of renal insufficiency. Semin Nephrol 3:335, 1983
83. Maschio G, Oldrizzi L, Lessitore N, et al: Effects of dietary protein and phosphorus restriction on the progression of early renal failure. Kidney Int 22:371, 1982
84. Ross LA, Finco DR, Crowell WA: Effect of dietary phosphorus restriction on the kidneys of cats with reduced renal mass. Am J Vet Res 43:1023, 1982
85. Polzin DJ, Osborne CA, Leininger JR: The influence of diet on the progression of canine renal failure. Compend Cont Ed Pract Vet 6:1123, 1984
86. Bovee KE, Kronfeld DS, Ramberg C, et al: Long-term measurement of renal function in partially nephrectomized dogs fed 56, 27 or 19% protein. Invest Urol 16:378, 1979
87. Polzin DJ, Osborne CA, Hayden DW, et al: Influence of modified protein diets on morbidity, mortality, and renal function in dogs with induced chronic renal failure. Am J Vet Res 45:506, 1984

88. Brenner BW, Meyer TW, Hostetter TH: Dietary protein intake and the progressive nature of kidney disease: The role of hemodynamically mediated glomerular injury in aging, renal ablation, and intrinsic renal disease. N Engl J Med 307:652, 1982
89. Osborne CA, Polzin DJ: Conservative medical management of feline chronic polyuric renal failure. p. 1008. In Kirk RW (ed): Current Veterinary Therapy VIII. WB Saunders, Philadelphia, 1983
90. Rogers QR, Morris JG, Freedland RA: Lack of hepatic enzyme adaptation to low and high levels of dietary protein in the adult cat. Enzyme 22:348, 1977
91. Peterson ME: Treatment of canine and feline hypoparathyroidism. J Am Vet Med Assoc 181:1434, 1982

7 Familial Renal Disease in the Dog and Cat

Deborah J. Davenport
Stephen P. DiBartola
Dennis J. Chew

A congenital renal disease is one that is present at birth (e.g., unilateral renal aplasia). Congenital defects may be genetically determined or may result from exposure to adverse environmental factors during development. The term *familial* refers to disorders that occur in related individuals with a higher frequency than would be expected by chance. In many of the familial renal diseases of dogs, the kidney is presumably normal at birth, with progressive structural and functional deterioration developing during the first few years of life.

During the 25 year period following the original description of renal cortical hypoplasia in cocker spaniel dogs, familial renal diseases have been observed in many other breeds of dogs. Familial renal disease is rare in the cat, with the exception of familial amyloidosis in Abyssinian cats. The modes of inheritance and pathogenesis for many of these diseases are unknown, but the associated clinical and pathologic features have been well documented. (The signalment of dogs and cats with familial renal disease can be found in Table 7-1.) The diseases discussed here are presented in the chronologic order in which they were recognized and described in the veterinary literature.

COCKER SPANIEL[1,2,3]

The first canine familial renal disease was recognized in cocker spaniels by Krook in 1957.[1] Renal cortical hypoplasia was described in 40 young cocker spaniels of both sexes. The age at diagnosis ranged from 6 to 24 months, with

Table 7-1. Signalment of Dogs and Cats with Familial Renal Disease

Breed	Age at Presentation	Sex Predisposition
Cocker spaniel	0.5–2 yr	None
Beagle	Birth	None
Norwegian elkhound	1–5 yr	None
Lhaso apso/Shih Tzu	1–2 yr	None
Basenji	1–5 yr	None
Samoyed	Males—1 yr Females—5 yr	Males > females
Doberman pinscher	1–2 yr	None
Domestic long-haired cats	6 wk	None
Cairn terrier	6 wk	None
Abyssinian cats	1–5 yr	Females > males
Standard poodles	0.25–2 yr	Unknown
Pembroke Welsh corgi	5–13 yr	Unknown
Soft-coated wheaten terriers	0.5–3 yr	None

the majority of dogs being presented around 12 months of age. Animals of both popular coat colors, solid and particolored, were affected.

Affected dogs exhibit a variable course of progressive anorexia, vomiting, polyuria, polydipsia, weight loss, lethargy, pallor, and uremic halitosis. Affected animals may have systemic hypertension, ocular disease such as retinal detachment, and fibrous osteodystrophy suggestive of renal secondary hyperparathyroidism. Laboratory findings typical of dogs in renal failure include azotemia, hyperphosphatemia, and isosthenuria. Proteinuria is a consistent finding. Hypercalcemia and glucosuria are variable features.

Gross necropsy findings in affected cocker spaniels include systemic evidence of uremia, as well as small kidneys with pitted surfaces and adherent capsules. Histologically, the hallmark of the disease is bilateral renal cortical hypoplasia. Although this disease has not been studied during its early stages, the kidneys are presumably normal at birth, with progressive degeneration during the first few years of life. Thus, the term hypoplasia is probably a misnomer. Cystic glomerular atrophy and glomerular sclerosis are consistent findings. Marked tubular changes, including tubular dilatation, tubular atrophy, and mineralization of tubular basement membranes, are frequently present. There is minimal interstitial inflammation. Immunofluorescence studies to detect complement and immunoglobulins have been negative.

A presumptive diagnosis of this disease is based on the signalment and typical history and clinical findings. Renal biopsy is required for confirmation of the diagnosis. Familial renal disease in the cocker spaniel appears to be uniformly progressive and therapy is limited to supportive measures.

BEAGLE[4,5,6]

Unilateral renal agenesis has been described in colonies of beagles maintained for research. The reported incidence of this defect in the beagle ranges from 1:100 to 1:400. This high incidence of unilateral renal agenesis is suggestive of a familial disorder, but no heritability pattern has been established.

In affected dogs, the ureter, renal artery, and bladder trigone on the ipsilateral side, as well as the kidney, are all absent. The solitary kidney is often grossly hypertrophied. Histologically, there appears to be an increase in the number of nephrons rather than hypertrophy of individual nephrons. In female dogs, there is often dysgenesis of the uterine horn and ovarian duct on the affected side. However, the gonads and adrenal glands in both sexes are normal. Polycystic renal disease has also been reported in a small group of beagles with solitary kidneys.

NORWEGIAN ELKHOUND[7,8,9]

A familial nephropathy has been observed in Norwegian elkhounds ranging from 8 months to 5 years of age and affecting both sexes. Based on common ancestry among spontaneously affected dogs and the results of breeding trials, a genetic basis for the disease is suspected, but the mode of inheritance has not been conclusively determined.

There is usually a history of anorexia, depression, weight loss, polydipsia, polyuria, and vomiting. Affected dogs often display stunted growth, signs of fibrous osteodystrophy, dehydration, and oral ulceration on physical examination. Systemic hypertension has not been reported. Laboratory findings include isosthenuria, azotemia, hyperphosphatemia, nonregenerative anemia, and variable serum calcium values. Proteinuria and glucosuria are variable. Severe metabolic acidosis is a frequent finding in dogs with terminal disease.

Breeding trials have established that familial nephropathy of Norwegian elkhounds is a progressive disease that varies in the severity and rate of progression. Periglomerular fibrosis, an early histopathologic lesion, may be detected in some dogs before the development of azotemia. The number and size of nephrons are normal at this stage. Pathologic findings in dogs with more advanced disease consist of generalized interstitial fibrosis with glomerular sclerosis and atrophy. Renal vascular lesions are not apparent. Tubular changes are mild except in extremely severe cases, in which tubular atrophy, saccular dilation of the distal tubule and collecting duct, and basement membrane mineralization are noted. Minimal inflammatory changes consisting of interstitial mononuclear infiltration are recognized only in dogs with advanced disease. Immunopathologic studies have been negative.

Unfortunately, early diagnosis of this disease by means other than renal biopsy is not reliable. Percutaneous renal biopsy at 3 to 14 months of age is usually diagnostic.

LHASA APSO AND SHIH TZU[10,11,12]

The widespread occurrence of a progressive, chronic, renal disease in the Lhaso apso and Shih Tzu breeds has been recognized since 1972. This syndrome is the most common renal disease of these breeds, and its high prevalence suggests a familial etiology. Studies of the mechanism of inheritance have not been completed, but the trait does not appear to be inherited in a simple autosomal recessive pattern.

Affected dogs of both sexes are usually presented at a young age (often 1 to 2 years) with a history of progressive weight loss or stunted growth, vomiting, diarrhea, polydipsia, and polyuria. There is marked variability in the severity of clinical signs and rate of progression of disease among affected dogs. Some animals develop renal failure before 6 months of age, whereas others remain clinically normal for many years prior to the development of renal failure. Pathologic fractures and fibrous osteodystrophy due to renal secondary hyperparathyroidism may occur. Systemic hypertension may also be present. Laboratory findings include nonregenerative anemia, azotemia, hyperphosphatemia, isosthenuria, and occasional hypercalcemia. Proteinuria and glucosuria may also be observed.

Gross pathologic findings consistently include small, irregular kidneys with thin renal cortices and capsular adhesions. The kidneys may have a so-called "dumb-bell" shape, with most cortical tissue being present at the renal poles. Other systemic findings associated with uremia include hemorrhagic gastroenteritis, soft tissue mineralization, fibrous osteodystrophy, and enlarged parathyroid glands. Microscopic findings inlcude a reduced number of glomeruli, glomerular atrophy, and small, immature glomeruli. Tubular changes include atrophy, dilation, and epithelial hyperplasia. Interstitial fibrosis is particularly severe in the renal medulla, while interstitial inflammation is minimal. Hypertrophy of the juxtaglomerular apparatus may also be observed.

Presumptive diagnosis of this disease is based on the signalment and typical historical and clinical findings. Definitive diagnosis requires renal biopsy.

BASENJI[13,14,15,16]

The basenji breed is predisposed to several presumably inherited defects, including pyruvate-kinase deficiency anemia, immunoproliferative small intestinal disease, endocrine abnormalities, and a renal tubular defect similar to Fanconi's syndrome in man. Fanconi's syndrome is a disorder of renal tubular transport resulting in aminoaciduria, glucosuria, hyperphosphaturia, uricosuria, and bicarbonaturia. In man, the disorder may be inherited or acquired. Clinical consequences of Fanconi's syndrome in man include metabolic acidosis, bone demineralization, impaired growth, polyuria, dehydration, and hypokalemia.

The renal tubular defects characterizing Fanconi's syndrome occur in basenjis of both sexes. Affected dogs are usually presented as adults from 1 to 5 years of age. Clinical signs include polydipsia, polyuria, weight loss, dehydration, and weakness. In addition, in advanced cases, signs consistent with renal failure may be present.

Routine laboratory analysis consistently reveals dilute urine and glucosuria in the absence of elevated blood glucose levels. Results of routine tests of renal function may be normal or abnormal, depending on the severity of the disease at presentation. Azotemia, hyperphosphatemia, and severe metabolic acidosis are common findings in dogs with advanced disease. Aminoaciduria is a consistent finding and may be generalized or selective for cystine. Other laboratory abnormalities include proteinuria, hypokalemia, and moderate metabolic acidosis, which may be associated with hyperchloremia.

Diagnosis of this disorder is based on the signalment, clinical signs, and demonstration of reduced tubular reabsorption of glucose, phosphate, sodium, potassium, and uric acid. The most sensitive indicator of the disease appears to be paper chromatography of urine and demonstration of aminoaciduria.

Histologic findings in kidneys of affected dogs have not been consistent. Nonspecific findings include tubular atrophy and interstitial fibrosis. Occasionally, affected dogs have been noted to have enlarged, hyperchromatic nuclei in renal tubular cells.

The course of the disease is variable, and affected animals may remain stable without treatment for months to years. Only uncommonly does chronic renal failure develop. Often animals die suddenly of acute renal failure with papillary necrosis or pyelonephritis.

SAMOYED[17,18]

A sex-linked heredofamilial progressive nephropathy has been described in Samoyeds. Males are more often affected than females, and males typically die earlier than females. Males are commonly presented at less than 1 year of age with severe renal failure, whereas females usually have a much later onset (average, 5 years) and a much milder form of the disease.

Clinical findings in affected dogs included anorexia, weight loss, and stunted growth. Laboratory findings consistently include isosthenuria, proteinuria, glucosuria, and azotemia. Animals frequently have inflammatory urine sediments, presumably reflecting urinary tract infection. Occasionally, urate or uric acid crystals have been observed in the urine of affected dogs.

Gross pathologic findings include small kidneys with a disproportionate loss of cortical mass. On microscopic examination, mesangial thickening, glomerular sclerosis, and periglomerular fibrosis are observed. Marked medullary interstitial fibrosis is present, along with tubular basement membrane mineralization. Mononuclear interstitial inflammation is minimal.

DOBERMAN PINSCHER[19,20]

A progressive renal disease has been described in young Doberman pinscher dogs. Affected animals may be presented at less than 1 year of age, but the majority are approximately 2 years old at the time of diagnosis. The duration of clinical signs prior to presentation is very variable, ranging from a few months to several years. Both males and females are affected.

Historical and clinical findings are usually compatible with advanced renal failure. Owner complaints include anorexia, weight loss, vomiting, lethargy, polydipsia, polyuria, diarrhea, epistaxis, and nocturia. Physical findings include emaciation, dehydration, hypothermia, oral ulcers, ascites or edema, palpably small kidneys, retinal detachment, and fibrous osteodystrophy.

Laboratory abnormalities frequently include azotemia, hyperphosphatemia, hypercholesterolemia, nonregenerative anemia. The urine specific gravity is variable but is usually in the isosthenuric range. Proteinuria and cylindruria are invariable findings. Glucosuria and pyuria are uncommon.

Affected Dobermans have consistent pathologic findings. Grossly, the kidneys appear pale, have irregularly pitted surfaces, and are smaller than normal. Spherical cysts may be noted in the renal cortices in some dogs. Unilateral renal aplasia has been observed in some affected females. Systemic pathologic findings are compatible with uremia and renal secondary hyperparathyroidism.

Histologically, renal glomerular, tubular, and interstitial lesions are found. Glomerular lesions are classified as predominantly sclerotic, predominantly cystic, or a combination of both. Additional glomerular lesions include thickened capillary loops and periglomerular fibrosis. Tubular dilation and atrophy, interstitial fibrosis, and interstitial infiltration by mononuclear inflammatory cells are commonly recognized. Epithelial hyperplasia of the collecting ducts and focal interstitial mineralization may also be observed. Complement and immunoglobulin deposits in glomeruli have been detected in some animals, leading to speculation that this disease may represent an example of a primary familial glomerular disease.

DOMESTIC LONG-HAIRED CATS[21]

Congenital cystic lesions of the kidney occur in man and many animal species. A kindred of domestic long-haired cats with frequent occurrence of multiple congenital renal and biliary cysts has been described. Affected kittens are of both sexes, have long hair, and usually die by 6 weeks of age. The predominant physical finding in affected animals is marked abdominal distension.

Necropsy findings include an absence of obstructive renal or biliary lesions; thus, the cystic lesions of these organs are considered spontaneous. Both kidneys contain multiple small cyst-like structures in both the cortex and the medulla. Microscopically, glomeruli are reduced in number and appear to be compressed by cystic channels that extend from the renal capsule to the medulla. These dilated channels are lined with flattened, cuboidal epithelium. The renal papilla has a more normal architecture, but the tubules appear dilated.

The liver contains multiple cystic bile ducts throughout the parenchyma. These dilated ducts are lined with hyperplastic columnar epithelium and often contain precipitated bile. The gallbladder and common bile duct appear grossly and microscopically normal. Hepatocytes themselves are normal, but portal fibrosis is often noted. No inflammatory component has been recognized. The heredofamilial and histologic aspects of this disease are similar to infantile polycystic disease in man.

CAIRN TERRIER[22]

A congenital polycystic disease affecting the liver and kidneys has been reported in related cairn terriers. This disease is similar to infantile polycystic disease in man and to that described in domestic long-haired cats. Pedigree analysis suggests an autosomal recessive mode of inheritance.

Both males and females are affected and usually present for abdominal distension at an early age (6 weeks). Affected puppies are alert and active and, on examination, abdominal distension can be attributed to marked enlargement of the liver and kidneys. No abdominal effusion is noted.

Pathologically, the hallmark of the disease is the presence of multiple cysts throughout all liver lobes and both kidneys. In the liver, the cysts are formed by proliferative biliary epithelium in a complex network of biliary ducts. Biliary structures are increased in number and diameter. Cystic bile ducts are lined by cuboidal epithelium. Vascular structures and hepatocytes appear normal. Marked hepatic fibrosis is noted in portal areas, accentuating the normal hepatic lobular architecture.

Multiple fusiform to cylindrical cysts are present in both the renal cortex and the medulla. These cysts radiate from the capsular surface to the medulla. The renal parenchyma appears normal except for a decrease in the total number of glomeruli.

ABYSSINIAN CAT[23,24,25,26]

Amyloidosis is uncommon in domestic cats, but spontaneous amyloidosis has been observed in many related Abyssinian cats. The disease has been detected in females twice as commonly as in males. Affected cats are usually presented at 1 to 5 years of age for evaluation of poor haircoat quality, weight loss, polydipsia, polyuria, lethargy, and chronic anorexia. Physical examination findings include dehydration, rough haircoats, marked gingivitis, and small irregular kidneys. There is marked variability in the severity and progression of renal amyloidosis in the Abyssinian cat. Some cats develop renal failure by 1 year of age, but affected cats have occasionally lived for 12 to 14 years with only small amounts of amyloid being found in the kidneys at necropsy. In a large number of affected cats, however, it was found that 90 percent had died or been euthanatized for renal failure by 5 years of age.

Laboratory evaluation reveals evidence of chronic renal failure, including azotemia, hyperphosphatemia, metabolic acidosis, mild hyperglycemia, non-regenerative anemia, isosthenuria, and cylindruria. Proteinuria is a variable finding. In some affected cats, serum protein electrophoresis has revealed marked hyperglobulinemia with elevations of α_2 globulins.

The principal pathologic lesions in Abyssinian cats include medullary amyloidosis, papillary necrosis, chronic tubulointerstitial nephritis, and variable glomerular amyloidosis. Glomerular amyloidosis is generally mild and often difficult to detect in many affected cats. Occasionally glomerular amyloid deposition is severe, resulting in marked proteinuria. Medullary interstitial amyloid deposits are believed to interfere with blood flow to the renal papilla via the vasa recta, resulting in papillary necrosis and secondary interstitial medullary fibrosis and mononuclear inflammation.

Amyloid deposition is not restricted to the kidneys: deposits are frequently found in other organs, including the adrenal, thyroid, spleen, stomach, small intestine, heart, liver, and tongue. The amyloid deposits in these organs do not appear to contribute importantly to the clinical syndrome, which is characterized by chronic renal failure.

Amyloid deposits in affected cats may be detected by the use of several different staining techniques. Tissues stained with alkaline Congo red and viewed under polarized light demonstrate birefringence and a characteristic green color if amyloid is present. When stained with thioflavine-T, the amyloid deposits show strong yellow-green fluorescence under ultraviolet light. Thioflavine-T, however, is not specific for amyloid.

An ongoing prospective study indicates that amyloid deposits first appear in the kidneys of affected cats between 9 and 24 months of age. Some cats develop renal failure and die or are euthanatized within 1 year of the appearance of amyloid in their kidneys. In others, deterioration of renal function appears to be slower. Isolation and characterization of the amyloid protein from the kidneys of affected Abyssinian cats has demonstrated that this disease is an example of reactive amyloidosis, based on the presence of amyloid protein AA.

Studies of pedigrees of affected cats and an ongoing prospective study indicate that this disease is inherited, but these studies do not yet allow differentiation between autosomal recessive inheritance and autosomal dominant inheritance with reduced expressivity. Difficulty in determining the exact mode of inheritance arises from the late age of onset of clinical disease in some cats and the difficulty of obtaining diagnostic renal medullary biopsies.

STANDARD POODLE[27]

A nephropathy has been recognized in related juvenile standard poodles. Affected animals were presented at 3 months to 2 years of age and five of eight affected dogs were females. The occurrence of renal failure at a young age in related standard poodles is suggestive of a genetic disorder, but confirmation would require breeding trials of similarly affected dogs.

The clinical and laboratory findings are typical of renal failure. Younger dogs display stunted growth, lethargy, uremic halitosis, polydipsia, polyuria, and bony deformities suggestive of fibrous osteodystrophy. Polydipsia, polyuria, anorexia, vomiting, and diarrhea occur in older dogs. Laboratory abnormalities include hyperphosphatemia, azotemia, and hypercholesterolemia, but serum albumin values are within normal limits. Hypercalcemia occurs in some dogs, and nonregenerative anemia is documented in approximately 50 percent of affected dogs. Urine abnormalities include isosthenuria and proteinuria.

Pathologic lesions in affected dogs are consistent and include cystic glomerular atrophy and large numbers of immature glomeruli, especially in dogs presented at 3 to 4 months of age. Tubular changes consist of focal to diffuse tubular dilation and atrophy. Tubular basement membrane mineralization is a frequent finding. The renal interstitium contains areas of fibrosis with more diffuse lesions in the medulla. Occasional interstitial mononuclear infiltrates are noted. These inflammatory infiltrates were minimal in younger dogs and more severe in older dogs.

PEMBROKE WELSH CORGI[26]

A syndrome of telangiectasia with multiple organ involvement has been described in the red Pembroke Welsh corgi. Dogs of both sexes are affected and range in age from 5 to 13 years. There is often a prolonged history of intermittent gross hematuria with occasional passage of blood clots. Additional clinical signs include abdominal pain, dysuria, and vomiting. Physical examination occasionally reveals renal pain or small, irregular kidneys.

The most consistent laboratory feature in these dogs is hematuria. Microscopic hematuria is present between episodes of gross hematuria. Additional laboratory features include urinary tract infection and anemia which may be severe. Abdominal radiography may demonstrate renal calculi or renal calcification in chronically affected dogs. Contrast radiography may reveal distortion of the renal pelvis and hydronephrosis secondary to ureteral obstruction by blood clots.

Bilateral renal involvement has been found on postmortem examination in all reported cases. Red to black nodules are visible on the capsular surfaces and in the renal medulla adjacent to the corticomedullary junction. Clotted blood is often identified in these lesions and in the renal pelvis. Hydronephrosis occurs in approximately 50 percent of affected dogs. Similar nodular lesions may be identified in other tissues, including the subcutis, spleen, duodenum, anterior mediastinum, thoracic wall, retroperitoneal space, and central nervous system. Histologically, these lesions are cavernous, blood-filled spaces lined with endothelium, and thrombosis is a frequent finding in the sinuses. These sinuses with their simple endothelial linings may represent vascular malformations rather than benign tumors of vascular origin.

SOFT-COATED WHEATEN TERRIER[29,30]

A familial nephropathy has been reported in soft-coated wheaten terriers. Dogs with this disease are usually presented at 7 to 30 months of age. Males and females are affected with equal frequency. Clinical signs are nonspecific and include stunted growth, weight loss, anorexia, vomiting, diarrhea, polyuria, polydipsia, and anemia. Laboratory abnormalities include azotemia, hyperphosphatemia, hypocalcemia, and hypoalbuminemia. On urinalysis, there is isosthenuria, but proteinuria is variable and glucosuria has not been observed.

Pathologic findings suggest a dysplastic disorder of renal maturation. Gross changes include small renal cortices with irregular surfaces and a thickened capsule. Numerous cystic lesions may be noted in the cortex. Histopathologically, cortical lesions are segmental, whereas medullary disease is more diffuse. Cortical lesions include interstitial fibrosis, periglomerular fibrosis, cystic glomerular atrophy, decreased numbers of glomeruli, and the presence of immature, fetal glomeruli. Medullary changes include tubular atrophy and dilatation, interstitial fibrosis, tubular basement membrane mineralization, and minimal mononuclear inflammatory cell infiltration. Adenomatous proliferation of the collecting duct epithelium is also a prominent feature.

DIAGNOSIS AND TREATMENT

Historical, physical, and laboratory abnormalities that can facilitate diagnosis for familial disease of dogs and cats are listed in Table 7-2. Pathologic findings that may be encountered following renal biopsy are listed in Table 7-3.

Most of the canine and feline familial renal diseases are progressive. Therapy of these patients is therefore limited to symptomatic measures and conservative medical management of chronic renal failure. The goals of this therapy include correction of initial fluid deficits and derangements of acid-base and electrolyte balance; dietary protein restriction (discussed in Ch. 8); restriction of phosphorus intake by the use of phosphorus-restricted diets and oral administration of phosphorus-binding agents; management of metabolic acidosis; management of anemia; control of uremic gastroenteritis; administration of water-soluble vitamins; reduction of stress; and prevention and treatment of urinary tract infection.

At the time of presentation, animals with chronic renal failure are often dehydrated and require appropriate parenteral fluid therapy to correct prerenal azotemia and restore fluid and electrolyte balance. Likewise, the owner should provide unlimited access to fresh water at home as a part of the long-term management of the small animal patient with polyuric chronic renal failure. Alternate-day administration of a preparation containing water-soluble vitamins is recommended to offset losses that may occur due to ongoing polyuria. In animals with severe metabolic acidosis, sodium bicarbonate in tablet or powder form is used at a dosage of 25 to 35 mg/kg/day. This dosage is adjusted based on repeated blood gas analyses, and an attempt is made to maintain a serum bicarbonate concentration above 18 mEq/L.

Oral phosphorus-binding agents have been used in conjunction with phosphorus-restricted diets to control hyperphosphatemia and to blunt renal secondary hyperparathyroidism. Such treatment may also lessen such detrimental histologic changes in the kidney as interstitial mineralization and fibrosis. Several formulations of phosphorus-binding agents are available, including cap-

Table 7-2. Historical, Physical, and Laboratory Abnormalities in Familial Renal Diseases of the Dog and Cat

Abnormality	Breed									
	Cocker Spaniel	Norwegian Elkhound	Lhaso Apso/ Shih Tzu	Basenji	Samoyed	Doberman Pinscher	Abyssinian	Standard Poodle	Pembroke Welsh Corgi	Soft-Coated Wheaten Terrier
Historical										
Anorexia	+	+	+	+/−	+	+	+	+		+
Depression	+	+	+	+/−	+	+	+	+		+
Weight loss	+	+	+	+/−	+	+	+	+		+
Stunted growth		+	+		+			+		+
Vomiting	+	+	+	+/−	+	+		+	+/−	+
PD/PU	+	+	+	+	+	+	+	+		+
Physical										
Bony deformities	+	+	+			+		+		
Ocular lesions	+					+				
Small kidneys	+	+	+		+	+	+/−	+		+
Hypertension	+/−		+/−							
Laboratory										
Anemia	+/−	+/−	+/−		+	+/−	+/−	+/−	+/−	+/−
Azotemia	+	+	+	+/−	+	+	+	+		+
Hyperphosphatemia	+	+	+	+/−		+	+	+		+
Hypercalcemia	+/−	+/−	+/−					+/−		
Hypercholesterolemia						+		+		
Isosthenuria	+	+	+	+	+	+	+	+		+
Cylindriuria						+	+			
Proteinuria	+	+/−	+/−		+	+	+/−	+		+/−
Glucosuria	+/−	+/−	+/−	+ +	+	+/−				
Hematuria									+ +	
Pyuria					+/−	+/−			+/−	
Crystalluria					+					

Key: + = abnormality present.
+/− = may or may not be present.
Blank = no data available.

Table 7-3. Pathologic Findings in Familial Renal Diseases of the Dog and Cat

	Glomerular Changes					Tubular Changes		Interstitial Changes			
Breed	Thickened BM	Sclerosis	Cystic Atrophy	Fetal Glomeruli	BM Mineralization	Atrophy	Dilatation	CD hyperplasia	Fibrosis	Inflammation	Other Changes
Cocker spaniel		+	+		+	+	+		+		
Beagle						+	+	+			Unilateral renal agenesis
Norwegian elkhound		+	+		+	+	+	+	+	+/−	
Lhaso apso/ Shih Tzu			+	+		+	+	+	+		Juxtaglomerular hypertrophy
Basenji						+			+		Papillary necrosis; pyelonephritis
Samoyed	+	+			+				+	+	
Doberman pinscher		+	+			+	+	+	+	+	Unilateral renal agenesis
Domestic long haired cats									+		Multiple cystic lesions of liver and kidney
Cairn terrier											Multiple cystic lesions of liver and kidney
Abyssinian									+	+	Medullary and glomerular amyloid deposition; papillary necrosis
Standard poodle			+	+	+	+	+		+	+	
Pembroke Welsh corgi											Renal telangiectasis, renal calculi, hydronephrosis
Soft-coated wheaten terriers		+	+	+	+	+	+	+	+		

BM = Basement membrane; CD = collecting duct.

sules, tablets, and suspensions of aluminum hydroxide and aluminum carbonate. These products are administered with food to maximize their phosphorus-binding potential, and their dosage is adjusted by frequent monitoring of the serum phosphorus concentration.

Animals with chronic renal failure also often have nonregenerative anemia due primarily to decreased renal activation or production of erythropoietin. Occasionally, such anemias are severe enough to necessitate blood transfusion. Often, however, anemia is mild to moderate in severity, and anabolic steroids are used in their management. Testosterone propionate (10 to 15 mg/day), nandrolone decanoate (1.0 to 1.5 mg/kg/wk), oxymetholone (1 to 2.5 mg/kg bid), and stanozolol (1 to 4 mg bid) are products which have been recommended. Additional potential effects of anabolic steroids which may be of benefit include promotion of protein anabolism, increased erythrocyte 2,3-diphosphoglyceric acid levels, and enhanced deposition of calcium in bone. The effects of anabolic steroids may not be evident for 2 to 3 months after initiation of therapy.

Chronic intermittent vomiting may also be a problem for animals with chronic renal failure and may be attributed to direct activation of the chemoreceptor trigger zone of the medulla by uremic toxins or to hypergastrinemia. Centrally acting antiemetics such as the phenothiazines (chlorpromazine 0.5 mg/kg or prochlorperazine 0.5 mg/kg) or trimethobenzamide (3.0 mg/kg) may be useful in the control of intractable vomiting. The recent demonstration of hypergastrinemia in dogs with renal failure has led to the use of the H_2 receptor blocker cimetidine in the management of uremic gastroenteritis. Cimetidine blocks the H_2 receptors of the acid-producing parietal cells of the stomach. It has been used in dogs with renal failure at a dosage of 5 to 10 mg/kg IV bid followed by 5 mg/kg qd to bid. An additional effect of cimetidine which may be of benefit in chronic renal failure is its ability to reduce the circulating level of parathyroid hormone in uremic dogs and man. It also may reduce serum phosphorus concentration, increase serum 1,25-dihydroxycholecalciferol, and promote positive calcium balance without a change in serum ionized calcium concentration.

Animals with chronic renal failure of any etiology may be predisposed to urinary tract infection due to impaired cell-mediated immunity and loss of concentrating ability. In addition, Pembroke Welsh corgi dogs with telangiectasia may be especially predisposed to urinary tract infection. As a result, frequent monitoring of the urine sediment is advisable, and appropriate antibiotics should be administered whenever urinary tract infection is detected.

REFERENCES

1. Krook L: The pathology of renal cortical hypoplasia in the dog. Nord Vet Med 9:161, 1957
2. Persson F, Persson S, Asheim A: Renal cortical hypoplasia in dogs. Acta Vet Scand 2:68, 1961
3. Steward AP, MacDougall DF: Familial nephropathy in the cocker spaniel. J Small Anim Pract 25:15, 1984

4. Robbins GR: Unilateral renal agenesis in the beagle. Vet Rec 77:1345, 1965
5. Vymetal F: Case reports: renal aplasia in beagles. Vet Rec 77:1344, 1965
6. Fox MW: Inherited polycystic mononephrosis in the dog. J Hered 55:29, 1964
7. Finco DR, Kurtz HJ, Low DG, Perman V: Familial renal disease in Norwegian elkhound dogs. J Am Vet Med Assoc 156:747, 1970
8. Finco DR: Familial renal disease in Norwegian elkhound dogs: physiologic and biochemical examinations. Am J Vet Res 37:87, 1976
9. Finco DR, Duncan JR, Crowell WA, Hulsey ML: Familial renal disease in Norwegian elkhound dogs: morphologic examinations. Am J Vet Res 38:941, 1977
10. Dr. D. Gribble, personal communication, Davis, CA, 1975
11. O'Brien TD, Osborne CA, Yano BL, Barnes DM: Clinicopathologic manifestations of progressive renal disease in Lhaso apso and Shih Tzu dogs. J Am Vet Med Assoc 180:658, 1982
12. Hawe RS, Loeb WF: Caudal vaginal agenesis and progressive renal disease in a Shih Tzu. J Am Anim Hosp Assoc 20:123, 1984
13. Easley JR, Breitschwerdt EB: Glucosuria associated with renal tubular dysfunction in three basenji dogs. J Am Vet Med Assoc 168:938, 1976
14. Bovee KC, Joyce T, Reynolds R, Segal S: The Fanconi syndrome in basenji dogs: A new model for renal transport defects. Science 201:1129, 1978
15. Bovee KC, Joyce T, Blazer-Yost B, Goldschmidt MS, Segal S: Characterization of renal defects in dogs with a syndrome similar to the Fanconi syndrome in man. J Am Vet Med Assoc 174:1094, 1979
16. Breitschwerdt EB, Ochoa R, Waltman C: Multiple endocrine abnormalities in basenji dogs with renal tubular dysfunction. J Am Vet Med Assoc 182:1348, 1983
17. Bernard MA, Vali VE: Familial renal disease in Samoyed dogs. Can Vet J 18:181, 1977
18. Bloedow AG: Familial renal disease in Samoyed dogs. Vet Rec 108:167, 1981
19. Wilcock BP, Patterson JM: Familial glomerulonephritis in Doberman pinscher dogs. Can Vet J 20:244, 1979
20. Chew DJ, DiBartola SP, Boyce JT, et al: Juvenile renal disease in Doberman pinscher dogs. J Am Vet Med Assoc 182:481, 1983
21. Crowell WA, Hubbell JJ: Polycystic renal disease in related cats. J Am Vet Med Assoc 175:286, 1979
22. McKenna SC, Carpenter JL: Polycystic disease of the kidney and liver in the Cairn terrier. Vet Pathol 17:436, 1980
23. Chew DJ, DiBartola SP, Boyce JT, Gasper PW: Renal amyloidosis in related Abyssinian cats. J Am Vet Med Assoc 181:139, 1982
24. Boyce JT, DiBartola SP, Chew DJ, Gasper PW: Familial renal amyloidosis in Abyssinian cats. Vet Pathol 21:33, 1984
25. DiBartola SP, Benson MD, Dwulet FE, Cornacoff JB: Isolation and characterization of amyloid protein AA in the Abyssinian cat. Lab Invest 52:485, 1985
26. DiBartola SP, Tarr MJ, Benson MD: Tissue distribution of amyloid deposits in Abyssinian cats with familial amyloidosis. (In preparation, 1985)
27. DiBartola SP, Chew DF, Boyce JT: Juvenile renal disease in related standard poodles. J Am Vet Med Assoc 183:693, 1983
28. Moore FM, Thorton GW: Telangiectasia of Pembroke Welsh corgi dogs. Vet Pathol 20:203, 1983
29. Nash AS, Kelly DF, Gaskell CJ: Progressive renal disease in soft-coated wheaten terriers: possible familial nephropathy. J Small Anim Pract 25:479, 1984
30. Eriksen K, Grondalen J: Familial renal disease in soft-coated wheaten terriers. J Small Anim Pract 25:489, 1984

8 Dietary Management of Canine Renal Failure

David J. Polzin
Carl A. Osborne

DEFINITIONS AND CONCEPTS

Azotemia

Azotemia is defined as abnormal concentration of urea, creatinine, or other nonprotein nitrogenous substances in blood, plasma, or serum. Azotemia is a laboratory finding and may or may not be caused by generalized lesions of the renal parenchyma. Azotemia resulting from generalized lesions of the kidneys is termed *primary renal azotemia.*

Prerenal azotemia may result from decreased renal blood flow or increased urea production. Renal blood flow may be decreased as a result of dehydration (e.g., from vomiting or diarrhea), poor filling of the vasculature (e.g., hypoproteinemia), or heart failure. Increased urea production may result from increased protein consumption or enhanced protein catabolism (e.g., following stress or corticosteroid administration). Prerenal azotemia may occur in patients with normal or abnormal kidneys. It may be detected in patients with normal kidneys by identifying azotemia in association with adequate urine concentrating ability (i.e., urine specific gravity $>$ 1.030 in dogs).

Postrenal azotemia occurs when urine is abnormally retained in the body as a result of obstruction of the urinary tract or following rupture of any portion of the urinary tract. Postrenal azotemia may occur in patients with normal or abnormal kidneys. Urine concentrating ability may or may not be normal in patients with postrenal azotemia.

Uremia

Uremia is the polysystemic toxic syndrome which occurs as a result of decreased renal function. Unlike azotemia, which is a laboratory finding, uremia is a clinical syndrome. Although uremia is always accompanied by azotemia and renal failure, azotemia and renal failure may or may not be associated with uremia.

Renal Failure

Failure is defined as the inability to perform. The kidneys perform multiple functions in maintaining homeostasis, including elimination of waste products of metabolism from the body, synthesis of a variety of hormones, and degradation of a variety of hormones and other metabolites. Failure to perform these functions may not be an all-or-none phenomenon. In slowly progressive renal diseases, for example, failure of the ability to concentrate or dilute urine according to body needs typically precedes failure to eliminate waste products of protein metabolism. In turn, laboratory detection of impaired ability to maintain electrolyte and nonelectrolyte solute balance typically precedes onset of polysystemic clinical signs caused by renal dysfunction. In some situations, renal disease may precede renal failure, and likewise, renal failure may precede uremia. In many instances, however, renal disease does not progress to a state of renal failure. By definition, dogs that have lost the ability to concentrate urine as a result of generalized renal lesions have primary renal failure. Inability to adequately concentrate urine (clinically manifest as polyuria and polydipsia) is usually the earliest clinical evidence of chronic renal failure.

The concept that adequate renal function is not synonymous with total renal function is of importance in (1) understanding the difference between renal disease and renal failure, (2) formulating meaningful prognoses, and (3) formulating specific, supportive, and symptomatic therapy.

Renal Disease

Renal disease indicates the presence of renal lesions of any size, distribution (focal or generalized), or cause (anomalies, infection, endogenous or exogenous toxins, neoplasms, ischemia, immune disorders, hypercalcemia, trauma) in one or both kidneys. The specific cause(s) of renal disease may not be known; however, quantitative information concerning renal function (or dysfunction) is not defined.

Renal disease should not be considered synonymous with renal failure because of the tremendous reserve capacity of the kidneys. Depending on the quantity of renal parenchyma affected and the severity and duration of lesions, renal disease may or may not cause renal failure and uremia. For example, following acute reduction of renal functional mass, impairment of renal concentrating and diluting capacities cannot be detected unless greater than two-thirds of the renal mass is surgically removed. Likewise, greater than three-quarters of the renal parenchyma must be nonfunctional before significant azotemia can be detected. However, because of the considerable ability of canine kidneys to develop compensatory hypertrophy, adequate concentrating ability is usually restored 8 to 12 weeks after removal of two-thirds to three-quarters (or more!) of the kidney mass. Furthermore, some ability to dilute urine (urine specific gravities between 1.004 and 1.007) may remain after development of azotemic chronic primary renal failure. Compensatory hypertrophy also results in an increase in glomerular filtration rate (GFR) from 25 percent of normal immediately after surgery to about 50 percent of normal 12 weeks after surgical removal of 75 percent of the renal mass.

Polyuria and Oliguria

Renal failure, regardless of whether it is acute or chronic, may be associated with polyuria, oliguria, or a normal urine production rate. In dogs, polyuria is defined as a urine production rate exceeding 50 ml/kg body wt/day. Oliguria is defined as production of urine at a rate of less than 0.66 ml/kg body wt/day.

Urine production rate may have a profound impact on the pathophysiologic changes occurring in patients with renal failure. Oliguric renal failure is more likely to be associated with retention of fluids and electrolytes, whereas polyuric renal failure is more likely to be associated with fluid and electrolyte deficits. Therefore, urine production rate profoundly influences formulation of symptomatic and supportive therapy of renal failure. In addition, patients with oliguric renal failure are typically more difficult to treat and tend to have a poorer short-term prognosis than patients with polyuric renal failure. For these reasons, urine production rate should be consistently determined during the initial diagnostic evaluation of patients suspected of having renal failure.

Acute Versus Chronic Renal Failure

Acute renal failure is a *potentially reversible* loss of renal function. In contrast, chronic renal failure (CRF) is an irreversible condition in which neither rapid improvement nor rapid deterioration of renal function occurs unless other factors intervene (e.g., prerenal or postrenal conditions). In general, patients with acute renal failure develop clinical signs of greater intensity at the onset of the disorder than do patients with CRF. Patients with acute renal failure have a much higher mortality rate during the initial period of hospitalization. However, patients that recover from acute renal failure may regain sufficient renal function to become asymptomatic. In general, patients with CRF do not recover their lost renal function. Most of these patients eventually die of uremia, although they may experience reasonably good health for months to years.

Table 8-1. Etiopathologic Basis of Canine Renal Disease

Disease Process	Specific Treatment Available?	References
Glomerular diseases		
Amyloidosis	Unlikely	58
Immune complex disorders	Possibly	1, 17, 59
Antiglomerular basement membrane disorders	Possibly	1, 17, 59
Congenital disorders	No	—
Hypercalcemic nephropathy	Sometimes	17, 60
Nephrotoxins	Sometimes	1, 61
Neoplasia	Sometimes	62
Urinary obstruction	Sometimes	17, 63
Pyelonephritis	Yes	64, 65
Leptospirosis	Yes	66
Systemic mycoses	Yes	67
Urolithiasis	Yes	17, 68
Hypertension	Yes	15
Idiopathic	No	—
Ischemia	Sometimes	—
Others	—	—

CAUSATIVE FACTORS

Etiologic Agents

Chronic renal failure may result from a wide variety of causes (Table 8-1). However, in most instances it has been difficult or impossible to determine the primary etiology of renal dysfunction once CRF has ensued. Inability to identify the inciting cause of renal failure derives, in part, from the fact that many distinctly different pathophysiologic entities are morphologically and clinically indistinguishable once renal disease has advanced to the point of CRF. In some cases, disease processes initially responsible for renal damage are no longer present or active in patients with CRF. For these reasons, it has become common usage to refer to small, fibrotic, irreversibly damaged kidneys as *end-stage kidneys*, a term that does not suggest any specific etiopathologic process.[1]

Significance of Specific Therapy Versus Conservative Medical Management

Conservative medical management primarily encompasses symptomatic and supportive therapy of patients with CRF. It is not designed to reverse or eliminate renal lesions, but rather is directed at minimizing clinical, metabolic, biochemical, endocrine, and nutritional abnormalities associated with the uremic state.

Specific therapy consists of therapy designed to slow, stop, or reverse development of renal lesions by influencing the etiopathogenic processes responsible for the lesions. Examples of specific treatment include correction of hypercalcemia that has caused calcium nephropathy, administration of antibiotics to eliminate bacterial infections, removal of lesions causing obstructive

Table 8-2. Partial List of Compounds Incriminated as Uremic Toxins

Urea	Aromatic compounds
Guanidinium compounds	Phenolic acid
Methylguanidine	Hydroxyphenobic acid
Dimethylguanidine	Aromatic amines
Guanidinosuccemic acid	Indoles
Guanidinoacetic acid	Aliphatic amines
Creatinine	Conjugated amino acids
Peptides	Middle molecules
Sulfates	Hydrogen ions

uropathy, and correction of abnormal renal perfusion that has caused ischemic renal lesions.

Although it is often difficult to determine the initiating disease process in dogs with CRF, the value of formulating specific therapy based on an etiologic/pathologic diagnosis should not be overlooked. By definition, CRF cannot be reversed by specific therapy. Nonetheless, progression of renal lesions and failure may be slowed or stopped by specific therapy. Therefore, diagnostic efforts directed especially at detecting treatable renal diseases should be performed prior to formulating plans for conservative medical management (Table 8-1).

PATHOPHYSIOLOGY OF RENAL FAILURE

Conceptual understanding of the seemingly complex manifestations of CRF may be enhanced by categorizing related events to one of three broad categories of dysfunction: (1) excretory failure, (2) regulatory failure, and (3) biosynthetic failure. All of the clinical and laboratory consequences of renal failure can be ascribed to one or more of these functional deficiencies.

Excretory Failure

Excretory failure consists of impaired ability of the kidneys to rid the body of metabolic waste products. Azotemia, as evidenced by elevated serum creatinine and urea nitrogen concentrations, is the hallmark of excretory failure; however, many other metabolites are also retained in renal failure (Table 8-2). Many of these compounds are considered uremic toxins and may contribute to clinical manifestations of uremia. However, in most cases, a definite cause and effect relationship between these so-called toxins and clinical signs of uremia have yet to be proved.

Regulatory Failure

Regulatory failure consists of impaired ability of the kidneys to maintain fluid, electrolyte, and acid-base balance. Failing kidneys become progressively less able to adapt to normal variations in water and electrolyte consumption, and thus the range of intakes over which the kidneys are able to maintain homeostatic balance becomes narrowed. Commonly, loss of adequate urine concentrating ability, often characterized by polyuria, is the earliest evidence of regulatory failure. Impaired urine concentrating ability and polyuria predispose the patient to dehydration should compensatory polydipsia become inadequate (e.g., with vomiting or lack of access to water).

Serum sodium and potassium concentrations generally remain within the normal range in dogs with CRF. Nonetheless, chronically diseased kidneys have an impaired ability to adapt to changes in consumption of these electrolytes.[2,3,4] Clinically this is manifest most clearly by reduced ability to adapt to abrupt changes in sodium intake.[3] Sudden restriction of sodium intake may result in transient negative sodium balance and acute deterioration of renal function. This effect appears to represent an adaptive phenomenon related to sodium intake rather than an intrinsic loss of ability to conserve sodium.

In contrast to sodium and potassium, the ability of the kidneys to maintain serum phosphorus concentrations within the normal range is more limited. In order to maintain phosphorus balance, dietary consumption must equal excretion. Because phosphorus excretion is primarily renal, phosphorus intake must approximate renal excretion. Renal phosphorus excretion is the sum effect of glomerular filtration and renal tubular reabsorption. As glomerular filtration rate declines in renal failure, the filtered load (i.e., the amount of phosphorus excreted by glomerular filtration) decreases, and phosphorus retention occurs. Phosphorus retention results in hypocalcemia as a result of the physiochemical interrelationship between calcium and phosphorus. (These early changes in plasma phosphorus and calcium concentrations are miniscule, transient, and undetectable by blood chemical methods.) Hypocalcemia stimulates parathyroid hormone (PTH) secretion. Parathyroid hormone and, possibly, increased plasma phosphorus concentrations, inhibit renal tubular reabsorption of phosphorus, thereby increasing renal excretion of phosphorus. By this mechanism, the kidneys and parathyroid glands maintain plasma phosphorus concentrations within normal limits until moderate to advanced renal failure develops. At that time, inhibition of tubular reabsorption of phosphorus no longer compensates adequately for the reduced filtered load of phosphorus, and hyperphosphatemia develops. Hyperphosphatemia is commonly first recognized at about the same time that azotemia is first recognized in dogs with CRF.

The compensatory adaptations responsible for maintaining plasma phosphorus concentrations within the normal range during the early phases of renal failure exact a pathophysiologic price from the patient, commonly referred to as the *trade-off phenomenon*.[5] The persistently elevated PTH levels required to maintain normocalcemia and normophosphatemia in patients with CRF ("renal secondary hyperparathyroidism") are ultimately responsible for development of renal osteodystrophy. In addition to causing renal osteodystrophy, PTH may act as a uremic toxin responsible for (1) neurologic dysfunction involving the brain and peripheral nerves, (2) bone marrow inhibition, (3) increased red blood cell fragility, (4) altered carbohydrate, lipid, and acid-base metabolism, (5) cardiomyopathy, (6) soft tissue calcification, and (7) impotence.[6,7]

Biosynthetic Failure

Biosynthetic failure consists of an impaired ability of failing kidneys to elaborate adequate quantities of hormones and other compounds as a result of reduced function. Compounds normally produced by the kidneys include erythropoietin, 1,25-dihydroxycholecalciferol (1,25-vitamin D_3; the most biologically active form of vitamin D), and ammonium. Insufficient production of these hormones and compounds is responsible for many abnormalities associated with uremia. For example, inadequate erythropoietin production contributes to the development of nonregenerative anemia in CRF.

Reduced renal conversion of 25-hydroxycholecalciferol to 1,25-dihydroxycholecalciferol contributes to development of renal secondary hyperparathyroidism and renal osteodystrophy. Inadequate production of 1,25-vitamin D_3 impairs gastrointestinal absorption of calcium and contributes to skeletal resistance to the action of PTH, thereby promoting hypocalcemia and hyperparathyroidism.

Metabolic acidosis develops in CRF in part because the kidneys' ability to excrete acid (hydrogen ions) is reduced. Hydrogen ions are excreted by the kidneys as titratable acids (primarily in the form of phosphate) or ammonium. Ammonia produced by the kidneys diffuses into the renal tubules where it combines with hydrogen ions forming ammonium. Hydrogen ions are thus effectively trapped in the renal tubules because ammonium cannot readily diffuse out of the renal tubules and must be excreted. As renal function deteriorates, renal ammoniagenesis is reduced, thereby promoting metabolic acidosis by reducing the capacity of the kidneys to excrete hydrogen ions.

DIAGNOSIS OF RENAL FAILURE

Criteria for Diagnosis of Primary Renal Failure

Renal failure is defined as impaired ability of the kidneys to perform normal excretory, regulatory, and biosynthetic functions. Impaired ability to regulate water balance is usually the earliest evidence of CRF in dogs and is manifest clinically as polyuria and polydipsia. However, dogs with primary glomerular diseases (e.g., amyloidosis or glomerulonephritis) may develop azotemia, edema, or clinical signs of uremia prior to marked loss of urine concentrating ability. When this occurs, it is known as *glomerular–tubular imbalance*. Moderate to marked proteinuria is a hallmark of these diseases.

Diagnosis of primary renal failure in *nonazotemic* dogs is based on demonstrating (1) impaired ability to concentrate urine in response to dehydration or exogenous administration of antidiuretic hormone and (2) reduced renal function in the absence of identifiable prerenal causes. Diagnosis of primary renal failure in *azotemic* dogs is based on demonstrating concurrent azotemia and inadequate urine concentrating ability.

In exceptional cases, other polyuric diseases may be associated with inadequate urine concentrating ability and azotemia, but only when azotemia results from prerenal causes (e.g., diabetes insipidus with inadequate compensatory water intake resulting in prerenal azotemia). In dogs with primary glomerular diseases and glomerulotubluar imbalance, diagnosis of primary renal failure is based on demonstrating reduced renal function in the absence of prerenal causes. In our experience, the disease most likely to be confused with azotemic primary renal failure is hypoadrenocorticism. Although characteristically associated with oliguria, hypoadrenocorticism may be characterized by normal to increased urine formation, azotemia, and inadequate urine concentrating ability. However, hypoadrenocorticism typically differs from primary renal failure in that the ratio of serum sodium to serum potassium concentration is usually less than 27:1. Unfortunately, the Na^+/K^+ ratio may not invariably differentiate hypoadrenocorticism from primary renal failure. Therefore, clinical signs, electrocardiographic findings, hematologic findings results of an adrenocorticotropic hormone (ACTH) response test, and response to therapy should be used to confirm the diagnosis of hypoadrenocorticism.

Differentiating of Chronic from Acute Primary Renal Failure

Chronic primary renal failure may be differentiated from acute renal failure on the basis of (1) onset and duration of clinical signs, (2) previous diagnosis of renal failure, (3) nonregenerative anemia, (4) radiographic evidence of renal osteodystrophy, and (5) bilateral reduction in kidney size. Patients with CRF may be predisposed to episodes of concurrent acute renal dysfunction due to unrelated causes which may be partially or completely reversible. In addition, combinations of primary renal failure, prerenal azotemia, and/or postrenal azotemia may occur simultaneously as part of the disease syndrome in a patient. It is of therapeutic and prognostic value to determine which of these syndromes are occurring in the patient (Table 8-3).

Diagnostic Tests

Determination of Glomerular Filtration Rate (GFR). Glomerular filtration rate may be estimated using serum creatinine (SC) and urea nitrogen (SUN) concentrations or may be determined more accurately by creatinine clearance studies. The usefulness of SC and SUN as estimates of GFR is limited to dogs that have lost approximately 75 percent or more of their functional nephrons. In dogs with CRF in which maximal compensatory hypertrophy has developed, loss of as much as 85 percent or more of the functional nephrons may occur before decreases in GFR are manifest as elevated SC and SUN concentrations. Measurement of GFR may reflect prerenal and postrenal influences, as well

Table 8-3. Comparison of Prerenal Azotemia, Acute Parenchymal Renal Failure, Chronic Parenchymal Renal Failure, and Postrenal Azotemia

Data	Prerenal Azotemia	Acute Parenchymal Renal Failure	Chronic Parenchymal Renal Failure	Postrenal Azotemia
BUN	↑	↑	↑	↑
Serum creatinine	↑	↑	↑	↑
Serum phosphorus	N, ↑	↑	↑	↑
Serum calcium	N	↓,N, ↑	↓,N, ↑	N
Serum sodium	N(↑)(↓)	↓,N, ↑	N	N, ↓
Serum potassium	N	N, ↑	N	N, ↑
Serum chloride	N	↓,N, ↑	N, ↑	N
Blood bicarbonate	↓,N	↓,N	↓,N	↓,N
Urine sp gr	>1.030[a] >1.035[b]	<1.030[a] <1.035[b]	<1.030[a] <1.035[b]	*
Urine sodium[c]	<10 mEq/L	>25 mEq/L	>25 mEq/L	*
FE_{na}[c]	<1.0	>1.0	>1.0	*
Urine/serum creatinine[+]	>20	<5	<5	*
Urine output	↓(N)	↓,N, ↑	↑,(↓,N)	↓(N, ↑)
PCV	N, ↑	N, ↑(↓)	↓,(N)	N
Previous history of polyuria/polydipsia	0	0	+(0)	0(+)
Previous history of oliguria/anuria	+(0)	+/0	0	+(0)
Previous history of uremic symptoms	0	0	+/0	0
Debilitation	0	0	+/0	0
Renal osteodystrophy	0	0	+/0	0
Renal size	N	N, ↑	↓,N, ↑	N, ↑

Key: ↑ = increased, N = normal range, ↓ = decreased
( ) = uncommon, * = no specific values characteristic of the condition
0 = absent, + = present.
[a] Canine
[b] feline
[c] extrapolated from data in human beings.
(Polzin DJ, Osborne CA: Diseases of the urinary tract. p. 333 In Davis L: Manual of Therapeutics in Small Animal Practice. Churchill Livingstone, New York, 1985.)

as changes resulting from primary renal dysfunction, regardless of whether SUN, SC, or creatinine clearance studies are used to evaluate GFR.

Serum urea nitrogen and creatinine determinations can be used (1) as screening tests of renal function, (2) for evaluating the need for and effectiveness of conservative medical management and diet therapy, and (3) for serially monitoring changes in GFR in azotemic patients. Because serum urea nitrogen concentration may be influenced by a variety of nonrenal factors, it is less desirable than SC as a measure of GFR. Nonrenal factors that may elevate SUN concentrations include increased dietary protein intake, decreased urine flow rate, hemorrhage into the gastrointestinal tract, infection, fever, burns, intake of corticosteroids, and other processes that enhance protein catabolism.[8] Nonrenal factors which may decrease SUN concentrations include: diminished protein intake, severe hepatic insufficiency, and possibly anabolic steroids.[8]

Serum urea nitrogen determinations are particularly useful for evaluating the influence of modified protein diets on retention of proteinaceous waste products in patients with renal failure. Although SC is minimally affected by nonrenal factors, studies in humans indicate that changes in SC are not consistently proportional to changes in creatinine clearance, possibly limiting its usefulness as a measure of changes in renal function.

Renal function may also be evaluated by endogenous or exogenous creatinine clearance (C_{cr}). A major indication for performing C_{cr} is to confirm preazotemic primary renal failure. Creatinine clearance may also be indicated in dogs with glomerular dysfunction and renal tubular imbalance and when accurate serial determination of GFR is desired (e.g., for determining progression of renal dysfunction). The concept of clearance and the methods used to determine it in dogs have been described elsewhere.[9,10,11]

Major factors influencing results of endogenous C_{cr} studies include (1) completeness of urine collection, (2) method of determination of SC, (3) systemic hemodynamics, and (4) status of renal function. Failure to empty the bladder completely at the beginning of the study will result in an erroneously high C_{cr} value, whereas failure to empty the bladder at the end of the study will result in an erroneously low value. The potential magnitude of these errors progressively increases as collection times and volumes decrease.

Methods used for determination of SC influence C_{cr} because of serum noncreatinine chromagens. The most commonly used methods of determining SC (including automated techniques) cannot differentiate between true creatinine and noncreatinine chromagens and therefore overestimate SC. However, noncreatinine chromagens do not appear in urine. Determination of C_{cr} by methods that are influenced by noncreatinine chromagens underestimate C_{cr}. The error is greatest when SC is within the normal range, because serum noncreatinine chromagens do not increase substantially when GFR decreases. Exogenous C_{cr} techniques (i.e., techniques utilizing an exogenous source of creatinine) are likely to be more accurate than endogenous techniques, especially in nonazotemic patients, because the influence of noncreatinine chromagens is minimized. A clinically applicable technique for determination of exogenous C_{cr} in dogs using a subcutaneous injection of sterile, pyrogen-free creatinine has been described.[10]

Normal 20-minute and 24-hour endogenous C_{cr} values have been reported. Normal values for 30-minute C_{cr} have been reported to be 2.8 $\pm$ 0.96 ml/min/kg (range 1.7 to 5.0 ml/min/kg).[12] Normal values for 24-hour C_{cr} have been reported to be 3.7 $\pm$ 0.77 ml/min/kg (approximate range 1.7 to 4.5 ml/min/kg).[9] Noncreatinine chromagens were included in the determination of the 24-hour study but not in the 20-minute study.

Adequate Urine Concentrating Ability. Several different types of studies designed to evaluate urine concentrating ability have been described.[13,14] Adequate urine concentrating ability in dogs is defined as a urine specific gravity of 1.030 or greater.

Failure to adequately concentrate urine is not proof of parenchymal renal failure. Diagnosis of renal failure as the cause of inadequate urine concentrating

Table 8-4. Conservative Medical Management of Chronic Renal Failure

1.	Maintain normal hydration (unlimited access to water)
2.	Avoid stress
3.	Institute diet therapy
4.	Administer water soluble vitamin supplements
5.	Administer sodium bicarbonate
6.	Control sodium intake
7.	Administer anabolic agents
8.	Administer intestinal phosphorus binders
9.	Give calcium and vitamin D supplements
10.	Avoid nephrotoxic drugs or drugs likely to cause adverse drug reactions; adjust drug dosages for drugs excreted primarily by the kidneys
11.	Institute antihypertensive therapy

ability must be based on assessment of other clinical and laboratory studies. In general, demonstration of reduced GRF in the absence of prerenal and postrenal causes supports parenchymal renal failure as the cause of reduced urine concentrating ability. *Caution: Water deprivation studies should not be performed on azotemic patients.*

DIETARY MANAGEMENT OF CHRONIC RENAL FAILURE

Conservative Medical Management of Renal Failure

Conservative medical management of CRF consists of symptomatic and supportive therapy designed to correct deficits and excesses in fluid, electrolyte, acid-base, endocrine, and nutritional balance and thereby minimize the clinical and pathological consequences of reduced renal function. The components of conservative medical management are outlined in Table 8-4. Diet therapy should be viewed as one component in the overall scheme of conservative medical management of renal failure. Details concerning nondietary components of conservative medical management of renal failure have been described elsewhere.[15,16,17,18]

Rationale of Diet Therapy

While a direct cause and effect relationship has not been proved in many instances, it is a well-accepted fact that retained protein catabolites contribute significantly to production of uremic signs and many of the laboratory abnormalities found in patients with renal failure. Catabolism of protein results in a variety of nitrogenous and nonnitrogenous waste products, including urea, creatinine, guanidinosuccinic acid, methylguanidine, hydrogen ions, potassium, phosphate, sulfate, and many others (Table 8-2). Many proteinaceous waste products are excreted primarily by glomerular filtration. Thus, patients with primary renal failure have an impaired ability to excrete protein catabolites because of marked reduction in glomerular filtration rate. Retention of metabolic waste may be further aggravated by alterations in tubular secretion and by extrarenal factors that cause a reduction in renal perfusion or increased catabolism of body tissues or both.

The rationale for nutritional management of patients with primary renal failure is based on the premise that controlled reduction of nonessential proteins will result in decreased production of nitrogenous wastes with consequent amelioration of clinical signs. This hypothesis has been supported by results of studies in dogs with experimental renal failure.[19] By formulating diets that contain a reduced quantity of high quality protein and adequate nonprotein calories, many of the signs associated with uremia may be reduced in severity or eliminated, even though renal function remains unchanged.

Indications for Diet Therapy

There are at least three potential benefits that may result from dietary protein restriction: (1) the quantity of proteinaceous waste products ("uremic toxins") in the body will be reduced, (2) progression of CRF may be delayed or stopped, and (3) abnormalities of divalent ion metabolism leading to renal secondary hyperparathyroidism and renal osteodystrophy may be minimized as a result of reduced dietary phosphorus (reduced-protein diets are generally also reduced-phosphorus diets). The major potential disadvantage of dietary protein restriction is protein malnutrition. Other less significant disadvantages of protein restriction are reduced palatability and inconvenience.

Influence of Dietary Protein Intake on Progression of Renal Failure. ***The Progressive Nature of Renal Failure.*** In some mammalian species, once a threshold loss of renal function has occurred, progression to end-stage renal failure invariably follows, regardless of whether the initiating cause of renal dysfunction persists. Removal of approximately 75 percent or more of functional renal tissue in rats results in a syndrome of progressive azotemia, proteinuria, arterial hypertension, and eventual death due to uremia.[20,21] In human beings with renal disease, renal insufficiency regularly progresses to end-stage renal failure without apparent regard to the initiating cause of renal damage.[20–22]

Clinical impression suggests that canine CRF spontaneously progresses in much the same way as that observed in rats and human beings. Most dogs with CRF eventually die or are euthanized as a result of uremia or its complications. However, conclusive data documenting the progressive nature of spontaneous canine renal failure is not yet available. Long-term studies of dogs with experimentally reduced renal mass have failed to document progressive deterioration of renal function during periods of 40 weeks to 48 months.[23,19] Therefore, the question as to whether spontaneous deterioration of renal function occurs in dogs in a fashion analogous to that observed in rats with reduced renal mass remains unresolved.

Modifying the Progressive Nature of Renal Failure. Recent studies in rats suggest that the progressive nature of renal failure may be modified by at least two dietary factors: protein and phosphorus. Consumption of normal or high protein diets by rats with experimental renal failure is associated with altered renal function, renal structure, and proteinuria. These physiologic and pathologic changes are associated with progressive deterioration of renal function, and, ultimately, death due to complications of the uremic syndrome. In contrast, development of proteinuria, renal structural lesions, and progressive deterioration of renal function may be largely prevented when rats are fed reduced-protein diets.[20–22,24–26]

Considerable data has been gathered in an attempt to ascertain the influence of protein intake on progression of renal failure in human beings with CRF. While results of these studies are not yet conclusive, available data strongly support a beneficial role of dietary protein restriction in slowing or preventing progression of CRF. In virtually every study in patients with renal failure where low-protein diets were prescribed, there appears to be a reduction in the rate of progression of renal failure.

Data on the influence of diet on progression of renal failure in dogs are lacking. However, data are available which demonstrate that some of the physiologic effects of protein restriction recognized in rats and people, including reduced glomerular hyperfiltration (see below) and reduced proteinuria, also occur in an analogous fashion in dogs.

The Hyperfiltration Theory. Studies in a variety of species, including dogs, have demonstrated that dietary protein has a direct effect on renal function. Increased protein consumption is associated with enhanced renal blood flow and glomerular filtration rate (GFR), whereas reduced protein consumption is associated with reductions in these functions. Dietary protein-enhancement of renal function appears to be mediated by hormonal mechanisms.

It has been shown that protein consumption also influences filtration rates in remaining functional nephrons of dogs and cats with experimental renal failure. Single nephron GFR (SNGFR) is enhanced when dietary protein intake is increased and is reduced when protein intake is reduced. When SNGFR exceeds levels found in normal kidneys, the increase is termed *hyperfiltration*. When high-protein diets are fed to dogs or rats with CRF, SNGFR of many functional nephrons exceed levels found in normal kidneys, yet total GFR remains reduced from normal because the total number of nephrons contributing to overall GFR is reduced.

It has been hypothesized that hyperfiltration may be responsible for the development of proteinuria and glomerular lesions in rats with reduced renal mass; thereby hyperfiltration serves as a link between high dietary protein intake and progression of renal failure. It is thought that sustained hyperfiltration resulting from consumption of high protein diets may damage the glomerular microvasculature, leading to increased passage of macromolecules into the glomerular mesangium and urinary space. The net result is proteinuria and mesangial proliferation leading to glomerular sclerosis. Hyperfiltration may therefore serve as the final common pathway for progression of renal failure after a threshold reduction in renal mass. Low-protein diets are thought to protect against progression of renal failure by mitigating the hemodynamic alterations resulting from high-protein intake.

High-Protein Diets versus the Canine Kidney. It has been proposed that "normal" and even high-protein diets are beneficial for dogs with early renal failure, because they sustain maximum renal function.[27] However, there is no clinical or experimental evidence to support the contention that sustaining maximum renal function by feeding high-protein diets is necessary or beneficial. The extent to which maximum function is sustained is dictated by physiologic requirements; artificially stimulating maximum function while increasing the excretory requirements of the failing kidneys appears to be illogical. In fact, studies indicate that consumption of high-protein diets by patients with early to moderate renal failure may be associated with increased retention of some uremic toxins, despite enhancement of renal function.

In contrast to studies in rats, long-term studies of dogs with experimentally reduced renal functions have generally not demonstrated progressive deterioration of renal function, regardless of whether high- or low-protein diets were fed. These findings have been interpreted to mean that dogs differ from rats in that no obvious association exists between consumption of high-protein diets and progressive deterioration of renal function. However, these studies failed to rule out the possibility that progressive nephron destruction occurred and that renal function remained stable as a result of functional modification (increased hyperfiltration) in remaining nephrons. If this were the case, progressive deterioration in overall GFR might not occur until the capacity of residual nephrons to undergo compensatory hyperfiltration is exceeded.

There is evidence that beneficial effects of reduced protein intake similar to those observed in rats with diminished renal function may also occur in dogs. As previously described, dogs fed reduced-protein diets have reduced glomerular hyperfiltration and reduced proteinuria. In addition, studies in our laboratory have demonstrated that glomerular lesions similar to those observed in uremic rats fed high-protein diets occur in dogs with reduced renal function. Furthermore, these lesions are more severe in dogs with demonstrable hyperfiltration.

In summary, available data do not conclusively demonstrate a protective effect of dietary protein restriction against progression of CRF. However, a beneficial role for dietary protein restriction is suggested by physiologic and pathologic findings in dogs with CRF. Additional studies are required before firm conclusions can be stated regarding the beneficial role of dietary protein restriction in preventing spontaneous progression of canine CRF.

Recommendations. Reduced-protein diets are clearly indicated for dogs with moderate to severe CRF that are azotemic, hyperphosphatemic, and not anorectic. Justification for use of these diets in this category of patients is based primarily on the need to control the clinical signs of uremia. Prescribing modified-protein diets for dogs with CRF which do not require reduction in their dietary protein intake for control of uremia remains controversial. We currently recommend that owners of azotemic dogs with CRF be offered the option of electing dietary protein restriction for their pet, regardless of the magnitude of the dog's azotemia. However, the decision as to whether modified-protein diets should be considered for use based solely on their potential for slowing progression of renal functional deterioration remains a matter of personal opinion.

Goals of Diet Therapy

The goals of diet therapy for patients with chronic primary renal failure are to: (1) ameliorate clinical signs of uremia by reducing production of protein catabolites, (2) minimize electrolyte, vitamin, and mineral disturbances associated with excessive consumption of protein and certain minerals, (3) supply daily protein, calorie, and mineral requirements, and (4) modify spontaneous progression of renal failure, if possible.

Modification of diets to minimize deficits and excesses of metabolites associated with generalized renal dysfunction is not an all-or-none phenomenon. The best results are achieved when other components of conservative medical management are also utilized. While diet therapy is often of value in controlling some of the polysystemic disturbances associated with uremia, it is not a panacea that can be expected to control or modify all dysfunctions associated with primary renal failure.

Methods of Diet Therapy

Protein Intake. ***Protein Requirements for Dogs with Renal Failure.*** The minimum requirement for high-biological-value protein for normal dogs has been reported to be approximately 1.25 to 1.75 g/kg body wt/day.[28,29,30] Optimum protein and amino acid requirements have not been established for dogs with CRF. Based on the assumption that nonessential amino acids could be synthesized using ammonium derived from urea nitrogen in the intestines, it has been suggested that patients with CRF may have reduced protein requirements.[31,32] However, current data suggests that intestinal urea nitrogen is not significantly utilized for protein synthesis in uremic human beings.[33–37]

There is evidence in humans and rats that protein requirements for uremic individuals may be greater than those for normal individuals.[38,33,39] Uremia is characterized by a catabolic state induced by a variety of endocrine and metabolic derangements.[40–43] Protein and amino acid requirements of uremic patients may be altered by a variety of pathophysiologic disturbances characteristic of the uremic syndrome, including any combination of the following: (1) glucose intolerance; (2) impaired intestinal absorption of amino acids; (3) impaired renal tubular reabsorption of amino acids; (4) decreased activities of intestinal dipeptidases and disaccharidases, which may result in impaired digestion of proteins and carbohydrates; (5) elevated serum concentrations of some hormones, such as glucagon, somatotropin, and parathyroid hormone.[39] In addition, acidosis may be associated with urea production, and total body potassium depletion (which may occur especially in anorectic renal failure patients) may promote protein catabolism.[30] Protein requirements may also be increased by external losses of protein, including albuminuria, hematuria, and gastrointestinal hemorrhage.

When dogs with a moderate degree of CRF were fed a diet containing 1.25 g of cooked egg protein/kg body wt/day for 40 weeks, clinical and laboratory evidence of malnutrition characterized by hypoalbuminemia, anemia, weight loss, and reduced body tissue mass developed.[44] In this same study, dogs fed 3.6 g of protein/kg body wt/day did not develop clinical or biochemical evidence of protein malnutrition. Studies performed in our laboratory have indicated that reduction of dietary protein intake from 2.0 to 0.7 g of protein/kg body wt/day may be associated with varying degrees of protein malnutrition, the severity of which is related to the degree of protein restriction. However, reduced consumption of dietary protein also consistently resulted in a proportional reduction of serum urea nitrogen concentrations. In a subsequent study, dogs with moderate CRF (mean serum creatinine concentration = 3.2 mg/dl) were fed 2.0 g of protein/kg body wt/day for 16 weeks without developing detectable evidence of protein malnutrition.

Because normal control dogs were not used in these studies, it is not possible to conclude that dogs with CRF require more protein than normal dogs. However, results of this study emphasize that excessive dietary protein restriction may be associated with development of protein malnutrition. Furthermore, these studies have indicated that maximum protein restriction (i.e., 1.25 g or less of high-biological-value protein/kg body wt/day) is not required for therapeutic efficacy in all dogs with CRF.

Recommended Dietary Protein Intake for Dogs with CRF. We currently recommend that dogs with mild to moderate CRF (mean serum creatinine concentration = 1.5 to approximately 4.5 mg/dl) be fed approximately 2.0 to 2.2 g of high-biological-value protein/kg body wt/day. However, we emphasize the intrinsic variability of protein requirements of normal dogs and the probable varied influence of uremia on protein requirements of uremic dogs. Therefore, dietary protein should be adjusted to meet the individual needs of the patient. If evidence of protein malnutrition occurs (hypoalbuminemia, anemia, weight loss, or loss of body tissue mass), dietary protein should gradually be increased until these abnormalities are corrected. Serial assessment of the patient's renal function and nutritional status is an integral component of diet therapy.

If diets designed to provide 2.0 g of protein/kg body wt/day do not result in amelioration of the clinical and biochemical manifestations of uremia, dietary protein intake may be cautiously reduced further. The decision to reduced dietary protein further must be based primarily on clinical assessment of the patient. *Dietary protein should not be reduced for the sole purpose of attaining a prescribed reduction in serum urea nitrogen concentration*! The goal of therapy in patients with advanced uremia should be to achieve the best attainable compromise between dietary control of the biochemical and clinical manifestations of uremia and prevention of malnutrition.

Caloric Intake. Dietary energy is as important as dietary protein for maintenance of nitrogen balance and prevention of protein malnutrition. Modification of diets for treatment of chronic primary polyuric renal failure should encompass provision of adequate calories in addition to reduction of protein. Caloric intake should be adjusted to optimize protein anabolism.

Minimum daily requirements for calories, carbohydrates, and fats have not been established for dogs with CRF. Because this information is unavailable, it has been necessary to make the unproved assumption that minimum requirements for these nutrients are the same as those that are required by normal dogs. Accordingly, most nephrologists have recommended that dogs receive 70 to 110 kcal/kg body wt/day. Since carbohydrate, fat, and caloric requirements for uremic dogs may be affected by metabolic disturbances characteristic of the uremic syndrome (including glucose intolerance, maldigestion, and elevated serum insulin and glucagon concentrations), these values should be used as guidelines only. Determination of caloric requirements should be individualized to patient needs, based on serial determinations of body weight. Unless the patient is markedly obese and weight reduction is deemed necessary, an attempt should be made to maintain stable body weight. If the patient is malnourished, caloric intake should be increased for an appropriate period.

Vitamins. ***Water-Soluble Vitamins.*** Uremic human beings have a tendency to develop deficiencies of water-soluble vitamins, especially folate, ascorbate, and pyridoxine.[45] This tendency to develop vitamin deficiencies is most apparent in patients with poor dietary intakes. Minimum daily requirements for water-soluble vitamins have not been established for dogs with renal failure. However, based on results of studies in uremic human beings, the possibility that vitamin deficiencies may develop in uremic dogs must be considered. Because of this concern, we recommend that B-complex and C vitamin supplements be administered to dogs with CRF, particularly during periods of reduced food consumption.

Vitamin D. Progressive loss of renal mass is associated with impaired conversion of vitamin D precursors to their most active form (1,25-vitamin D). Even though the need for oral or parenteral administration of 1,25-vitamin D increases as renal function decreases, oral or parenteral administration of vitamin D without consideration of serum and dietary concentrations of calcium and phosphorus is extremely hazardous. Therapeutic elevation of the plasma concentration of calcium in patients with hyperphosphatemia may result in soft tissue calcification and further deterioration of renal function. Therefore, supplementation of the diet with vitamin D must be carefully individualized to the patient.

Vitamin A. Although the minimum daily requirement for vitamin A has not been determined for dogs with CRF, human patients with renal failure often develop an excess of vitamin A.[39] Excess vitamin A may directly or indirectly increase parathormone release and therefore aggravate renal osteodystrophy and acidosis.[47]

Phosphorus Intake. ***Adverse Effects of Excessive Phosphorus Intake.*** Dietary phosphorus is absorbed from the gastrointestinal tract and excreted primarily by the kidneys via glomerular filtration. In patients with CRF, reduced glomerular filtration rate results in phosphorus retention and subsequent hyperphosphatemia. Hyperphosphatemia is a primary cause of renal secondary hyperparathyroidism, which in turn promotes renal osteodystrophy and soft tissue calcification. In addition, parathyroid hormone (PTH) appears to be a uremic toxin which may contribute to neurotoxicity, anemia, hemorrhagic diathesis, susceptibility to infection, and a variety of other disorders characteristic of the uremic syndrome.[7]

It has also been proposed that excessive dietary phosphorus intake may predispose to progression of renal failure. Studies performed in rats with experimentally induced CRF suggest that dietary phosphorus restriction may prevent proteinuria, renal calcification, renal histologic alterations, and the renal functional deterioration and death due to uremia which occur when higher-phosphorus diets are fed.[48] However, the precise role of dietary phosphorus in the progression of renal dysfunction in rats with experimental renal failure is currently unresolved, in part because the extent of phosphorus restriction used in this and similar studies caused phosphate depletion.

Studies performed in cats with experimentally induced renal failure revealed that normal dietary phosphorus consumption was associated with microscopic evidence of renal mineralization, fibrosis, and mononuclear cell infiltration.[49] Restriction of dietary phosphorus prevented these abnormalities. However, evidence of renal functional deterioration was not detected in either normal or restricted-phosphorus groups.

The role of phosphorus in the progression of renal failure in dogs is unclear. Results of long-term studies of dogs with mild to moderate renal failure indicate that normal dietary phosphorus intake does not appear to be associated with progressive renal dysfunction.[19,23]

Recommendations for Phosphorus Intake in Dogs with CRF. It is desirable to attempt to normalize phosphorus balance in patients with CRF in order to minimize hyperparathyroidism (and possibly to retard the progression of renal failure). Therapeutic options include (1) maintaining body fluid balance, blood vascular volume, and renal perfusion; (2) feeding reduced-protein/reduced-phosphorus diets; (3) enhancing intestinal loss of phosphorus by administering nonabsorbable phosphorus-binding agents; and/or (4) a combination of these techniques.

We prefer to utilize reduced-protein/reduced-phosphorus diets in properly hydrated patients. This therapy is supplemented with phosphorus-binding agents if diet alone fails to normalize serum phosphorus concentrations. We do not recommend use of intestinal phosphorus-binding agents unless dietary restriction has failed to reduce serum phosphorus concentrations to normal. Our preference for dietary management is related to the fact that most oral phosphorus-binding agents (except capsules) are poorly tolerated by dogs and owners. In addition, the use of oral phosphorus-binding agents requires greater patient monitoring to prevent hypophosphatemia and other complications. Severe hypophosphatemia can produce debility, weakness, and anorexia, which may be confused with signs of uremic syndrome. Some phosphorus-binding agents may be less effective than was initially thought. Administration of 1,500 to 2,500 mg of aluminum carbonate to dogs with moderate CRF failed to consistently correct hyperphosphatemia when dogs were fed diets containing greater than 1.0 percent phosphorus on a dry matter basis.[50] Aluminum oxide has been found to be more effective than aluminum hydroxide or aluminum carbonate in phosphorus-binding agents in dogs.[51] However, this product is not currently available because of production and marketing difficulties.

Phosphorus restriction should clearly be employed to achieve normal serum phosphorus concentrations; however, the degree to which dietary phosphorus must be reduced to prevent the adverse effects of phosphorus retention is unknown. Some nephrologists have suggested that perhaps phosphorus intake should be restricted sufficiently to maintain normal renal tubular reabsorption of phosphorus. This magnitude of reduction would require extremely low phosphorus intakes, which might result in phosphorous depletion. Pending the results of further studies, we prefer to attempt to normalize serum phosphorus concentration. Phosphorus consumption and/or the dosage of oral phosphorus binder should be adjusted in response to results of serial determinations of serum phosphorus concentrations. Samples obtained for determinations of serum phosphorus concentration should be collected after a 12-hour fast to avoid postprandial influence.

Available oral phosphorus-binding agents include aluminum hydroxide and aluminum carbonate. These agents should be mixed with the food to achieve optimum benefit. Dosage of these drugs should be individualized to patient needs. An initial dose of 30 to 90 mg/kg/day is recommended. The effect should be monitored by serial evaluation of serum phosphorus concentrations at 10- to 14-day intervals until the desired effect is achieved. Constipation, a common side effect, may require laxative therapy.

Dietary Sodium. ***Rationale for Increased Sodium Intake.*** In the past, high-sodium diets were recommended for dogs with CRF because: (1) sodium-induced diuresis was hypothesized to minimize tubular reabsorption of potential uremic toxins, (2) pathologic sodium-wasting was thought to routinely accompany generalized renal dysfunction, mandating therapeutic sodium replacement; and (3) reduced sodium intake might promote metabolic acidosis in dogs with CRF by reducing renal tubular capacity to reabsorb bicarbonate. Results of pilot studies performed in our laboratory support the concept that high-sodium intakes (approximately 1,200 mg sodium/100 g dry wt) may enhance urinary excretion of nitrogenous waste products and thereby decrease the magnitude of azotemia.

It has recently been shown that increased urinary fractional excretion of sodium in dogs with one form of experimentally induced CRF is a compensatory physiologic response to sodium intake rather than an obligatory pathologic loss of sodium associated with renal dysfunction.[3] Whether or not this data can be extrapolated to dogs with all forms of spontaneously occurring renal failure has not yet been determined. However, certain forms of renal disease recognized in human beings (especially diseases that affect primarily the renal medulla) may be associated with a pathologic, irreversible sodium-wasting tendency.

Pilot studies performed in our laboratory have not revealed substantial metabolic acidosis when diets containing 250 mg sodium/100 g of dry food were fed to dogs with moderate experimental CRF. (Typical sodium content for commercial canned dog foods is 750 mg sodium/100 g dry wt). Whether or not clinically significant metabolic acidosis would result from more profound dietary sodium restriction is unknown.

Sodium and Hypertension. In humans, hypertension is an established cause of renal dysfunction and may aggravate the polysystemic signs of uremia. In addition, hypertension may be a major factor involved in self-perpetuation of renal failure. It has recently been recognized that high sodium intake may contribute to hypertension in dogs with CRF.[15] The role of hypertension in development and progression of renal dysfunction in dogs is currently under investigation.

Recommendations—Sodium Intake. Because of the apparent link between sodium intake, hypertension, and renal disease, we recommend that dogs with CRF be fed normal- (as opposed to high-) or restricted-sodium diets. The establishment of sodium requirements for dogs with polyuric CRF will have to be based on future controlled experimental and clinical studies designed to evaluate sodium balance and its impact on hypertension and hypertension-related complications associated with chronic primary renal failure. Until such data becomes available, dietary sodium should be individualized on the basis of knowledge of current disease processes (e.g., hypertension, congestive heart failure, hypoproteinemia, edema, and so on) and response to modification of dietary sodium intake.

Dietary sodium may be modified in an attempt to achieve the following goals: (1) minimize or prevent sodium-associated hypertension, (2) prevent negative sodium balance and volume depletion, and (3) avoid inducing metabolic acidosis. *Changes in sodium intake should always be made gradually.* Patients with CRF may adapt to a wide range of dietary consumption patterns; however, adaptation occurs gradually. Abrupt changes in dietary sodium may be associated with transient imbalances between intake and urinary loss. Sudden reduction in dietary sodium may reduce extracellular fluid volume, which in turn may lead to poor renal perfusion and further reduction in renal function. We recommend that changes in dietary sodium be made over at least a 2-week period.

The response to adjustments in dietary sodium may be determined by monitoring body weight, hydration, renal function, and acid-base status during and for several weeks after reducing dietary sodium. Progressive loss of body weight, progressive azotemia, and/or dehydration suggest that the patient may be unable to adapt to reduced sodium intake. In this event, a more gradual and lesser reduction of sodium intake may be considered.

Monitoring Diet Therapy

Before initiating diet therapy, the patient's renal function, nutritional status, the need for supplemental therapy (e.g., sodium bicarbonate therapy for acidosis, calcium supplementation for hypocalcemia, and anabolic steroid therapy for anemia) should be evaluated. Minimum patient evaluation should include: physical examination; subjective evaluation of nutritional status and hydration; determination of body weight, serum creatinine, urea nitrogen, albumin, calcium, and phosphorus concentrations; plasma bicarbonate concentration or total CO_2 content; complete blood count; and urinalysis. This evaluation should be repeated at appropriate intervals. Initially, we routinely recommend monthly evaluations after initiating diet therapy. Patient reevaluation at regular intervals is necessary to assess the response to therapy. Diet formulation and other forms of symptomatic and supportive therapy may be altered on the basis of these reevaluations.

COMPLICATIONS OF DIET THERAPY

Protein Malnutrition

Inadequate protein nutrition is probably the most significant potential adverse effect associated with feeding low-protein diets. In our experience, protein malnutrition has not been a substantial problem when dogs with CRF are fed 2.0 or more g of high-biological-value protein/kg body wt/day. However, dogs fed less than this quantity of protein may develop clinical and laboratory evidence of protein deficiency. Signs of protein malnutrition include: (1) reduced muscle mass, (2) progressive loss of body weight, and (3) progressive reductions in packed cell volumes and/or serum albumin concentrations. If malnutrition is detected prior to or after initiating diet therapy, consideration should be given to increasing dietary protein intake. Conversely, if diet therapy does not result in amelioration of clinical signs of uremia, consideration may be given to further reducing protein intake. Reductions in dietary protein intake, however, should only be undertaken after considering the potential adverse nutritional effects of this action. It is sometimes necessary to seek a balance between the adverse nutritional effects and the beneficial clinical effects of protein restriction.

Anorexia in Renal Failure

Anorexia and poor appetite are common impediments to successful conservative medical management of dogs with CRF. The pathogenesis of anorexia in uremic patients has not been fully elucidated; however, it appears to result, at least in part, from retention of uremic toxins. The hypothesis that retained uremic toxins contribute to anorexia is supported by the observations that modified-protein diets and/or dialysis improve or correct anorexia. Studies in dogs indicate that anorexia may occur in association with stimulation of the medullary emetic chemoreceptor trigger zone by uremic toxins.[52] Ablation of this area in nephrectomized dogs suppressed the onset of anorexia. Altered taste perception may also contribute to anorexia.

Treatment of anorexia may involve (1) feeding several smaller meals throughout the day, (2) enhancing the palatability of the diet, or (3) pharmacologic appetite stimulation. Feeding several smaller meals rather than a single large meal generally increases daily food consumption. In addition, the timing of feeding may influence consumption. Despite an initially good appetite, uremic humans sometimes experience nausea and loss of appetite after starting to eat breakfast. These same patients are often able to eat later in the day without developing nausea and anorexia. Some dogs appear to experience a similar syndrome of waxing and waning appetite throughout the day. By offering fresh food several times each day, the probability of encountering an interval during which the appetite is good is enhanced. As noted above, observations in humans suggest that failure to consume a meal after showing initial interest should not necessarily be interpreted as a palatability problem; it may represent food-induced nausea or anorexia which may not persist throughout the day.

Diets containing reduced quantities of protein and sodium are often unpalatable. Palatability may be enhanced by warming the food to create an appetizing aroma; the food should not be served hot. The food can also be flavored with small quantities of meat, animal fat, or other flavor enhancers. However, avoid creating nutritional imbalances by adding excessive quantities of these substances (e.g., addition of too much meat may increase dietary protein consumption, promoting uremia; excessive addition of fat may reduce dietary protein content, thereby promoting protein malnutrition). Sometimes palatability can be improved by fomulating homemade diets based on known dietary preferences of the patient.

As a general rule, we prefer to attempt to stimulate eating by the methods described above before attempting pharmacologic management. Treatment with drugs designed to stimulate the appetite is generally reserved for patients that have failed to respond to more conservative forms of therapy or for patients developing malnutrition as a result of chronic lack of appetite.

Diazepam and other benzodiazepines have been used successfully as appetite stimulants in a variety of animal species, including dogs and cats.[53] In uncontrolled clinical trials in uremic dogs and cats, we have used diazepam as an appetite stimulant with variable success. In some cases, a dramatic improvement in food consumption has followed initiation of diazepam therapy. The onset of eating is rapid, but the duration of effect from an individual dose is brief.

The recommended dosage of diazepam in anorectic cats is 0.05 to 0.4 mg/kg given orally, intravenously, or intramuscularly.[53] Dogs have been reported to require higher doses than cats.[54,55] We have used doses of from 1 to 5 mg given orally one to three times daily. Diazepam is available in 2, 5, and 10 mg scored tablets. It may be used on a short-term basis to initiate eating, then withdrawn if the patient continues to eat spontaneously. Sometimes the drug must be continued long-term to sustain adequate food consumption.

Diazepam is metabolized in the liver to active metabolites, which are excreted in the urine. Diazepam and other benzodiazepines are usually well tolerated by humans and dogs with renal failure; when used for sedation, the dosage is generally not reduced.[56] However, administration to patients with renal failure may lead to excessive sedation, as well as other central nervous system side effects.[56] Sedation and ataxia have been noted in some of our patients. Because the efficacy may be best at higher doses and because renal failure patients may be more sensitive to the sedative effects of these drugs, it may be necessary to seek a balance between these effects, based on patient response.

Although administered primarily for treatment of the anemia of CRF, anabolic steroids have been advocated as appetite stimulants for dogs with renal failure. In a recent study designed to evaluate the efficacy of one anabolic steroid in treatment of dogs with experimental renal failure, the anabolic steroid tested did not appear to enhance food consumption.[57] Clinical studies designed to evaluate the effectiveness of this and other anabolic steroids in promoting appetite in dogs with spontaneous CRF have apparently not been performed.

REFERENCES

1. Cowgill LD: Diseases of the kidney. p. 1793. In Ettinger S, Textbook of Veterinary Internal Medicine. 2nd Ed. Philadelphia, WB Saunders, 1983
2. Bourgoignie JJ, Kaplan M, Pincus J, et al: Renal handling of potassium in dogs with chronic renal insufficiency. Kidney Int 20:482, 1981
3. Schmidt RW, Bourgoignie JJ, Bricker NS: On the adaptation in sodium excretion in chronic uremia: The effects of proportional reduction of sodium intake. J Clin Invest 53:1736, 1974
4. Wagnild JP, Wen S-F: Sodium transport in dogs with acute remnant and glomerulonephritic kidneys. J Lab Clin Med 91:911, 1978
5. Bricker NS, Fine LG: The renal response to progressive nephron loss. p. 1056. In Brenner BM, Rector FC, The Kidney. WB Saunders, Philadelphia, 1981
6. Finco DR: The role of phosphorus restriction in the management of chronic renal failure in the dog and cat. p. 131. 7th Annual Kal Kan Symposium for the Treatment of Small Animal Diseases, Columbus, OH, 1983
7. Massry SG: The toxic effects of parathyroid hormone in uremia. Semin Nephrol 3:306, 1983
8. Finco DR: Clinical evaluation of renal function. p. 95. 7th Annual Kal Kan Symposium for the Treatment of Small Animal Diseases, Columbus, OH, 1983
9. Bovee KC, Joyce T: Endogenous creatinine clearance in the dog. J Am Vet Med Assoc 174:488, 1979
10. Finco DR, Coulter DB, Barsanti JA: Procedure for a simple method of measuring glomerular filtration rate in the dog. J Am Anim Hosp Assoc 18:804, 1982
11. Finco DR: Kidney Function. p. 337. In Kaneko JJ (ed): Clinical Biochemistry of Domestic Animals. 3rd Ed. Academic Press New York, 1980
12. Finco DR: Simultaneous determination of phenosulfonphthalein excretion and endogenous creatinine clearance in the normal dog. J Am Vet Med Assoc 159:336, 1971
13. Hardy RM: Disorders of water metabolism. Vet Clin North Am 12:353, 1982
14. Hardy RM, Osborne CA: Water deprivation test in the dog. Maximal normal values. J Am Vet Med Assoc 174:479, 1979
15. Cowgill LD, Kallet AJ: Recognition and management of hypertension in the dog. p. 1025. In Kirk RW (ed): Current Veterinary Therapy VIII. Philadelphia, WB Saunders, 1983
16. Polzin DJ, Osborne CA: Update—Conservative medical management of chronic

renal failure. In Kirk RW (ed): Current Veterinary Therapy IX. Philadelphia, WB Saunders, (In press)
17. Polzin DJ, Osborne CA: Diseases of the urinary tract. p. 333. In Davis L: Manual of Therapeutics in Small Animal Practice. Churchill Livingstone, New York, 1985
18. Polzin DJ, Osborne CA: Conservative medical management of canine chronic polyuric renal failure. p. 997. In Kirk RW (ed): Current Veterinary Therapy VIII. Philadelphia, WB Saunders, 1983
19. Polzin DJ, Osborne CA, Hayden DW, Stevens JB: Influence of reduced protein diets on morbidity, mortality, and renal function in dogs with induced chronic renal failure. Am J Vet Res 45:506, 1984
20. Hostetter TH, Olson JL, Renke HG, et al: Hyperfiltration in remnant nephrons: A potentially adverse response to renal ablation. Am J Physiol 241:F85, 1981
21. Hostetter TH, Brenner BM: Glomerular adaptations to renal injury. p. 1. In Brenner BM, Stein JH (eds): Contemporary Issues In Nephrology. 7. Chronic Renal Failure. Churchill Livingstone, New York, 1981
22. Hostetter TH, Renke HG, Brenner BM: Compensatory renal hemodynamic injury: A final common pathway of residual nephron destruction. Am J Kidney Dis 1:310, 1982
23. Bovee KC, Kronfeld DS, Bomberg C, et al: Long-term measurement of renal function in partially nephrectomized dogs fed 56, 27 or 19% protein. Invest Urol 16:378, 1979
24. Olson JL, Hostetter TH, Renke HG, et al: Altered glomerular permselectivity and progressive sclerosis following extreme ablation of renal mass. Kidney Int 22:112, 1982
25. Purkerson ML, Hoffsten PE, Klahr S: Pathogenesis of the glomerulopathy associated with renal infarction in rats. Kidney Int 9:47, 1976
26. Shimamura T, Morrison AB: A progressive glomerulosclerosis occurring in partial five-sixth nephrectomized rats. Am J Pathol 79:95, 1975
27. Kronfeld DS, Bovee KC: Geriatric diets for dogs. Compend Con Ed 5:136, 1983
28. Corbin JE, Lehrer WP, Newberne PM, et al: Nutrient requirements of domestic animals: Nutritional requirements of dogs. No. 8. Nat Acad Sci, Nat Res Coun, Washington, DC, 1972
29. Morris ML, Doering GG: Dietary management of renal failure in dogs. Canine Pract 5:46, 1978
30. Rice EE, Allison JB, Corbin JE, et al: Nutrient requirements of domestic animals: Nutrient requirements of dogs. Nat Acad Sci, Nat Res Coun, Publ 989, Washington, DC, 1962
31. Bovee KC: The uremic syndrome: Patient evaluation and treatment. Compend Cont Ed 1:279, 1979
32. Giordano C: Use of exogenous and endogenous urea for protein synthesis in normal and uremic subjects. J Lab Clin Med 62:231, 1963
33. Kopple JD, Coburn JW: Metabolic studies of low protein diets in uremia. I. Nitrogen and Potassium. Medicine 52:583, 1973
34. Mitch, WE, Leitman PS, Walser M: Effects of oral neomycin and kanamycin in chronic uremia patients. I. Urea metabolism. Kidney Int 11:116, 1977
35. Pennisi AJ, Wang M, Kopple JD: Effects of protein amino acid diets in chronically uremic and control rats. Kidney Int 13:472, 1978
36. Varcoe AR, Holliday D, Carson ER, et al: Anabolic role of urea in renal failure. Am J Clin Nutr 31:1601, 1978
37. Varcoe AR, et al: Efficiency of utilization of urea nitrogen for albumin synthesis by chronically uremic and normal man. Clin Sci Mol Med 48:379, 1975

38. Delaporete C, Bergstrom J, Broyer M, et al: Variations in muscle cell protein of severely uremic children. Kidney Int 10:239, 1976
39. Walser M, Mitch WE: Dietary management of renal failure. The Kidney 10:13, 1977
40. Abitbol CL, Holiday MA: Effect of energy and nitrogen intake upon urea nitrogen production in children with uremia and undernutrition. Clin Nephrol 10:9, 1978
41. Bagade JD, Yee E, Shafrir E: Evidence for an accelerated adaptation to starvation in chronic uremia. Metabolism 26:1107, 1977
42. Kopple JD, Jones M, Fukuda S, et al: Amino acid and protein metabolism in renal failure. Am J Clin Nutr 31:1532, 1978
43. Walser M: The conservative management of the uremic patient. p. 1613. In Brenner BM, Rector,FC: The Kidney. Philadelphia, WB Saunders Co, 1976
44. Polzin DJ, Osborne CA, Stevens JB, Hayden DW: Influence of modified protein diets on the nutritional status of dogs with induced chronic renal failure. Am J Vet Res 44:1694, 1983
45. Kopple JD: Chronic renal failure: Nutritional and nondialytic management. p. 252. In Glassock RJ (ed): Current Therapy in Nephrology and Hypertension 1984–85. CV Mosby, St. Louis, 1984
46. Osborne CA, Polzin DJ: Strategy in the diagnosis, prognosis, and management of renal disease, renal failure, and uremia. p. 559. Proceedings of the 46th Annual Meeting, Am Anim Hosp Assoc 1979
47. Avioli LV, Tietelbaum SL: The renal osteodystrophies. p. 1542. In Brenner BM, Rector FC: The Kidney. Philadelphia, WB Saunders, 1976
48. Ibels LS, Alfrey AC, Haut L, et al: Preservation of function in experimental renal disease by dietary restriction of phosphate. N Eng J Med 298:122, 1978
49. Ross LA, Finco DR, Crowell WA: Effect of dietary phosphorus restriction on the kidneys of cats with reduced renal mass. Am J Vet Res 43:1023, 1982
50. Finco DR, Crowell WA, Barsanti JA: Effects of three diets on dogs with induced chronic renal failure. Am J Vet Res 46:646, 1985
51. Rutherford WE, Mercado A, Hruska K, et al: An evaluation of a new and effective phosphorus binding agent. Trans Am Soc Artif Intern Organs 19:446, 1973
52. Borison HL, Herbertson LM: Role of medullary emetic chemoreceptor trigger zone in post-nephrectomy vomiting dogs. Am J Physiol 197:850, 1959
53. Macy DW, Gasper PW: Diazepam-induced eating in anorexic cats. J Am Anim Hosp Assoc 21:17, 1985
54. Della Fera MA, Baile CA, McLaughlin CL: Benzodiazepine-like chemicals and feeding behavior in puppies. Physiologist 20:21, 1978
55. Randall LO: Pharmacology of methaminodiazepoxide. Dis Nerv Syst 21:7, 1960
56. Anderson RJ, Bennet WM, Gambertoglio JG, Schreirer RW: Fate of drugs in renal failure. p. 2659. In Brenner BM, Rector FC (eds): The Kidney. Philadelphia, WB Saunders, 1981
57. Finco DR, Barsanti JA, Adams D: Effects of an anabolic steroid on acute uremia in the dog. Am J Vet Res 45:2285, 1984
58. Chew DJ, DiBartola SP: Feline renal amyloidosis. p. 976. In Kirk RW (ed): Current Veterinary Therapy VIII. Philadelphia, WB Saunders, 1983
59. Scott RC: Immune-mediated renal disease. p. 966. In Kirk RW (ed): Current Veterinary Therapy VIII. Philadelphia, WB Saunders, 1983
60. Chew DJ, Capen CC: Hypercalcemic nephropathy and associated disorders. p. 1067. In Kirk RW (ed): Current Veterinary Therapy VII. Philadelphia, WB Saunders, 1980
61. Thornhill JA: Toxic nephropathy. p. 1047. In Kirk RW (ed): Current Veterinary Therapy VII. Philadelphia, WB Saunders, 1980

62. Caywood DD, Osborne CA, Johnston GR: Neoplasms of the canine and feline urinary tracts. p. 1203. In Kirk RW (ed): Current Veterinary Therapy VII. Philadelphia, WB Saunders, 1980
63. Barsanti JA, Finco DR: Management of postrenal uremia. Vet Clin North Am 14:609, 1984
64. Finco DR, Barsanti, JA: Bacterial pyelonephritis. Vet Clin North Am 9:645, 1979
65. Ling GV: Treatment of urinary tract infections with antimicrobial agents. p. 1051. In Kirk RW (ed): Current Veterinary Therapy VIII. Philadelphia, WB Saunders, 1983
66. Greene CE: Leptospirosis. p. 588. In Greene CE (ed): Clinical Microbiology and Infectious Diseases of the Dog and Cat. Philadelphia, WB Saunders, 1984
67. Attleberger MH: Systemic mycoses. p. 1180. In Kirk RW (ed): Current Veterinary Therapy VIII. Philadelphia, WB Saunders, 1983
68. Osborne CA, Abdullahi S, Krawiec DR, et al: Medical dissolution and prevention of canine struvite uroliths. p. 1066. In Kirk RW, (ed), Current Veterinary Therapy VIII. Philadelphia, WB Saunders, 1983

9 Renal Manifestations of Neoplastic Disease

Edward B. Breitschwerdt
Rodney L. Page

Many factors have contributed to the increased longevity of canine and feline companion animals. Nutrition, vaccination, parasite control, general and specialized surgical and medical care, and improved client education represent important factors which have been directly influenced by the veterinary profession. Due to the increased life expectancy of our patients, the category of neoplastic disease has become an increasingly prominent and important aspect of veterinary care.

The purpose of this chapter is to review renal manifestations of neoplastic disease. Cancer may directly or indirectly alter renal structure or function (Table 9-1). The kidney can be directly involved, as with renal carcinoma, nephroblastoma, lymphosarcoma, or other primary or metastatic neoplasias. Glomerulonephritis, amyloidosis, renal tubular dysfunction, acute renal failure, urinary tract infection, and obstructive uropathy represent examples of indirect kidney involvement secondary to neoplastic disease. Renal function can be altered in association with a variety of paraneoplastic syndromes that induce metabolic abnormalities, such as hypercalcemia, blood hyperviscosity, hyponatremia, and others. Finally, nephrotoxicity can occur during cancer treatment with various forms of antineoplastic therapy (Fig. 9-1).

With the exception of primary and metastatic renal neoplasia, few cases documenting indirect renal damage secondary to neoplastic disease, renal involvement in paraneoplastic syndromes, and chemotherapy-induced renal damage have been reported in the dog or cat. For this reason, we will occasionally reference the human literature, where documentation of these problems is more complete. It is our hope that, in addition to reviewing current information, this

Table 9-1. Differential Diagnosis of Intrinsic Renal Disease in Cancer

Tumor infiltration or replacement of parenchyma
Indirect renal involvement
Immune complex glomerulonephritis
Amyloidosis
Renal tubular dysfunction
Acute renal failure
Urinary tract infection
Obstructive uropathy
Renal involvement in paraneoplastic syndromes
Hypercalcemic nephropathy
Hyperviscosity syndromes
Polycythemia
Paraproteinemia
Hyponatremia
Hypernatremia
Hypokalemia
Hyperkalemia
Treatment-related nephropathy
Antineoplastic drugs
Methotrexate
Cisplatin
Streptozotocin
Others
Antibiotics
Aminoglycosides
Radiation nephritis
Immunotherapy

chapter will stimulate the development of prospective clinical studies to address questions regarding the frequency, severity, and pathophysiology of renal involvement in various canine and feline neoplastic diseases.

RENAL NEOPLASIA

The clinical and pathologic spectrum of renal neoplasia is diverse. Many malignant tumors and most benign masses are clinically indolent and diagnostically elusive. The clinical diagnosis is often made late in the natural course of these tumors, when invasion and metastasis have already occurred. The insidious nature of these neoplasms, the nonspecific clinical signs, and the relatively ineffective adjunctive therapy challenge the clinician to earlier detection, since successful treatment can only be accomplished when there is resectable disease.

Tumors involving the kidney are uncommon in animals. Feline renal neoplasia is extremely rare, most reported tumors being lymphosarcoma.[1–3] Canine renal neoplasms occur at a rate of 0.3 to 1.7 percent of all tumors,[1–5] which is very similar to the incidence of human renal neoplasia.[5] The most common renal tumor in dogs is adenocarcinoma; others are carcinoma of unclassified type, nephroblastoma, and various sarcomas.[2,5–8] Benign renal masses include adenoma, angioma, fibroma, and lipoma, as well as renal cysts.

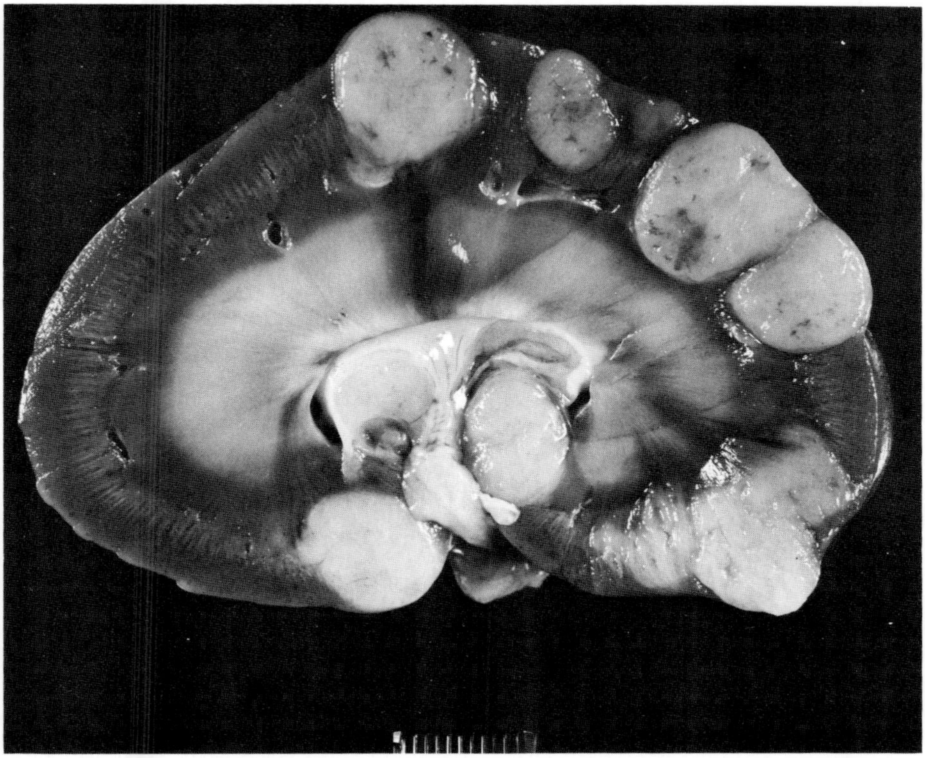

Fig. 9-1. Gross appearance of a kidney obtained at necropsy from a 9-year-old spayed female Labrador retriever with metastases from an anaplastic fibrosarcoma. Depression, polydipsia, and polyuria had existed for 2 weeks. Serum creatinine was normal. Isosthenuria (specific gravity 1.012), proteinuria (2.6 g/24 hr), and glucosuria (negative to 3+ on urine dipstick evaluation) were identified by urinalysis. Renal hisopathology identified glomerular and tubular degeneration. The clinical and pathologic data suggest high output renal failure, protein-losing glomerulopathy, and renal tubular dysfunction secondary to renal metastatic disease. This case illustrates the diversity of renal pathophysiologic mechanisms which might be encountered in animals with neoplastic disease.

Several reviews of renal neoplasia have been published in recent years.[2,6,7] This information will be summarized so as to consider a general description of new diagnostic approaches, relevant prognostic factors, staging systems, and treatment. Tumors of the renal pelvis will not be discussed.

Renal Carcinomas

Table 9-2 summarizes the clinical data from several recent reviews of canine renal neoplasia. There is a remarkably good correlation among these reviews for most information. Approximately 60 to 65 percent of canine renal

Table 9-2. Canine Renal Carcinoma

Study	Percent Carcinomas (# in study)	Sex M:F	Median Age (yr)	Presenting Clinical Signs			Metastasis		
				Abdominal Mass	Anorexia Wt Loss	Hematuria	Incidence	Lung	Liver
Preister & McKay[2]	64.5% (106)	2.3:1	7.9	45%	32%	20%	38%	75%	44%
Fein[8]	60% (10)	1.0:1	9.1	75%	33%	33%	NR	NR	NR
Lucke & Kelly[6]	100% (33)	1.8:1	6.0	22%	33%	22%	77%	85%	20%
Goldschmidt[7]	100% (118)	2.0:1	8.0	NR	NR	<10%	>50%	NR	NR

NR = Not reported.
Reference numbers refer to list at end of chapter.

tumors are carcinomas, which is slightly less than the percentage of human carcinomas of the kidney (85 percent).[9] Male dogs are almost twice as likely to develop renal carcinoma as females. This sex-related tendency is slightly less than that reported in the human literature.[9] The median age of occurrence in dogs is approximately 8 years; both kidneys have equal frequency of carcinoma; and no breed predisposition has been identified.

The biological behavior of renal carcinomas is incompletely understood. It is generally accepted that renal adenocarcinomas develop from the proximal convoluted tubule. Both de novo genesis and transformation from adenomatous hyperplasia have been proposed as pathogenic mechanisms. Specific agents, such as nitrosamines and hormones, have been used in laboratory animals to induce renal carcinomas.[9] In addition, several reports have shown a positive correlation between tobacco smoke and renal carcinomas in people.[9,10] To date, no etiopathogenic event or substance has been associated with canine renal carcinomas. The clinical time course of renal carcinoma in the dog is not known. Numerous reports in the human literature document both rapid progression and death, as well as prolonged survival or spontaneous regression.[10–12] Most cases of canine and human renal carcinoma are extremely invasive and are associated with frequent, widespread metastasis (Table 9-2).

The diagnosis of renal cancer is an intriguing challenge. In 30 to 45 percent of human patients, there are no clinicial signs referrable to the primary tumor.[10] Therefore, the diagnosis is rarely made early in the course of the disease. The earliest clinical manifestations of renal carcinomas are anorexia, weight loss, and a palpable abdominal mass. All recent reports agree that the "classical triad" of signs—hematuria, palpable mass, and flank pain—occur in less than 15 percent of the cases and portend advanced disease.[7,10,12] Gross or microscopic hematuria has been reported in 10 to 33 percent of canine renal neoplasia (Table 9-2). Gross hematuria has been associated with vascular invasion, involvement of the pelvis, or disseminated intravascular coagulopathy secondary to the malignancy.

Unless paraneoplastic syndromes or advanced disease exist, laboratory findings are usually inconclusive or within normal limits. Many paraneoplastic syndromes have been reported in humans with renal carcinomas.[13] These include hypercalcemia, polycythemia, immune complex glomerulonephritis, hepatic dysfunction, and hypertension. Polycythemia has been reported in dogs with renal carcinoma.[14,15] The other syndromes have not yet been reported in association with canine renal carcinoma.

Numerous radiographic and related studies are useful in establishing the diagnosis and prognosis for renal masses. Benign renal cysts are a primary differential of renal neoplasia. A recent review of human cases demonstrated that ultrasound techniques will accurately differentiate benign cysts from renal carcinomas.[16] Computed tomography (CT) also provides noninvasive information regarding tumor invasion of local tissue and vascular structures.[17] CT scans appear to be more accurate than angiography or ultrasound in assessing prognosis and establishing the extent of surgical resection.

Although CT scans and ultrasound equipment are not available to most

Table 9-3. Tumor Stages of Robson et al.[18]

Stages	5-Year Survival Rate (%)
Stage 1—Tumor confined within kidney	60–76
Stage 2—Involvement of perinephric fat	45–65
Stage 3—Involvement of renal vein, vena cava, or lymphatics	35–51
Stage 4—Involvement of adjacent organs or distant metastasis	18

veterinarians, routine and contrast radiographic evaluations can provide valuable diagnostic information. Highly vascular renal masses are likely to be tumors, whereas avascular lesions with smooth borders are probably cysts. Contrast radiographic evaluation of the caudal vena cava may demonstrate vascular invasion in advanced cases and should be regarded as a poor prognostic sign. As in all cases of malignant neoplasia, chest radiographs should be made to rule out pulmonary metastasis.

Further diagnostic, prognostic, and therapeutic information can be obtained only at surgery. If complete resection cannot be accomplished, the prognostic factors that affect the survival of humans include capsular invasion, regional or distant metastasis, and renal vein or vena cava involvement.[10–12]

Clinical staging has been recommended for accurate evaluation of treatment protocols and prognosis. Most cases are staged according to the plan of Robson et al[18] (Table 9-3).

Although total extirpation of the visible neoplastic masses is advantageous, partial nephrectomy has not decreased survival time. Partial nephrectomy may be indicated if tumor-free margins are achievable or if bilateral involvement has occurred.[19] In people, palliative nephrectomy is indicated in the face of distant metastasis if the patient is experiencing severe pain or hemorrhage or if a paraneoplastic endocrinopathy is producing systemic signs. Similar indications seem reasonable for canine or feline renal neoplasia.

Adjunctive therapy following surgery in human patients has been disappointing. Vinblastine sulfate has the highest reported response rate (25 percent) for single or combined agents.[18] Radiation therapy has not altered survival times, although preoperative radiation has delayed recurrence.[20]

Currently, renal neoplasia is a surgical disease. Protocols employing adjuvant therapy are being evaluated. Future protocols may include biologic response modifiers, new chemotherapeutic agents, and radiation therapy in combination with other treatment modalities.

Nephroblastoma (Embryonal Nephroma, Wilms' Tumor)

Nephroblastomas account for approximately 13 to 17 percent of all canine renal tumors.[2,3,7] The tissue components of nephroblastomas arise from combinations of embryonic metanephric blastoma and stromal and epithelial elements. These neoplasms are clinically distinct from other renal tumors in that the median age of occurrence is 8 months. Nephroblastomas are the second most common solid tumor in children.[21] No sex-related predilection has been reported in people or dogs.[7,21]

Canine nephroblastoma has recently been reviewed.[7] According to this review, as well as individual case descriptions, nephroblastomas are highly malignant. The most common clinical sign is abdominal distension (65 percent of all cases). Anorexia, lethargy, and hematuria are also reported. Metastasis is present in the majority of cases at the time of diagnosis, the most frequent metastatic sites being the omentum, lymph nodes, and lungs.

The clinical diagnosis of nephroblastoma is usually not difficult to establish. The age of occurrence, the large anterior abdominal mass, and likely radiographic evidence of pulmonary metastasis support the diagnosis. Differential diagnosis for localized nephroblastomas includes hydronephrosis and polycystic kidneys. Contrast radiographs, ultrasound, or computed tomography can be used to determine the nature of the mass (cystic versus solid) and the extent of disease. Definitive diagnosis requires biopsy.

The prognosis for children with nephroblastoma is based on the tumor size, capsular invasion, lymph node involvement, and distant metastasis.[21,22] In addition, the histologic pattern is of great prognostic value, with 90 percent of the tumors being of "favorable histology."[22] Favorable histology implies well-differentiated elements in all tissues. An unfavorable histology is determined by anaplastic characteristics in any or all of the three cell types *or* a predominantly monotypic, poorly differentiated sarcomatous cell type. No such histologic or clinical correlation has yet been made in veterinary medicine.

Treatment has not been aggressive. Most cases of canine nephroblastomas have been treated with surgical resection only. Aggressive therapy is recommended in children and involves surgery, radiation therapy, and chemotherapy.[21] Complete surgical resection is advised, unless distant metastasis is too extensive or the tumor invades surrounding vital structures. If resection is not possible, radiotherapy markers are placed, and biopsies are obtained. Nephroblastomas are very radiosensitive, and local control of the tumor is enhanced by postoperative radiation. Chemotherapy has dramatically improved survival rates in people with nephroblastomas.[21] Actinomycin D combined with vincristine are the chemotherapeutic agents of choice in human beings. With favorable histology and aggressive therapy, the overall cure rate is 85 to 90 percent, even with disseminated disease.[22] There is one report of prolonged survival of a dog with nephroblastoma following nephrectomy, radiation, and chemotherapy.[23]

Other Primary Renal Neoplasias

A wide variety of tumors have been reported to arise from the canine kidney. Benign neoplasms include hamartoma, hemangioma, lipoma, and adenoma.[2,7,8] Benign tumors of vascular origin may cause hematuria following erosion of large vessels or rupture into the renal collecting system. Other benign masses are generally incidental findings at necropsy.

Malignant mesenchymal tumors of primary renal origin have also been reported.[7,8] It is difficult to prove that tumors originate from the kidney, especially with highly metastatic cancer. A thorough investigation for other primary tumors should be performed. Hemangiosarcomas are one of the most commonly reported primary mesenchymal tumors of the kidney.[7,8] Other sarcomas of renal origin include myxosarcoma, liposarcoma, fibrosarcoma, and lymphosarcoma (Fig. 9-1).

Metastatic and Infiltrative Renal Neoplasia

Metastatic renal disease is reported to be more common than primary renal neoplasia.[24,25] Metastatic renal neoplasia is rarely associated with any specific physical or laboratory findings unless the tumor has reached advanced stages.

Metastasis to the kidney can occur through three mechanisms.[24] Embolization can occur via hematogenous or lymphatic routes, as with secondary carcinomas or sarcomas. Secondly, diffuse renal infiltration is commonly associated with leukemia, lymphoma, and plasma cell neoplasia. Finally, direct invasion can occur from adjacent neoplastic structures (i.e., adrenal glands or pancreas).

The incidence of renal involvement in lymphoproliferative disorders is poorly characterized in the dog. It is difficult to diagnose lymphomatous renal involvement, since only a small percentage of patients have laboratory evidence or clinical signs suggestive of renal disease. In large human autopsy studies, a lymphoid infiltrate was found in the kidneys of 67 percent of patients with acute leukemia and 46 percent of patients with non-Hodgkin's lymphoma.[24]

Neoplasms originating from many areas of the body spread as discrete emboli. Metastatic osteosarcoma, hemangiosarcoma, mast cell tumor, and malignant melanoma are often found in the canine kidney.[7] Epithelial tumors which spread to the kidney most often arise from lungs, mammary gland, intestine, or the contralateral kidney.[7,25]

Feline Renal Neoplasia

The rate of primary renal cancer in cats is extremely low and is reported to be approximately half the canine renal cancer rate.[3] There have been isolated reports of feline renal neoplasms and a recent review.[23] However, there is a paucity of information regarding the clinical and pathologic behavior of these tumors. Of 43 primary tumors, approximately 40 percent were renal carcinomas, 20 percent were nephroblastomas, and 40 percent were miscellaneous benign and malignant tumors of epithelial and mesenchymal origin.[23] There does not appear to be a sex predilection in cats for renal carcinoma, which is generally found in older cats.

Lymphosarcoma is the most common renal neoplasm in cats. Several recent reviews have debated whether renal lymphosarcoma is a diffuse or localized disease.[26,27] In the former syndrome, the kidneys may be only incidentally affected, in spite of widespread, bulky disease. With the latter syndrome, extensive renal cortical obliteration ensues, with invasion of local structures. Widespread, clinically detectable disease may not occur until late in the course of the localized form of renal lymphoma.

The prognosis for renal lymphosarcoma depends on several factors. Widespread neoplastic involvement, persistent feline leukemia virus infection, and azotemia are considered poor prognostic signs. However, in many cases, appropriate antineoplastic therapy may improve renal function and induce clinicial remission, but the long-term prognosis is guarded. Rapid initiation of supportive and antineoplastic therapy may facilitate a positive patient response.

INDIRECT RENAL INVOLVEMENT

In addition to direct invasion, tumors can involve the kidneys indirectly by inducing glomerulopathies, amyloidosis, renal tubular dysfunction, acute renal failure, urinary tract infection, or obstructive uropathy. Several of these pathophysiologic mechanisms may occur simultaneously in some patients with neoplastic disease.

Glomerulopathies

Tumor-associated injury to the glomerulus can be related to immune complex deposition, amyloidosis, aggregation of macroglobulins or cryoimmunoglobulins or excretion of excessive myeloma proteins.[28,29] Clinical identification of proteinuria or the nephrotic syndrome may precede discovery of the predisposing neoplasm. For example, carcinoma is eventually discovered in 11 percent of adult human nephrotics with membranous glomerulopathy.[28] This emphasizes the importance of routine urinalysis in the evaluation of geriatric or critically ill patients.

In people, glomerulopathies of neoplasia can be generally classified as (1) those occurring in association with carcinomas, (2) those occurring in association with lymphoma and other lymphoproliferative diseases, and (3) a miscellaneous category, including miscellaneous benign and malignant neoplasms.[28] A similar classification appears applicable to the canine and feline species. In a survey of 42 cases of canine glomerulonephritis, neoplasia was found in 40 percent of the dogs and represented the single most frequent predisposing cause of glomerulonephritis.[30] In this study, lymphosarcoma, myeloid leukemia, mastocytoma, and carcinoma of the urinary bladder comprised the majority of the neoplasms which predisposed to glomerulonephritis. Malignant lymphoid tumors comprised 65 percent of all neoplasms in dogs with glomerulonephritis. A similar rate of neoplastic involvement (33 percent) has been identified in additional studies of canine glomerulonephritis.[31,32] Glomerulonephritis is frequent in dogs with mastocytoma. In one report involving 29 dogs with mastocytoma, 66 percent had glomerulonephritis.[33] Both proliferative and membranous glomerulonephritis have been recognized in dogs with neoplastic disease.[30,31] Segmental or diffuse proliferative glomerulonephritis represents the major morphologic type of glomerular injury in the dog, regardless of cause.

Feline leukemia virus (FeLV) may represent the most frequent cause of glomerulonephritis in cats.[34,35,36] The nephrotic syndrome has been documented in some FeLV-positive cats.[34,36] The association of feline leukemia virus with lymphosarcoma and a variety of myeloproliferative disorders is well recognized.[35] In a study involving 45 cats with hematopoietic neoplasms, glomerulonephritis was documented in approximately one-third of the cases.[37] Electron and immunofluorescence microscopy identified subepithelial, subendothelial, and mesangial dense deposits and reticular aggregates indicative of immune complex glomerulonephritis. It has been suggested that the feline leukemia virus may cause immune complex glomerulonephritis in humans, but documentation is lacking.[37] However, the association of feline leukemia virus and immune complex glomerulonephritis deserves additional investigation because of a similar association in mice and human patients with lymphoid malignancies. Documentation of proteinuria of renal origin, nephrotic syndrome, or glomerulonephritis in a cat should initiate evaluation of the feline leukemia status of the animal.

Although spontaneous remission has been reported, treatment of glomerulonephritis carries a guarded prognosis.[38] Identification and subsequent elimination of the predisposing cause of glomerular injury markedly improves the prognosis. Partial resolution of proteinuria occurred following cancer chemotherapy in a dog with lymphocytic leukemia and glomerulonephritis.[39] Chemotherapy, if effective, would be expected to decrease tumor-associated antigen, thereby decreasing immune complex deposition and progressive glomerular injury. Identification and quantitation of tumor-specific circulating immune complexes in animals with glomerular disease may be used in the near future for tumor detection early in the course of malignancy. In human medicine, serologic evaluation for carcinoembryonic antigen (CEA) represents an example of current use of this methodology.[28,40] Remission of nephrotic syndrome associated with minimal change of glomerulopathy or immune complex glomerulopathy is expected in the majority of human patients effectively treated for Hodgkin's disease.[28] In some cases of Hodgkin's disease, subsequent exacerbations and remissions of the tumor have been associated with parallel changes in proteinuria. Although the prognosis is generally considered grave, remission of nephrotic syndrome has been reported in human patients following successful resection of carcinomas.[28] Few reports of canine or feline patients with glomerulopathy secondary to neoplasia are available for analysis of the clinical course and response to therapy.

Amyloidosis

Amyloid is an amorphous, homogenous, proteinaceous substance which accumulates in extracellular spaces.[41] Due to poor immunogenicity, amyloid elicits minimal inflammatory response. Organ dysfunction due to amyloidosis is related to vascular luminal encroachment. This leads to cellular ischemia, necrosis, and depression of cellular function due to restriction of fluid and gas exchange across cell membranes.

Proteinuria, often of sufficient magnitude to induce nephrotic syndrome, is a well-recognized sequela of amyloidosis in the dog and cat.[42–44] In the canine species, renal amyloidosis is most frequently encountered, whereas systemic amyloidosis with glomerular and peritubular involvement has been reported more commonly in cats. In the cat, the greatest renal accumulation of amyloid occurs in the medulla.[44]

Amyloidosis is characterized clinically as either primary or secondary. Primary amyloidosis develops in association with immunoglobulin-producing plasma cell dyscrasias, such as multiple myeloma or macroglobulinemia.[44] Secondary amyloidosis occurs in association with chronic infection, necrosis, and nonlymphoid neoplasia. In man, systemic amyloidosis occurs in 5 to 15 percent of patients with IgG and IgA myeloma and over 40 percent of patients with IgD myeloma.[29] Amyloidosis occurs in association with other human neoplasms, most notably Hodgkin's disease and renal carcinoma. The occurrence of amyloidosis in patients with Hodgkin's disease has diminished in recent years, due to more effective cancer chemotherapy.[27]

In one study, 6 of 44 dogs with renal amyloidosis had malignant neoplasms. Thromboembolic phenomena, a well-recognized sequela of amyloidosis, occurred in 14 dogs. The major site of renal deposition of amyloid in these dogs was the glomerulus. Amyloidosis has been documented in dogs with lymphosarcoma, lymphocytic leukemia, squamous cell carcinoma, thyroid carcinoma, adrenal cortical carcinoma, and malignant hepatoma.[43,44] Although the pulmonary arteries are the most frequent sites of embolization, renal vein thrombosis secondary to amyloidosis may precipitate episodes of acute renal failure in dogs.[43]

Renal amyloidosis carries a grave prognosis in the dog and cat. Diagnosis requires histopathologic examination of renal tissue. Management considerations include elimination of the predisposing cause of amyloid deposition, supportive care for the nephrotic patient, and, if present, treatment of the uremic syndrome.

Renal Tubular Dysfunction

Renal tubular dysfunction is characterized by selective defects in tubular secretion, reabsorption, urine concentration, or urine dilution, which are disproportionate to the reduction in glomerular filtration rate. Examples of tubular reabsorption defects in dogs include cystinosis, Fanconi's syndrome, and renal glycosuria. Excessive uric acid excretion in dalmation dogs is the only recognized renal secretory disorder.

Acquired renal tubular dysfunction secondary to neoplastic disease has received little attention in the dog and cat. Tumor-related defects in urine concentration and dilution will be considered later in this chapter. In humans, proximal renal tubular dysfunction (Fanconi's syndrome) has been reported in association with multiple myeloma or increased light chain excretion.[45] Proximal and distal renal tubular acidosis has also been reported in association with excessive light chain excretion.[45,46]

Acute Renal Failure

Neoplasia may contribute to the development of acute renal failure by causing dehydration, acidosis, electrolyte disturbances, massive hemorrhage, renal arterial obstruction, or obstructive uropathy, or by predisposing to urinary tract infection. Hypercalcemia secondary to malignancy represents an important cause of acute renal failure in dogs and will be considered under pareneoplastic syndromes. Cancer chemotherapy–induced renal damage will be considered later in the chapter. The use of other potentially nephrotoxic drugs, such as aminoglycoside antibiotics, tetracyclines, anesthetics, diuretics, phenytoin, phenylbutazone, or radiocontrast agents, may induce acute renal failure in animals with cancer. Avoidance of factors which might predispose an animal to acute renal failure represents a most important management consideration.[47]

Urinary Tract Infection

Neoplasia may contribute to the development of urinary tract infection, may coexist with infection in the urinary tract, or perhaps may evolve as a result of altered host defense mechanisms secondary to chronic infection. Bacterial infection is frequently documented in association with transitional cell carcinoma of the urinary bladder or canine prostatic adenocarcinoma.[48,49] Tumors may contribute to the development of urinary tract infection by altering local mucosal defense barriers, by inducing urine retention secondary to partial or total obstruction, by causing a neurogenic bladder secondary to spinal cord compression, by decreasing urine osmolality, or by depressing the animal's systemic immune response. Chronic renal or bladder hemorrhage due to cancer provides a good medium for bacterial growth within the urinary tract. In addition, tumor-induced myelophthisis, ineffective myeloma immunoglobulins, or defective leukemic cell function contribute to systemic as well as urinary tract infection.[29]

Recognition and concurrent management of urinary tract infection may be required in animals with cancer. Management considerations would include characterization of the extent of urinary tract involvement, determination of renal function, relief of urinary tract obstruction, cautious use of antimicrobial nephrotoxic drugs, and avoidance of urinary tract catheterization. In animals with recurrent urinary tract infection, sequential urinalysis, contrast radiography, and percutaneous or surgical biopsy may be necessary to rule out cancer as a predisposing factor.

Obstructive Uropathy

Urinary obstruction may be classified as intrarenal or extrarenal. Intrarenal obstruction associated with acute hyperuricemic nephropathy is a well-recognized syndrome in humans.[50,51] Increased urinary excretion of uric acid is associated with excessive neoplastic metabolism of purine nucleic acids by some malignant tumors. Intranephronal obstruction occurs due to intratubular crystallization and aggregation of uric acid. Chemotherapy or radiation therapy markedly increases uric acid excretion. Acute hyperuricemic nephropathy is not a major clinical concern in dogs, most likely due to an enhanced ability to metabolize uric acid.[52]

Extrarenal obstruction is characterized clinically as acute or chronic. Cancer generally causes insidious urinary obstruction, affecting one or both kidneys. Obstructive tumors may originate from within the urinary tract or may cause external compression of the urinary tract. Tumors involving the renal pelvis or ureter will cause unilateral renal dysfunction with minimal, subtle clinical findings, due to the functional capacity of the unaffected kidney. Tumors involving the trigone region of the bladder or urethra may cause retrograde hydroureter and hydronephrosis.[48] Polydipsia and polyuria due to defective urine concentration occurs in association with partial bilateral urinary tract obstruction.[53] Survey radiography, excretory urography, contrast cystography, urethrography, and ultrasound are useful in determining the site of urinary tract obstruction.

RENAL INVOLVEMENT IN PARANEOPLASTIC SYNDROMES

Hypercalcemic Nephropathy

Hypercalcemia secondary to neoplasia has been documented in dogs in association with lymphosarcoma, apocrine adenocarcinoma, nasal adenocarcinoma, thyroid adenocarcinoma, multiple myeloma, lymphocytic leukemia, mammary adenocarcinoma, squamous cell carcinoma, fibrosarcoma, interstitial cell tumor, and parathyroid adenocarcinoma.[54–56] In dogs and cats, lymphosarcoma represents the most frequently reported cause of neoplasia-induced hypercalcemia. Several mechanisms, including excessive parathormone secretion, release of parathormone-like substances, secretion of an osteoclast-activating factor, excessive serum 1,25-dihydroxycholecalciferol, and direct tumor osteolysis have been proposed to explain the pathogenesis of hypercalcemia.[56] In most instances, the mechanism responsible for hypercalcemia related to specific tumors requires additional clarification.

Hypercalcemia causes diverse clinical manifestations related to calcium's important role in cell membrane stability and excitability. In addition to a variety of gastrointestinal signs, muscle weakness, cardiac arrhythmias, and coma, hypercalcemia affects the kidney by interfering with water reabsorption and by direct damage to renal tubular epithelial cells.[55] Increased serum calcium blocks antidiuretic hormone–induced, cyclic AMP–mediated water resorption in the distal tubule and collecting duct. Despite progressive dehydration due to anorexia, vomiting, and polyuria, the hypercalcemic animal is unable to conserve water due to defective urine concentrating ability. Rapidly progressive dehydration will result in decreased glomerular filtration, prerenal azotemia, and metabolic acidosis. This sequence of events, plus direct renal tubular damage secondary to hypercalcemia, can result in severe oliguric acute renal failure.[55] This emphasizes the importance of treating a hypercalcemic cancer patient (serum calcium ≥ 13 mg/dl) immediately, to return serum calcium values to the normal range. Polydipsia and polyuria secondary to the hypercalcemia of malignancy can precede other clinical signs by days to weeks. Hyposthenuria, hematuria, renal tubular casts, or renal epithelial cells may be present prior to the development of azotemia. Treatment should be initiated despite the absence of clinical signs, urine abnormalities, azotemia, or uremia.[55] Saline diuresis may effectively lower serum calcium in some patients. Furosemide (2 mg/kg every 12 hours) will reduce renal tubular calcium resorption and can be used to enhance calciuresis, once the animal has been rehydrated. Glucocorticoids (prednisolone, 1 mg/kg every 12 hours) are most effective in correcting hypercalcemia secondary to hematologic malignancies, such as lymphosarcoma and myeloma. Glucocorticoids cause lympholysis, inhibit lymphocyte production, and decrease the production and release of osteoclast-activating factor. Glucocorticoids may be effective in treating nonhematologic malignancies. This beneficial effect may be due to the fact that glucocorticoids decrease intestinal calcium absorption and increase renal calcium excretion. A single intravenous dose of mithramycin (25 μg/kg) has been recommended for treatment of hypercalcemia that is unresponsive to a combination of fluid, diuretic, and corticosteroid therapy.[54] Tumor-specific chemotherapy, surgical debulking, and other anticancer treatment modalities are used for the treatment of refractory hypercalcemia.

Hyperviscosity Syndromes

Serum viscosity may be abnormally increased in association with excessive production of erythrocytes (polycythemia) or elevated production of serum proteins (monoclonal gammopathy).[57,58] Blood hyperviscosity causes microcapillary sludging, decreased perfusion, and tissue hypoxia, which results in multiorgan system dysfunction. Clinical signs may include visual disturbances, hemorrhage, cardiac decompensation, polyuria, and a variety of neurologic abnormalities ranging from depression to seizures or coma. The kidneys may be involved in polycythemic syndromes in one of two ways. Direct or indirect renal neoplastic involvement can result in polycythemia, and, regardless of cause, polycythemia can decrease renal concentrating ability.[57] Polycythemic hyperviscosity may occur as a result of excessive production of erythropoietin or erythropoietin-like substances by a renal neoplasia. Inappropriate renal erythropoietin production has been reported in dogs with renal carcinoma and renal lymphosarcoma.[14,15,59] Renal hypoxia secondary to tumor-related impairment of renal circulation can also cause polycythemia. In these cases, release of renal erythropoietin is an appropriate compensatory response to hypoxemia. Polyuria and polydipsia are frequently reported clinical findings in dogs with polycythemia vera, a chronic myeloproliferative disease characterized by erythropoietic bone marrow hyperplasia and increased total red blood cell mass.[60,61] Blood hyperviscosity causes circulatory impairment in the vasa recta, which interferes with removal of reabsorbed water from the renal medulla. This results in decreased medullary tonicity, inability to maximally concentrate urine, and polyuria. Management of polycythemia requires appropriate classification, so that therapy can be directed toward the predisposing cause of the increased hematocrit.

Polydipsia and polyuria occurs in some canine patients with monoclonal gammopathy secondary to various plasma cell dyscrasias.[62–65] In addition to causing defective urine concentrating ability due to hyperviscosity syndrome, monoclonal gammopathies may cause acute or chronic renal insufficiency. Altered coagulability, glomerular injury, renal tubular degeneration, interstitial plasma cell infiltration, amyloidosis, cryoimmunoglobulinemia, hypercalcemia, and urinary tract infection are factors which contribute to progressive renal insufficiency in human patients.[29] Acute renal insufficiency, proteinuria, renal tubular dysfunction, or defective renal concentrating ability should initiate evaluation of serum proteins for detection of monoclonal gammopathy and of urine for detection of Bence-Jones protein. It should be emphasized that Bence-Jones proteins are not detected by standard urine dipstick procedures. Serum and urine immunoelectrophoresis is preferred for documentation of Bence-Jones proteins. Plasmapheresis can be utilized to remove abnormal serum proteins and thereby eliminate serum hyperviscosity.[64] Combination chemotherapy is the currently recommended therapy for canine and feline myeloma.[64,65]

Hyponatremia

Inappropriate secretion of antidiuretic hormone (SIADH) induces hyponatremia secondary to excessive water retention and is most frequently associated with undifferentiated carcinoma of the lung in human beings.[66] Hodgkin's disease and carcinomas of the esophagus, duodenum, colon, pancreas, ovary, and nasopharynx have produced antidiuretic hormone.[29,66] SIADH has been reported in a dog with heartworm disease but has not been reported in association with neoplasia at this time.[67] Diagnostic criteria for SIADH include (1) hyponatremia, (2) serum hypoosmolality, (3) urine osmolality higher than blood osmolality, (4) elevated urinary sodium excretion, (5) normal renal function, (6) lack of evidence of dehydration or adrenal or cardiovascular disease, and (7) a therapeutic response to water restriction. In humans, complete removal of the tumor results in correction of fluid and electrolyte abnormalities associated with SIADH.

Hypernatremia

Hypernatremia may occur in association with sodium retention (hyperaldosteronism), inadequate water intake, or excessive loss of solute-free water.[68] Hypokalemia and hypertension are the most consistent findings in human patients with hyperaldosteronism (see hypokalemia). Adipsia may occur in association with neoplastic damage to the thirst center in the hypothalamus, defective osmoreceptor function as a result of severe debilitation secondary to cancer cachexia, or oropharyngeal neoplastic obstruction. In these instances, dehydration and hypernatremia develop despite normal urine concentrating ability. Adipsia, not related to neoplasia, has been reported in a dog due to impaired thirst and defective osmoreceptor function.[68]

Hypernatremia may develop in animals with antidiurectic hormone deficiency (central diabetes insipidus) or renal tubular unresponsiveness to antidiuretic hormone (nephrogenic diabetes insipidus).[69] Neoplasia of the diencephalopituitary region may cause antidiuretic hormone deficiency due to destruction of neurons responsible for production, transport, or release of antidiuretic hormone.[70]

Tumors may cause acquired nephrogenic diabetes insipidus in human patients due to hypercalcemia, hypokalemia, renal amyloidosis, and excessive production of prostaglandin E_1.[29,71] Hypercalcemia and postobstructive diuresis are the best characterized tumor-associated causes of nephrogenic diabetes insipidus in the dog and cat.

Hypokalemia

Hypokalemia has been reported in man in association with a wide variety of tumors which produce adrenocorticotropic hormone (ACTH), renin, or aldosterone.[29] These hormones directly or indirectly enhance distal tubular sodium reabsorption and potassium excretion into the urine. Hypokalemia, hypernatremia, and hypertension are generally features of disease associated with excessive production of these hormones. Hyperaldosteronism has been reported in a dog manifesting hypokalemia, hypernatremia, and hypertension in association with zona glomerulosa hyperplasia.[72] Hyperaldosteronism has not been reported in the dog in association with adrenal neoplasia.

Hyperkalemia

Acute renal failure and adrenal cortical insufficiency are well-recognized causes of hyperkalemia in the dog and cat.[73] The contribution of neoplastic disease to the development of acute renal failure has been considered previously in this chapter. Metastasis of tumors to the adrenal glands or adrenal deposition of amyloid secondary to neoplastic disease could contribute to the development of adrenal insufficiency.

RENAL CONSIDERATIONS OF ANTINEOPLASTIC THERAPY

The design of optimal therapeutic regimens for anticancer therapy is dependent upon several important pharmacologic principles. The pharmacokinetics of antineoplastic agents are influenced by clinical situations which cause reduced volume of distribution (vascular shunting, altered protein binding), as well as changes in biotransformation and degradation (hepatic dysfunction). The kidneys eliminate most drugs via glomerular filtration and tubular transport. Therefore, during renal failure, the elimination of many classes of drugs is reduced. The pharmacokinetics of antineoplastic agents during disease states has been incompletely investigated. In general, the kidneys play a small role in the elimination of drugs that require extensive metabolism prior to cytotoxic effectiveness. Therefore, doxorubicin, vincristine, cytosine arabinoside, and cyclophosphamide doses are not adjusted unless severe renal dysfunction exists. Bleomycin, although not specifically nephrotoxic, progressively increases in blood concentration as creatinine clearance deteriorates. It has been suggested that dosage modification for bleomycin should be based on glomerular filtration rate.[74] Methotrexate (MTX), streptozotocin, and cisplatin (cis-DDP) are nephrotoxic and will be discussed separately.

Methotrexate (MTX) is an analog of folic acid. It exerts cytotoxic activity as a consequence of dihydrofolate reductase binding and subsequent depletion of reduced folate (tetrahydrofolate).[75,76] This limits the amount of thymidine and purine nucleotide synthesis. All actively proliferating cells are susceptible to the toxic effects of MTX, including bone marrow stem cells and cells of the gastrointestinal tract. Although the kidney has a low percentage of actively cycling cells, MTX-induced nephrotoxicity will occur at high doses.

The pharmacokinetics of MTX have been examined extensively.[75–79] Following an intravenous dose of MTX, 50 percent is weakly bound to albumin. Little metabolic modification of MTX occurs, with 90 percent of the drug excreted unchanged by glomerular filtration, as well as active tubular transport. In man, the clearance of MTX is greater than inulin clearance at high MTX doses. In dogs, one report indicates that tubular reabsorption of MTX predominates.[80] Although there is active enterohepatic circulation of MTX, less than 10 percent is excreted in the feces.

Several theories have been proposed to explain the pathogenesis of MTX-induced renal disease. At low or moderate doses of MTX (5 to 75 mg/m^2), renal toxicity is rare. Nephrotoxicity is associated with high-dose MTX (1 to 15 g/m^2) and citrovorum factor rescue. Citrovorum factor is a competitive inhibitor of MTX that is administered with high-dose MTX protocols. Approximately 20 percent of the deaths associated with high-dose MTX are due to renal failure.[77] Acute renal failure is believed to result from either precipitation of MTX crystals in the tubules, direct tubular toxicity, or reduced glomerular blood flow.[77,79,81] MTX crystal precipitation in the distal convoluted tubule produces oliguric or anuric acute renal failure. Urinary alkalinization and adequate urine flow enhance solubility and excretion of the drug.[82] Tubular epithelial necrosis and cast formation without evidence of crystal precipitation has been associated with increased plasma MTX concentrations.[83] Nonoliguric acute renal failure results from direct renal tubular toxicity. Diuresis or dialysis generally results in recovery. Several cases of subclinical reduction of GFR have been documented.[81] Afferent arteriole constriction is the most likely mechanism, since amelioration of this effect was shown with adequate fluid therapy during administration of MTX.

Nephrotoxicity due to high-dose MTX therapy has not been evaluated adequately in dogs and cats. Toxicity, expense, and the need for intensive therapeutic monitoring limit its use. Low- or moderate-dose MTX has been utilized for many types of canine and feline neoplasia. Gastrointestinal and bone marrow toxicity are limiting factors, even at these lower doses. Coincident renal disease may exacerbate systemic toxicities, as well as predispose to primary MTX nephrotoxicity. Therefore, renal function should be carefully evaluated before administering MTX.

Cis-diaminedichloroplatinum (cis-DDP) is a platinum coordination complex with significant antineoplastic activity. Preclinical trials in dogs have been performed to study various pharmacologic and toxicologic aspects of administration regimens. This information has recently been reviewed.[84] The mechanism of action is similar to the bifunctional alkylating agents such as cyclophosphamide and is considered phase nonspecific within the cell cycle.[85] Cis-DDP preferentially binds to purine nucleotides on DNA strands and prevents replication. Although the overall response rate to cis-DDP alone is less than doxorubicin, encouraging results have been shown with several historically resistant forms of neoplasia. The spectrum of cis-DDP activity includes germ cell neoplasia, bladder, prostate, and squamous carcinomas, and several sarcomas.[86] When cis-DDP is combined with other chemotherapeutic agents, radiation, or hyperthermia, there seems to be a significant synergistic effect.[86–89]

Pharmacokinetic studies of cis-DDP predicted several pertinent clinical problems. The rapid disappearance of cis-DDP in plasma is due to protein binding, tissue distribution, and renal excretion. Cis-DDP is freely filtered and actively secreted by the tubular epithelium, accounting for 60 percent recovery of the administered dose within 4 hours.[90,91] Nephrotoxicity was the dose-limiting side effect in preclinical studies. It is believed that nephrotoxicity occurs soon after the cis-DDP infusion, when plasma and urinary platinum levels are extremely elevated.

The pathophysiology of platinum-induced nephrotoxicity has not been fully explained. Direct tubular epithelial damage is associated with excessive intracytoplasmic accumulation of platinum. The pathologic event is suspected to be uncoupling of oxidative phosphorylation, leading to energy depletion and necrosis.[93] A second theory of cis-DDP-induced nephrotoxicity suggests a profound decrease in GFR and renal blood flow secondary to activation of the renin-angiotensin system.[93,94]

The clinical progression of cis-DDP-induced renal dysfunction is predictable, in most cases. Dogs given toxic doses of cis-DDP have peak elevations in serum creatinine and BUN values approximately 7 to 10 days post-infusion, with elevated values persisting for 14 to 17 days.[95] The majority of acute renal failure cases respond to appropriate fluid diuresis and cessation of cis-DDP therapy. Repeated platinum infusions of excessive doses may induce permanent renal disease.

Patient prehydration with saline and mannitol diuresis have independently been shown to ameliorate the nephrotoxic effects of cis-DDP in dogs given toxic doses.[95] This beneficial effect has been confirmed clinically in humans. The mechanism of mannitol's nephrotoxic-sparing effect is not known. Most protocols still employ both prehydration and osmotic diuresis. One report, however, suggests that mannitol may actually be contraindicated.[96] Cumulative nephrotoxicity was not a problem in most clinical protocols which were reviewed.[97]

Cis-DDP is undergoing continued clinical and laboratory investigation. There have not been any clinical trials utilizing cis-DDP reported in the veterinary literature. Several institutions, however, are evaluating cis-DDP for treatment of several types of canine tumors. Pretreatment prophylactic measures and awareness of potential toxicities should prevent renal injury from compromising the therapeutic outcome in the majority of cases. Cis-DDP should be omitted from the treatment regimen if adequate fluid therapy cannot be maintained or if there is preexisting renal dysfunction.

Streptozotocin is a nitrosourea antibiotic that alkylates and methylates DNA, thus inhibiting its synthesis. It has a lesser effect on RNA and protein synthesis.[98] Streptozotocin has proven efficacy in islet cell carcinomas, colorectal carcinoma, and carcinoid tumors in humans.[98] In the dog, use of streptozotocin therapy for islet cell carcinoma results in severe nephrotoxicity and hepatotoxicity.[99,100]

Functional and morphologic alterations of the kidney are the most significant toxic side-effects of streptozotocin.[98] The most common renal abnormalities include Fanconi's syndrome, renal glycosuria, proteinuria, and electrolyte abnormalities. Dogs treated with streptozotocin also developed renal tubular defects in association with acute tubular necrosis and atrophy and interstitial connective tissue proliferation.

As with other nephrotoxic chemotherapeutic drugs, prophylactic therapy has been attempted. Pretreatment hydration and osmotic diuresis have been added to most human protocols. Prolonged low-dose streptozotocin infusions have also been shown to reduce toxicity.[101]

There are numerous isolated reports of nephrotoxicity secondary to other forms of antineoplastic drugs. These reports consider rare idiosyncratic reactions or agents which are infrequently utilized. However, a recent report has documented glomerular and tubular damage from repeated doxorubicin administration in cats.[102]

The use of *Corynebacterium parvum* as an immunotherapeutic agent has been associated with renal damage in human patients.[103] Renal biopsies show proliferative glomerulonephritis with subendothelial basement membrane deposits of IgG, IgA, IgM, and C_3. The renal abnormalities resolve following withdrawal of immunotherapy. A case of proliferative glomerulonephritis has been reported in a dog following *C. parvum* therapy for malignant melanoma.[104]

Radiation nephropathy is a predictable and well-documented consequence of radiotherapy.[105–106] Following radiation exposure, structural changes in renal architecture are considered early or late changes. Early changes include vascular, parenchymal, and tubular damage which occur within the first several months of radiation exposure. The severity and onset of the pathologic change depends on the fractionation scheme and the total radiation dose. Late changes involve progressive fibrous connective tissue proliferation into the renal parenchyma, which occurs months to years following radiation therapy. The clinical signs of radiation nephropathy develop slowly and include hematuria, proteinuria, and azotemia. The differential diagnosis should include recurrent cancer or acute glomerulonephritis.

Direct radiation exposure to the kidney occurs in cases of total abdominal irradiation for carcinomatosis or more intense exposure for renal and perirenal tumors. Radiation nephropathy can be minimized by a thorough pretreatment renal evaluation, intravenous pyelography, and computerized tomography to focus the radiation precisely, and dynamic treatment planning to provide appropriate radiation shielding. The rate of radiation exposure may also be controlled. Dosages below 2,000 rads administered during 2 weeks has been recommended to prevent radiation nephropathy.[107] However, individual variability does exist, due to radiation sensitizers, tumor type, and the extent of disease.

The potential for direct or indirect renal involvement exists in all patients with neoplastic disease. The effect of treatment on renal function must be considered prior to cancer therapy. Increased awareness and characterization of renal manifestations of neoplastic disease will compliment the rapidly expanding knowledge of cancer therapy.

REFERENCES

1. Preister WA, McKay FW: The occurrence of tumors in domestic animals. p. 59. NCI Monograph #54. US Dept of Health and Human Resources Publication #80-2046, 1980
2. Baskin GB, DePaoli A: Primary renal neoplasms of the dog. Vet Pathol 14:591, 1977
3. Moulton JE: Tumors of the urinary system. p. 288. In Moulton JE (ed): Tumors in Domestic Animals. U of Cal Pr, Berkeley, CA, 1978
4. Dorn CR, Taylor DO, Frye FL, Hibbard HH: Survey of animal neoplasms in Alameda and Contra Costa Counties, California. J Natl Cancer Inst 40:295, 1968
5. Hayes HM, Fraumeni JF: Epidemiological features of canine renal neoplasms. Cancer Res 37:2553, 1977
6. Lucke VM, Kelly DF: Renal carcinoma in the dog. Vet Pathol 13:264, 1976
7. Goldschmidt MH: Renal neoplasia. p. 687. In Bovee KC (ed): Canine Nephrology. Harwal Pub Co, 1984
8. Fein K: Unpublished data, 1984
9. Bennington JL: Cancer of the kidney—Etiology, epidemiology and pathology. Cancer 32:1017, 1973
10. Holland JM: Cancer and the kidney—Natural history and staging. Cancer 32:1030, 1973
11. Skinner DG, Colvin RB, Vermillion CD, et al.: Diagnosis and management of renal

cell carcinoma—A clinical and pathologic study of 309 cases. Cancer 28:1165, 1971
12. Dikernian JB, Berry D: The diagnosis and treatment of renal cell carcinoma. Cancer 45:1947, 1980
13. Altaffer LA, Chenault OW: Paraneoplastic endocrinopathies associated with renal tumors. J Urol 122:573, 1979
14. Scott RC, Patnaik AK: Renal carcinoma associated with secondary polycythemia in the dog. J Am Vet Med Assoc 8:275, 1972
15. Peterson ME, Zanjoni ED: Inappropriate erythropoietin production from a renal carcinoma in a dog with polycythemia. J Am Vet Med Assoc 179:995, 1981
16. Laymann RV, Surya V, Miller RP, et al: Pursuit of the renal mass—Is ultrasound enough? Am J Med 77:218, 1984
17. Weymann PJ, McClennan BL, Stanley RJ, et al: Comparison of computed tomography and angiography in the evaluation of renal cell carcinomas. Radiology 137:417, 1980
18. Robson CJ, Churchill BM, Anderson W: The results of radical nephrectomy for renal cell carcinoma. J Urol 101:297, 1969
19. Palmer JM: Role of partial nephrectomy in solitary or bilateral renal tumors. JAMA 249(17):2357, 1983
20. Van der Werf-Messing: Carcinoma of the kidney. Cancer 32:1056, 1973
21. Richie JP, Garnick MB: Primary renal and ureteral cancer. p. 689. In Rieselbach RE, Garnick MB (eds): Cancer of the Kidney. Lea & Febiger, Philadelphia, 1982
22. Beckwith JB, Palmer NF: Histopathology and prognosis of Wilms' Tumor. Cancer 41:1937, 1978
23. Caywood D, Osborne CA, Johnston GR: Neoplasms of the canine and feline urinary tract. p. 1203. In Kirk RW (ed): Current Veterinary Therapy VIII. WB Saunders Co, Philadelphia, 1980
24. Mayer RJ: Infiltrative and metastatic disease of the kidney. p. 707. In Reiselbach RE, Garnick MB (eds): Cancer and the Kidney. Lea & Febiger, Philadelphia, 1982
25. Wagle DG, Moore RH, Murphy GP: Secondary carcinomas of the kidney. J Urol 114:30, 1975
26. Loar A: The management of feline lymphosarcoma. Vet Clin North Am 14:1299, 1984
27. Cotter SM: Treatment of lymphoma and leukemia with cyclophosphamide, vincristine, and prednisone: II. Treatment of cats. J Am Anim Hosp Assoc 19:166, 1983
28. Eagen JW, Lewis EJ: Glomerulopathies of neoplasia. Kidney Int 11:297, 1977
29. Glasscock RJ, Friedler RM, Massry SG: Kidney and electrolyte disturbances in neoplastic diseases. Contrib Nephrol 7:2, 1977
30. Murray M, Wright NG: Morphologic study of canine glomerulonephritis. Lab Invest 30:213, 1974
31. Muller-Peddinghaus R, Trautwein G: Spontaneous glomeruloneprhitis in dogs. II. Correlation of glomerulonephritis with age, chronic interstitial nephritis, and extrarenal lesions. Vet Pathol 14:121, 1977
32. DiBartola SP, Spaulding GL, Chew DJ, et al: Urinary protein excretion and immunopathologic findings in dogs with glomerular disease. J Am Vet Med Assoc 177:73, 1980
33. Hottendorf GH, Nielsen SW: Pathologic report of 29 necropsies on dogs with mastocytoma. Pathol Vet 5:102, 1968
34. Cotter SM, Hardy WD, Essex M: Association of feline leukemia virus with lymphosarcoma and other disorders in the cat. J Am Vet Med Assoc 166:449, 1975

35. Hardy WD: The feline leukemia virus. J Am Anim Hosp Assoc 17:951, 1981
36. Anderson LJ, Jarrett WFH: Membranous glomerulonephritis associated with leukemia in cats. Res Vet Sci 12:179, 1971
37. Glick AD, Horn RG, Holscher M: Characterization of feline glomerulonephritis associated with viral-induced hematopoietic neoplasms. Am J Pathol 92:321, 1978
38. Lewis RM, Carter SA: Primary diseases affecting glomeruli. p. 461. In Bovee KC (ed): Canine Nephrology. Harwal Publishing, Philadelphia, 1984
39. Willard MD, Krehbiel JD, Schmidt GM, et al: Serum and urine protein abnormalities associated with lymphocytic leukemia in a dog. J Am Anim Hosp Assoc 17:381, 1981
40. Baldwin RW, Price MR: Tumor antigens and tumor-host relationships. p. 151. In Creger WB, Coggins CH, Hancock EW (eds): Annual Reviews Inc. Vol. 27. Palo Alto, CA, 1976
41. Glenner GG: Amyloid deposits and amyloidosis. N Engl J Med 302:1283, 1333, 1980
42. Slauson DO, Gribble DH, Russell SW: A clinicopathologic study of renal amyloidosis in dogs. J Comp Pathol 80:335, 1970
43. Slauson DO, Gribble DH: Thombosis complicating renal amyloidosis in dogs. Vet Pathol 8:352, 1971
44. Chew DJ, DiBartola SP: Feline renal amyloidosis. p. 976. In Kirk RW (ed): Current Veterinary Therapy VIII. WB Saunders, Philadelphia, 1983
45. Costanza DJ, Smoller ML Multiple myeloma with Fanconi's syndrome. Am J Med 34:125, 1963
46. Walker BR, Alexander F, Tannenbaum PJ: Fanconi syndrome with renal tubular acidosis and light chain proteinuria. Nephron 8:103, 1971
47. Cowgill LD: Acute renal failure. p. 405. In Bovee KC (ed): Canine Nephrology. Harwal Publishing, Philadelphia, 1984
48. Osborne CA, Low DG, Perman V: Neoplasms of the canine and feline urinary bladder: Clinical findings, diagnosis, and treatment. J Am Vet Med Assoc 152:247, 1968
49. Hargis AM, Miller LM: Prostatic carcinoma in dogs. Compend Cont Ed 5:647, 1983
50. Ultman JE: Hyperuricemia in disseminated neoplastic diseases other than lymphomas and leukemias. Cancer 15:122, 1962
51. Kjellstrand C, Campbell DC, Hartitzch B, et al: Hyperuricemic acute renal failure. Arch Intern Med 133:349, 1974
52. Page RL, Leifer CE, Matus RE: Uric acid and phosphorous excretion in canine lymphosarcoma. Am J Vet Res (in press)
53. Bovee KC: Urinary obstruction disease. p. 385. In Bovee KC (ed): Canine Nephrology. Harwal Publishing, Philadelphia, 1984
54. Weller RE: Cancer-associated hypercalcemia in companion animals. Compend Cont Ed Pract Vet 6:639, 1984
55. Osborne CA, Stevens JB: Hypercalcemic nephropathy. p. 1080. In Kirk RW (ed): Current Veterinary Therapy VI. WB Saunders, Philadelphia, 1977
56. Meuten DJ, Kociba GH, Capen CC, et al: Hypercalcemia in dogs with lymphosarcoma: Biochemical, ultrastructural, and histomorphometic investigations. Lab Invest 49:553, 1983
57. Bloch KJ, Maki DG: Hyperviscosity syndromes associated with immunoglobulin abnormalities. Semin Hemat 10:113, 1973
58. Wells RW: Syndromes of hyperviscosity. N Engl J Med 283:183, 1970

59. Nelson RW, Hager D, Zanjani ED: Renal lymphosarcoma with inappropriate erythropoietin production in a dog. J Am Vet Med Assoc 182:1396, 1983
60. Peterson ME, Randolph JF: Diagnosis of canine primary polycythemia and management with hydroxyurea. J Am Vet Med Assoc 180:415, 1982
61. McGrath CJ: Polycythemia vera in dogs. J Am Vet Med Assoc 164:1117, 1974
62. MacEwen EG, Hurvitz AI, Hayes A: Hyperviscosity syndrome associated with lymphocytic leukemia in three dogs. J Am Vet Med Assoc 170:1309, 1977
63. Shull RM, Osborne CA, Barrett RE, et al: Serum hyperviscosity syndrome associated with IgA multiple myeloma in two dogs. J Am Anim Hosp Assoc 14:58, 1978
64. Matus RE, Leifer CE, Gordon BR, et al.: Plasmapheresis and chemotherapy of hyperviscosity syndrome associated with monoclonal gammopathy in the dog. J Am Vet Med Assoc 183:215, 1983
65. Drazner FH: Multiple myeloma in the cat. Compend Cont Ed 4:206, 1982
66. Cooke CR, Turin MD, Walker WG: The syndrome of inappropriate antidiuretic hormone secretion (SIADH): Pathophysiologic mechanisms in solute and volume regulation. Medicine 58:240, 1979
67. Breitschwerdt EB, Root CR: Inappropriate secretion of antidiuretic hormone in a dog. J Am Vet Med Assoc 175:181, 1979
68. Crawford MA, Kittleson MD, Fink GD: Hypernatremia and adipsia in a dog. J Am Vet Med Assoc 184:818, 1984
69. Breitschwerdt EB: Clinical abnormalities of urine concentration and dilution. Compen Cont Ed 3:414, 1981
70. Madewell BR, Osborne CA, Norrdin RA: Clinicopathologic aspects of diabetes insipidus in the dog. J Am Anim Hosp Assoc 11:497, 1975
71. Hays RM, Levine SD: Pathophysiology of water metabolism. p. 553. In Brenner BM, Rector FC (eds): The Kidney. WB Saunders, Philadelphia, 1976
72. Breitschwerdt EB, Meuten DJ, Greenfield CL, et al: Idiopathic hyperaldosteronism in a dog. J Am Vet Med Assoc 187:841, 1985
73. Schaer M: Disorders of potassium metabolism. Vet Clin North Am 12:399, 1982
74. Major P, Kufe D, Frei E: Role of the kidney in the pharmacokinetics of anticancer agents. p. 263. In Reiselbach RE, Garnick MB (eds): Cancer and the Kidney. Lea & Febiger, Philadelphia, 1982
75. Huffman DH, Wan SH, Azarnoff DL, et al: Pharmacokinetics of methotrexate. Clin Pharmacol Ther 14:572, 1973
76. Bleyer WA: The clinical pharmacology of methotrexate: New applications of an old drug. Cancer 41:36, 1978
77. Von Hoff DD, Penta JS, Helman LJ, et al: Incidence of drug related deaths secondary to high dose methotrexate and citrovorum factor administration. Cancer Treat Rep 61:745, 1977
78. Kristeasen LO: Renal function and the rate of disappearance of methotrexate. Eur J Clin Pharmacol 8:849, 1975
79. Pratt C, Roberts O, Shanks E, et al: Response toxicity, and pharmacokinetics of high-dose MTX with citrovorum factor rescue for children with osteosarcoma and other malignant tumors. Cancer Chemother Rep 6:13, 1975
80. Huang KC, Wenczak BA, Liu YE: Renal tubular transport of methotrexate in the Rhesus monkey and dog. Cancer Res 39:4843, 1979
81. Link DA, Fosburg MT, Ingelfinger JR, et al: Renal toxicity of high dose methotrexate. Pediat Res 10:455, 1976
82. Romolo JL, Goldberg NH, Hande KR, et al: Effect of hydration on plasma methotrexate levels. Cancer Treat Rep 61:1393, 1977

83. Pinedo HM, Chabner BA: The role of drug concentration, duration of exposure, and endogenous metabolites in determining methotrexate cytotoxicity. Cancer Treat Rep 61:709, 1977
84. Page RL, Matus RE, Leifer CE: Cisplatin: A new antineoplastic drug in veterinary medicine. J Am Vet Med Assoc 186:288, 1985
85. Zwelling LA, Kohn KW: Mechanisms of action of cis-dichlorodiammine platinum (II). Cancer Treat Rep 63:1439, 1979
86. Connors P: Platinum compounds. p. 843. In Holland JF, Frei E (eds): Cancer Medicine. Lea & Febiger, Philadelphia, 1982
87. Herman TS, Sweets CS, White DM: Effect of heating on lethality due to hyperthermia and selected chemotherapeutic drugs. J Natl Cancer Inst 68:487, 1982
88. Hahn G: Potential for therapy of drugs and hyperthermia. Cancer Res 39:2264, 1979
89. Double EB, Richmond RC: A review of interactions in platinum coordination complexes and ionizing radiation: Implications for cancer therapy. p. 125. In Prestayko AW, Crooke ST, Carter SK (eds): Cisplatinum: Current Status and New Developments. Academic Press, New York, 1980
90. Litterst CL, Torres IJ, Guarino AM: Plasma levels and organ distributions of platinum in the rat, dog and dogfish shark following single intravenous administration of cis-DDP (II). J Clin Hematol Oncol 7:169, 1976
91. Litterst CL, Gram TE, Dedrich RL: Distribution and disposition of platinum following intravenous administration of cis-diamminedichloroplatinum (II) (NSC-119875) to dogs. Cancer Res 36:2340, 1976
92. Jacobs C, Kalman SM: Renal handling of cis-DDP. Cancer Treat Rep 64:1223, 1980
93. Madias NE, Harrington JT: Platinum nephrotoxicity. Am J Med 65:307, 1978
94. Flowenbaum W: Pathophysiology of acute renal failure. Arch Intern Med 131:911, 1973
95. Cvitkovic E, Spaulding J: Improvement of cis-dichlorodiammineplatinum (NSC119875): Therapeutic index in an animal mode. Cancer 39:1357, 1977
96. Lehane D: Effect of diuretic pretreatment on DDP nephrotoxicity. Int J Radiat Oncol Phys 5:1393, 1979
97. Chiuten D, Vogl S, Kaplan B: Is there cumulative or delayed toxicity from cisplatinum? Cancer 52:211, 1983
98. Weiss RB: Streptozotocin: A review of its pharmacology, efficacy, and toxicity. Cancer Treat Rep 66:427, 1982
99. Meyer DJ: Pancretic islet carcinoma in a dog treated with streptozotocin. Am J Vet Res 37:1221, 1976
100. Meyer DJ: Temporary remission of hypoglycemia in a dog with an insulinoma after treatment with streptozotocin. Am J Vet Res 38:1201, 1977
101. Moertel CG, Hanley JA, Johnson LA: Streptozotocin alone compared with streptozotocin plus fluorouracil in the treatment of advanced islet cell carcinoma. N Engl J Med 303:1189, 1980
102. Cotter SM, Kanki PJ, Simon M: Renal disease in five tumor-bearing cats treated with Adriamycin. J Am Anim Hosp Assoc 21:405, 1985
103. Dasik GM: Nephrotoxicity from cancer immunotherapy. Ann Intern Med 89:41, 1978
104. Leifer CE, Page RL, Matus RE, et al: *C. Parvum* induced glomerulonephritis in a dog. J Am Vet Med Assoc (in press)

105. Sagerman RH: Radiation nephritis. J Urol 91:332, 1976
106. Keane WF, et al: Radiation-induced renal disease: A clinicopathologic study. Am J Med 60:127, 1976
107. Cassady JR: Considerations in the radiation therapy of Wilms tumor. Cancer 32:598, 1973.

10 Radiographic Evaluation of the Urinary Tract in Dogs and Cats

Gary R. Johnston
Daniel A. Feeney

Survey and contrast radiography of the urinary system can provide information towards the diagnosis of upper or lower urinary tract disease. Radiography is too frequently excluded as a diagnostic modality for evaluation of the urinary system because of prior experience or unfulfilled expectations. However, negative radiographic findings encountered on survey or contrast radiographs should not be considered an inherent defect of the modality. Some upper and lower urinary tract diseases may have no radiographic abnormalities. A thorough understanding of the technical and interpretative pitfalls inherent in survey radiography and special radiographic procedures will prevent the skilled clinician from misinterpreting the false-negative or -positive roentgen signs associated with special radiographic procedures.

Valuable information can be obtained on the size, shape, location, and radiographic density of the kidneys and urinary bladder. However, in cases of emaciation and retroperitoneal and/or free peritoneal fluid, the radiographic identification of the abdominal structures provided by retroperitoneal and peritoneal fat may not be adequate for identifying the kidneys and urinary bladder. Special radiographic procedures are designed to increase the radiographic contrast and detail of these structures to gain additional information not available from survey radiographs.

The maximum amount of information can only be obtained from survey or contrast radiographs of the urinary system if one approaches film evaluation in a systematic fashion. The roentgen-signs approach is a description of basic terms of radiographic density, geometry, and function of the affected organ encountered on the radiographs. The roentgen signs associated with organ density include the five subject densities: air, fat, soft tissue (water), bone, and metal. Geometric signs include size, shape, position/location, number, and margination. The roentgen signs appropriate to organ function include excretion and concentration (renal function), patency, integrity, motility, and distensibility (of ureters, urinary bladder, and urethra). Following careful evaluation of the survey and contrast radiographs, the abnormal roentgen signs should be compared with the expected normal signs. These abnormal roentgen signs should then be combined with the history, physical findings, clinical laboratory data, and cytology, and a list of radiographic differential diagnoses (gamuts) should then be constructed in order of decreasing likelihood. Based on the ranking of the gamuts, additional tests (laboratory, radiography, surgical biopsy, or ultrasonography) should be performed until a definitive diagnosis has been achieved. Information obtained from survey and contrast radiographs will frequently not identify a definitive diagnosis. The ultimate goal in radiology is to define the site(s) of involvement and the extent of involvement. Additional laboratory tests to include a surgical biopsy are necessary for a definitive diagnosis and prognosis.

The goal of this chapter is to provide diagnostic radiographic information that can be obtained from survey and contrast radiographs for evaluation of the kidneys, ureters, urinary bladder, prostate, and urethra. Perspectives on the sequential use of survey or contrast radiographs, indications, limitations, contraindications, technical and interpretative pitfalls, and complications will be described where applicable. We will describe each of the structures within the urinary system considering both normal and abnormal survey radiography. This will be followed by a description of the special radiographic procedures used for evaluation of the kidneys, ureters, urinary bladder, and urethra. Normal and abnormal examples of each of the special procedures will be described and illustrated. An approach to the interpretation of the abnormal roentgen signs will follow.

SURVEY RADIOGRAPHY

Lateral and ventrodorsal survey radiographs should be the initial step of the radiograhpic sequence for evaluation of the upper and lower urinary tracts. Survey radiographs will provide information relative to renal and urinary bladder silhouettes pertaining to size, shape, location, margination, position, and radiographic density. If insufficient retroperitoneal or peritoneal contrast exists, visualization of these structures may not be possible. Inadequate patient preparation resulting in superimposing intestinal contents over urinary structures will also impair the ability to identify the kidneys and urinary bladder on survey radiographs. Abnormal roentgen signs on survey radiographs are nonspecific and may indicate congenital anomalies or inflammatory, infectious, neoplastic, or traumatic diseases. The abnormal roentgen signs must be evaluated relative to the history, physical findings, and clinical laboratory data before a list of differentials can be identified. Subsequent examinations, including special contrast procedures or a surgical biopsy, will be necessary before a definitive diagnosis can be obtained. Clinical signs frequently associated with renal, ureteral, or retroperitoneal disease include dysuria, pollakiuria, arched back, tender abdomen, and fever of undetermined origin.[1,2] Since these clinical signs are nonspecific, the categories of diseases previously mentioned might apply to any set or sets of clinical signs.

To obtain the maximum information from survey radiographs, proper patient preparation should include withholding food for 24 hours and a cleansing enema 1 to 3 hours prior to survey radiography. Survey radiographs should be taken in both lateral and ventrodorsal recumbency since each radiograph provides only a two-dimensional image of a three-dimensional object. The right lateral recumbent radiograph is recommended because it allows greater separation of the left and the right kidneys.[3,4] Additional lateral and ventrodorsal oblique radiographs may be necessary if abnormal roentgen signs are encountered with the renal or urinary bladder silhouettes.

Normal and Abnormal Radiographic Findings

Kidneys. In normal dogs, the two kidneys are located retroperitoneally, with the right kidney cranial to the left (Fig. 10-1).[3,5] The cranial pole of the right kidney is approximately at the level of T13-L1 but may not be identifiable radiographically because of its association with the renal impression of the caudate lobe of the liver.[3,5] The left kidney is more variable in position than the right but is more easily identifiable radiographically and is located at the level of L2 and L3.[3] On lateral survey radiographs, the nondependent kidney appears to be more rounded because of the influence of gravity, whereas the dependent kidney appears more oval.[3] Superimposition of the caudal pole of the right kidney and the cranial pole of the left kidney is frequently encountered on lateral survey radiographs and must be differentiated from a renal mass lesion or retroperitoneal mass lesion (Fig. 10-1).

The kidneys of the adult feline are more easily identifiable radiographically than in a dog (Fig. 10-2). Cat kidneys are more caudally located and are more loosely attached in the retroperitoneal space than in dogs.[5–7] In cats, the right kidney is approximately at the level of the L1–L4, and the left kidney is approximately at the level of L2–L5.[6,7] Variations in the location of dog or cat kidneys can be normal and related to the phase of respiration, the degree of gastric distention, and patient positioning.[3] Intrarenal and extrarenal mass lesions may cause displacement of the kidneys. The direction of displacement is dependent upon the origin of the mass lesion.

The normal dog kidney is somewhat bean-shaped, whereas the cat kidney is more oval.[6,7] Renal borders should be smooth, regular, and distinct. Ab-

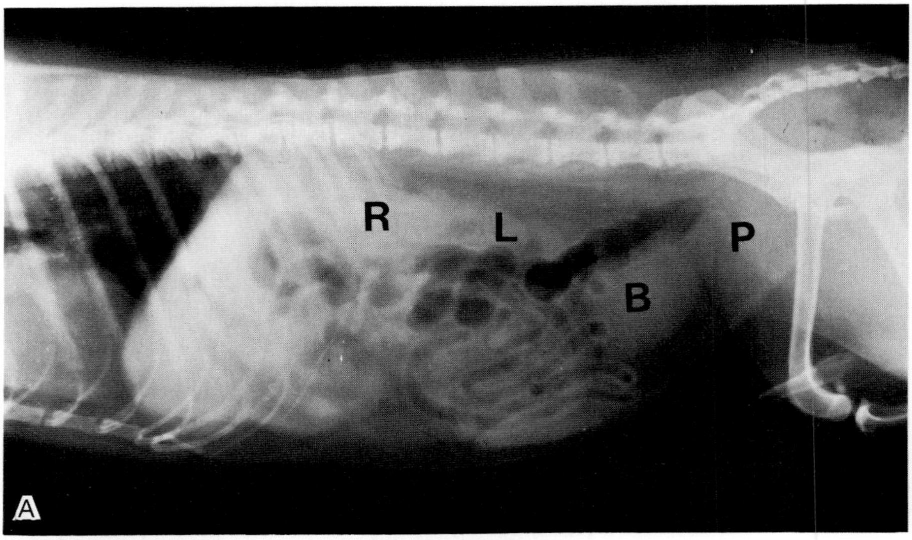

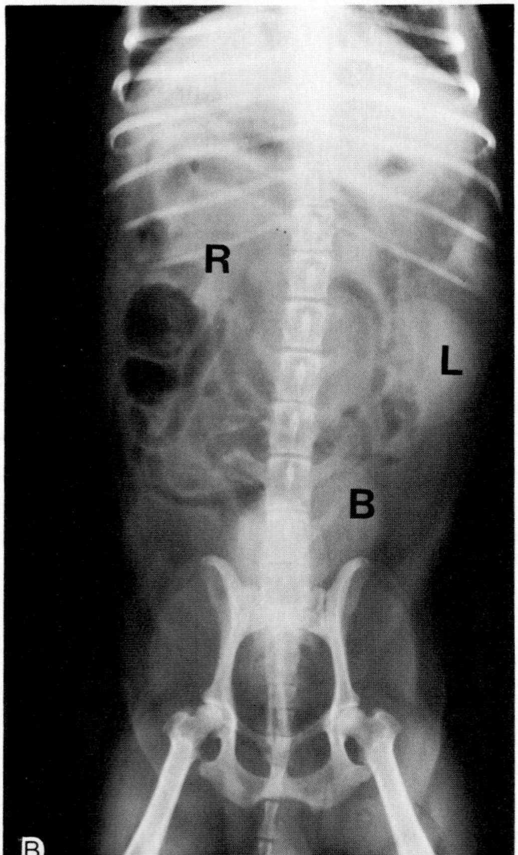

Fig. 10-1. Lateral (A) and ventrodorsal (B) survey abdominal radiographs from a normal 11-year-old male miniature poodle. The left (L) and right (R) kidneys, urinary bladder (B), and prostate gland (P) are illustrated.

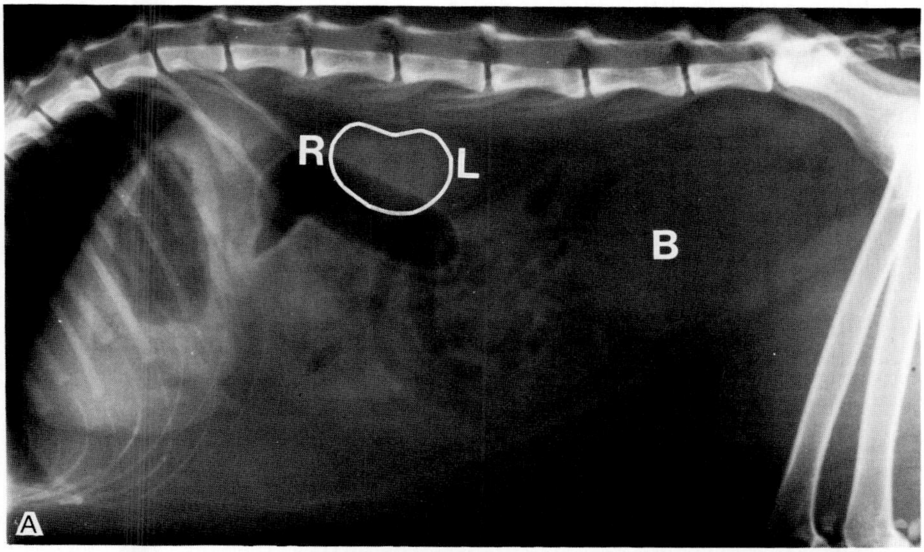

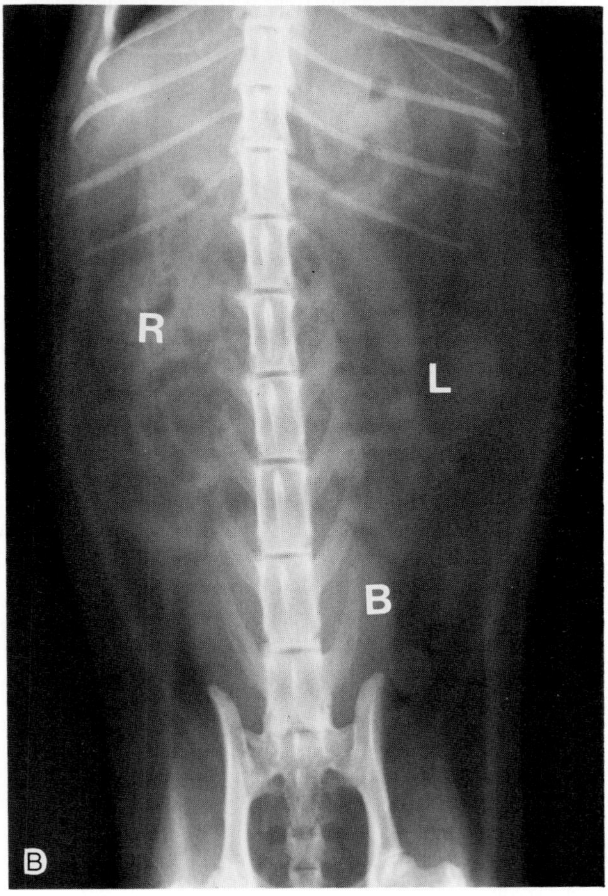

Fig. 10-2. Lateral (A) and ventrodorsal (B) survey abdominal radiographs from a normal 2-year-old spayed female domestic shorthair cat. Left (L) and right (R) kidneys and the urinary bladder (B) are illustrated. The encircled area in the lateral survey radiographs shows a normal increased soft tissue density because renal silhouettes are partially superimposed.

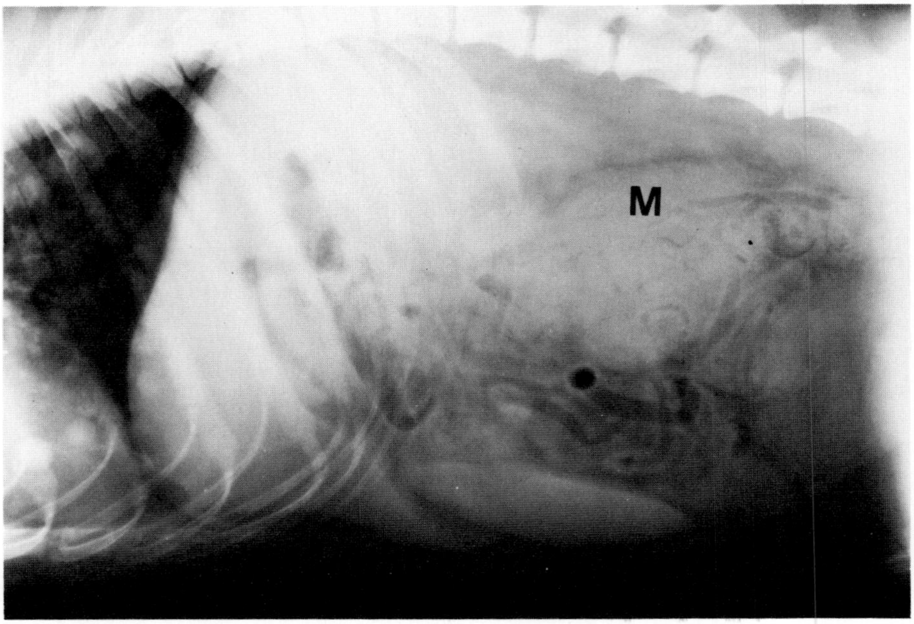

Fig. 10-3. Lateral survey radio graph from 5-year-old German shepherd dog with anorexia of 1 month's duration. Physical examination revealed a palpable abdominal mass (M) in the midabdomen. Postmortem diagnosis was renal adenocarcinoma of the left kidney. Note interstitial nodular lung disease. Compare to Figure 10-17.

normalities in the shape of the kidneys may be related to congenital, inflammatory, infectious, traumatic, or neoplastic disease.

In general, the canine kidney is approximately $2\frac{1}{2}$ to $3\frac{1}{2}$ times the size of the second lumbar vertebra on the ventrodorsal radiograph.[8] The normal adult cat kidney is 2.4 to 3 times the length of the second lumbar vertebra on the ventrodorsal radiograph.[9] The kidney which is smaller than normal may be the result of end-stage renal disease from any etiology.[1,2,10] Congenital anomalies and hypoplasia must also be considered for small, irregularly shaped kidneys.[1,2,10] A normal-sized kidney, whether symmetrically or asymmetrically shaped could be caused by a variety of diseases except hypoplasia.[1,2,10,11,12] Markedly enlarged kidneys may be indicative of obstructive uropathy, inflammation, or traumatic or neoplastic disease (Fig. 10-3).[1,2,4,10,11,13,14] Inability to identify the kidneys on survey radiographs of a young animal may be normal and related to inadequate quantities of retroperitoneal and peritoneal fat or may be related to poor patient preparation. However, inability to define the kidneys on survey radiographs may be abnormal and related to blood, urine, inflammatory or neoplastic infiltrate in the retroperitoneal space, or free peritoneal fluid (Fig. 10-4).

The normal radiographic density of the kidney is that of soft tissue (water). On a lateral recumbent projection, the renal pelvis may appear radiolucent

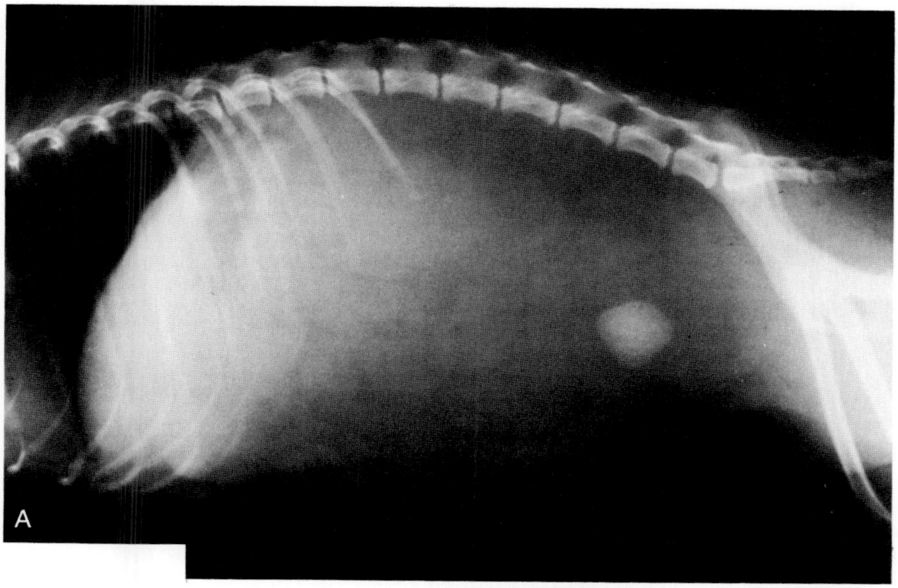

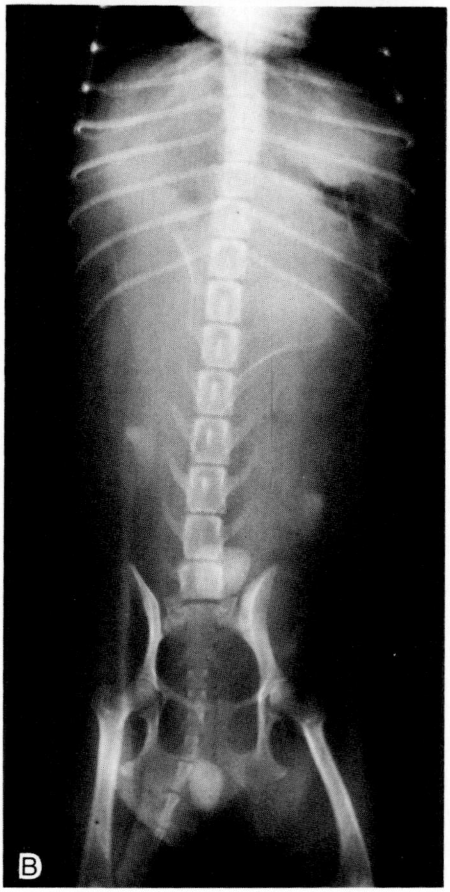

Fig. 10-4. Lateral (A) and ventrodorsal (B) survey radiographs from a 2-year-old female Yorkshire terrier with anorexia, depression, abdominal pain, and abdominal distension of 3 days duration. Poor retroperitoneal and peritoneal contrast and detail associated with a cystic and urethral (ventrodorsal radiograph) calculi are encountered radiographically. Ureteral, urinary bladder, and/or urethral rupture were suspected. Compare to Figure 10-23.

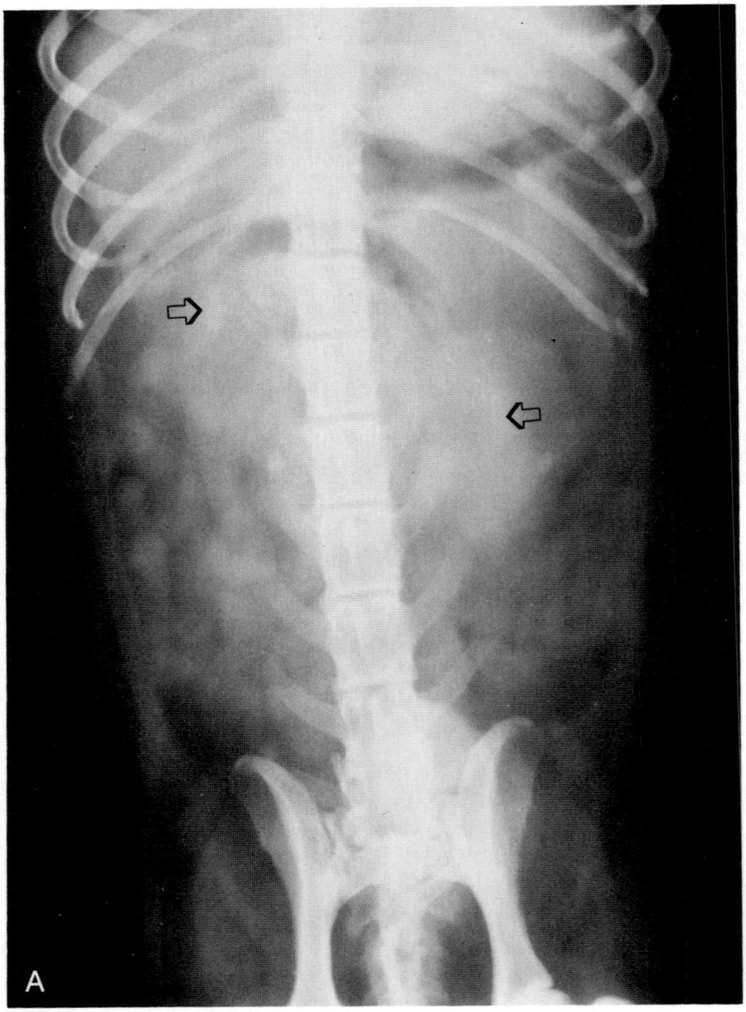

Fig. 10-5. Focal mineralization associated with the renal silhouettes may be encountered on survey radiographs and may result from dystrophic calcification of the renal parenchyma or renal pelvic calculi. (A) Ventrodorsal survey radiograph from a 2-year-old male dalmation dog with chronic hematuria, dysuria, and blood dripping from the prepuce. Bilateral focal mineralizations of the renal hilus (arrows) indicate renal pelvic calculi. Compare to Figure 10-18. (*Figure continues.*)

because of perihilar fat. Abnormal densities associated with the kidneys may be focal or diffuse radiopacities or radiolucencies.[4,5,10] Focal mineralization associated with the renal silhouette may be dystrophic calcification within the renal parenchyma associated with inflammatory, infectious, noninfectious, or neoplastic disease or renal pelvic calculi (Fig. 10-5). Nephrocalcinosis is a diffuse opacification of the kidneys but is not pathognomonic for a specific

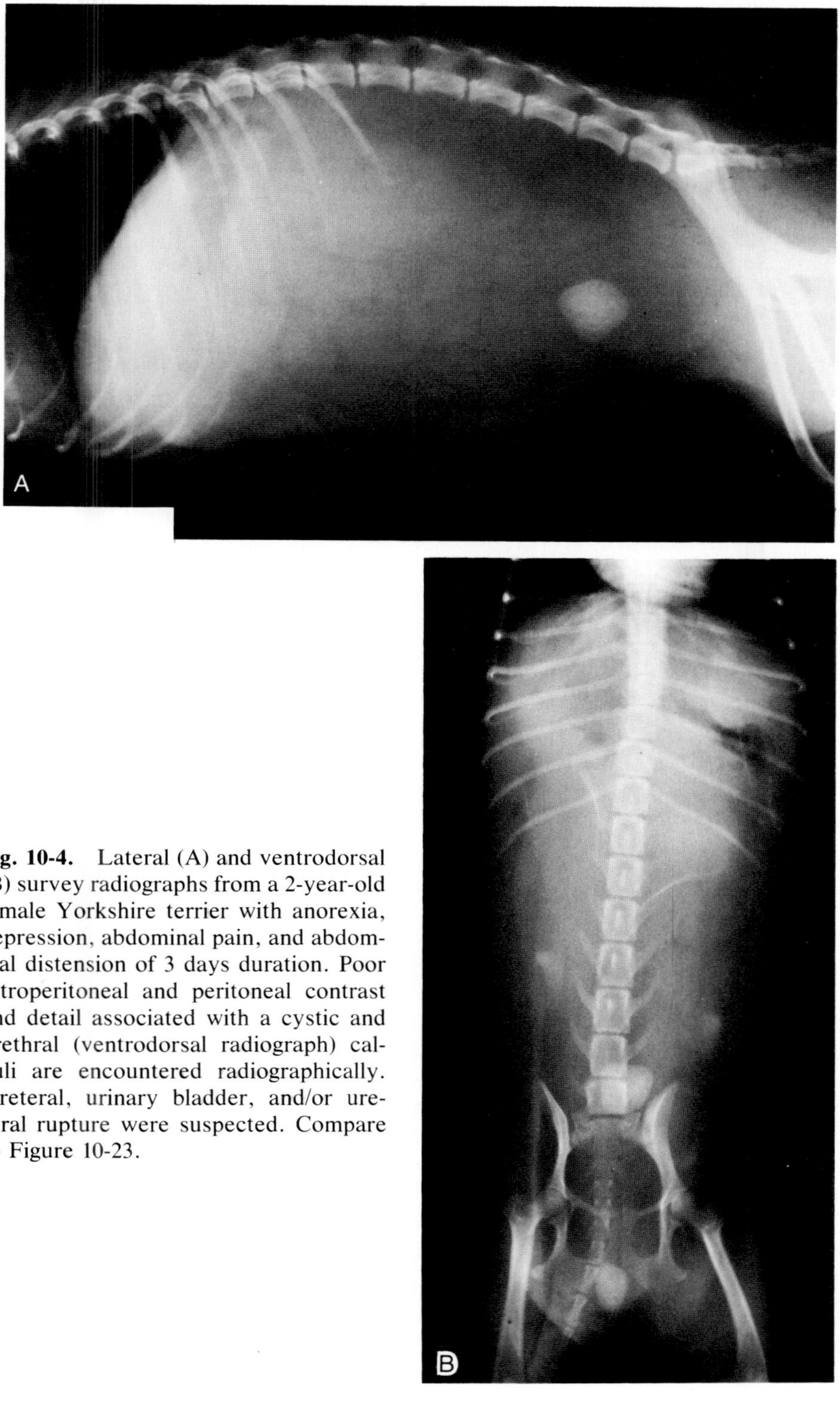

Fig. 10-4. Lateral (A) and ventrodorsal (B) survey radiographs from a 2-year-old female Yorkshire terrier with anorexia, depression, abdominal pain, and abdominal distension of 3 days duration. Poor retroperitoneal and peritoneal contrast and detail associated with a cystic and urethral (ventrodorsal radiograph) calculi are encountered radiographically. Ureteral, urinary bladder, and/or urethral rupture were suspected. Compare to Figure 10-23.

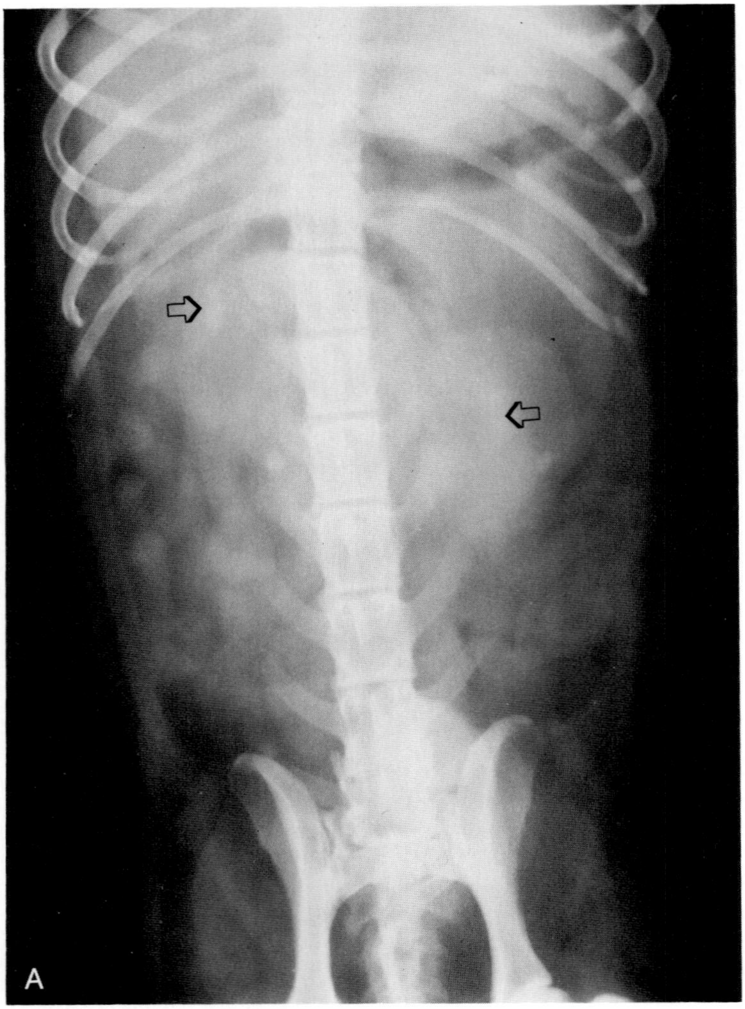

Fig. 10-5. Focal mineralization associated with the renal silhouettes may be encountered on survey radiographs and may result from dystrophic calcification of the renal parenchyma or renal pelvic calculi. (A) Ventrodorsal survey radiograph from a 2-year-old male dalmation dog with chronic hematuria, dysuria, and blood dripping from the prepuce. Bilateral focal mineralizations of the renal hilus (arrows) indicate renal pelvic calculi. Compare to Figure 10-18. (*Figure continues.*)

because of perihilar fat. Abnormal densities associated with the kidneys may be focal or diffuse radiopacities or radiolucencies.[4,5,10] Focal mineralization associated with the renal silhouette may be dystrophic calcification within the renal parenchyma associated with inflammatory, infectious, noninfectious, or-neoplastic disease or renal pelvic calculi (Fig. 10-5). Nephrocalcinosis is a diffuse opacification of the kidneys but is not pathognomonic for a specific

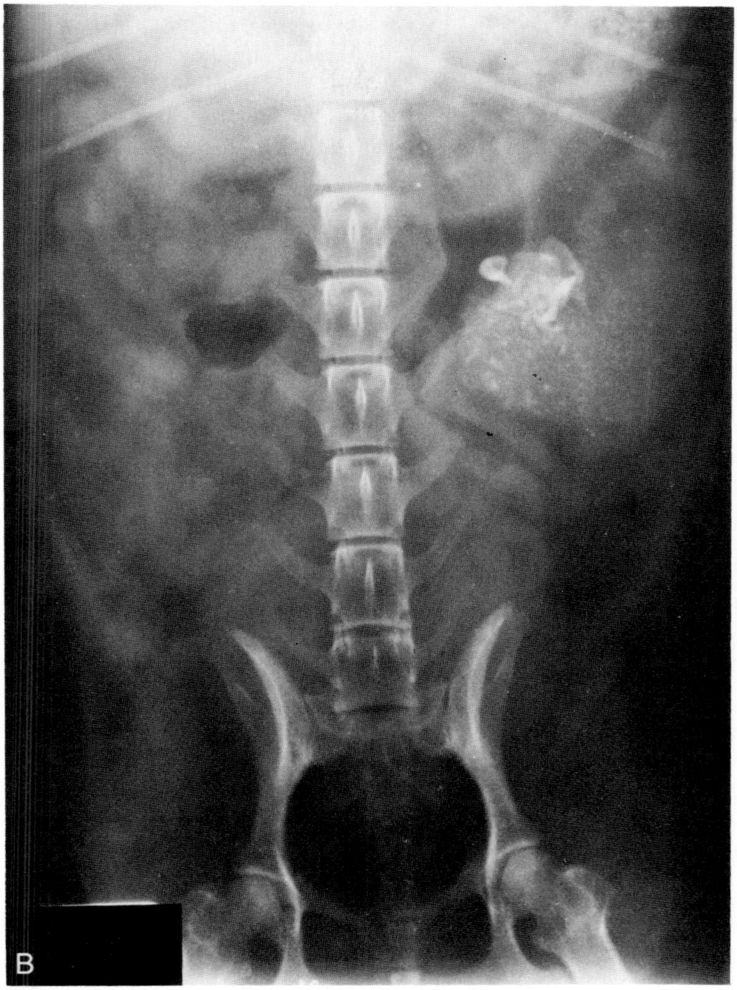

Fig. 10-5 (*continued*). (B) Multifocal mineralizations of the left renal hilum and caudal pole with focal enlargement of the caudal pole of the left kidney were encountered in an 11-year-old female miniature poodle with chronic gross hematuria. Compare to Figure 10-16.

disease. Nephrocalcinosis may be associated with calcium oxalate precipitation secondary to ethylene glycol toxicity, chronic end-stage renal disease, secondary hyperparathyroidism, and Cushing's syndrome.[5,15-17] Nephrocalcinosis has also been reported secondary to conditions that can result in hypercalcemia.[18] Radiolucent densities (gas) associated with the renal silhouette may be encountered on survey radiographs and may be located within the renal parenchyma, the renal pelvis, or both. Gas produced by bacteria, vesicoureteral reflux of gas during pneumocystography, double contrast cystography or emphysematous cystitis, and direct extension of gas from intra-abdominal or extra-abdominal diseases may result in radiolucent densities of the perirenal tissues or renal pelvis.[5]

Ureters. The ureters are fibromuscular tubular structures that connect the renal pelvis with the trigone of the urinary bladder. The function of the ureters is to transport urine produced by the kidneys to the urinary bladder. In normal dogs and cats, the ureters cannot be defined on survey radiographs. However, in animals with excessive amounts of retroperitoneal fat, the ureters have reportedly been identified.[5] The most common survey radiographic abnormality associated with the ureters is focal radiopacification caused by ureteral uroliths (Fig. 10-6). Because of the inability to define the ureters on survey radiographs, opacification of these structures by excretory urography is the most direct method for obtaining information about their size, patency, and site(s) of termination.

Urinary Bladder. The urinary bladder is a muscular tubular structure located in the caudal abdomen. The function of the urinary bladder is to collect and store urine that is produced by the kidneys and to void the contents to the exterior through the urethra. The ability to identify the urinary bladder on survey radiographs depends upon the degree of urinary bladder distension (Figs. 10-1 and 10-2). In dogs, the urinary bladder can be located partially or totally within the pelvis when empty.[19,21] As the urinary bladder distends, it will assume a more cranial location within the abdomen. A partially intrapelvic bladder has been reported following urinary bladder distension in normal male and female dogs.[22] In cats, the urinary bladder is intra-abdominally located regardless of the degree of urinary bladder distention.[7,23]

The shape of the urinary bladder is variable, depending upon the degree of urinary bladder distension and has been reported to be round to oval in dogs and more elipsoid or tear-drop shaped in cats.[19,24]

An abnormal position or location for the urinary bladder may be caused by abdominal, inguinal, or perineal hernias or by displacement from caudal abdominal masses (Fig. 10-7).[19] The direction of displacement is related to the origin of the mass and its relationship to the urinary bladder. Testicular tumors, prostatic cysts, lymphadenopathy, pelvic neoplasia, and retroperitoneal abscesses may cause urinary bladder displacement (Fig. 10-8). Cystography should follow survey radiography for identification of the location of the urinary bladder.

An abnormal shape to the urinary bladder, indicative of a urachal diverticulum, may be encountered on lateral survey radiographs and is characterized by a cranioventral wedge-shaped soft tissue protuberence from the urinary bladder (Fig. 10-9).

Abnormal radiographic densities (radiopaque or radiolucent) may be associated with the urinary bladder. Radiopaque calculi are a common cause of abnormal radiodensities associated with the urinary bladder silhouette. Uroliths may be solitary or multiple and may vary in size (Figs. 10-4, 10-6, 10-9, and 10-10). The common uroliths encountered in dogs and cats within the lower urinary tract, their composition, relative radiographic density, and other dis-

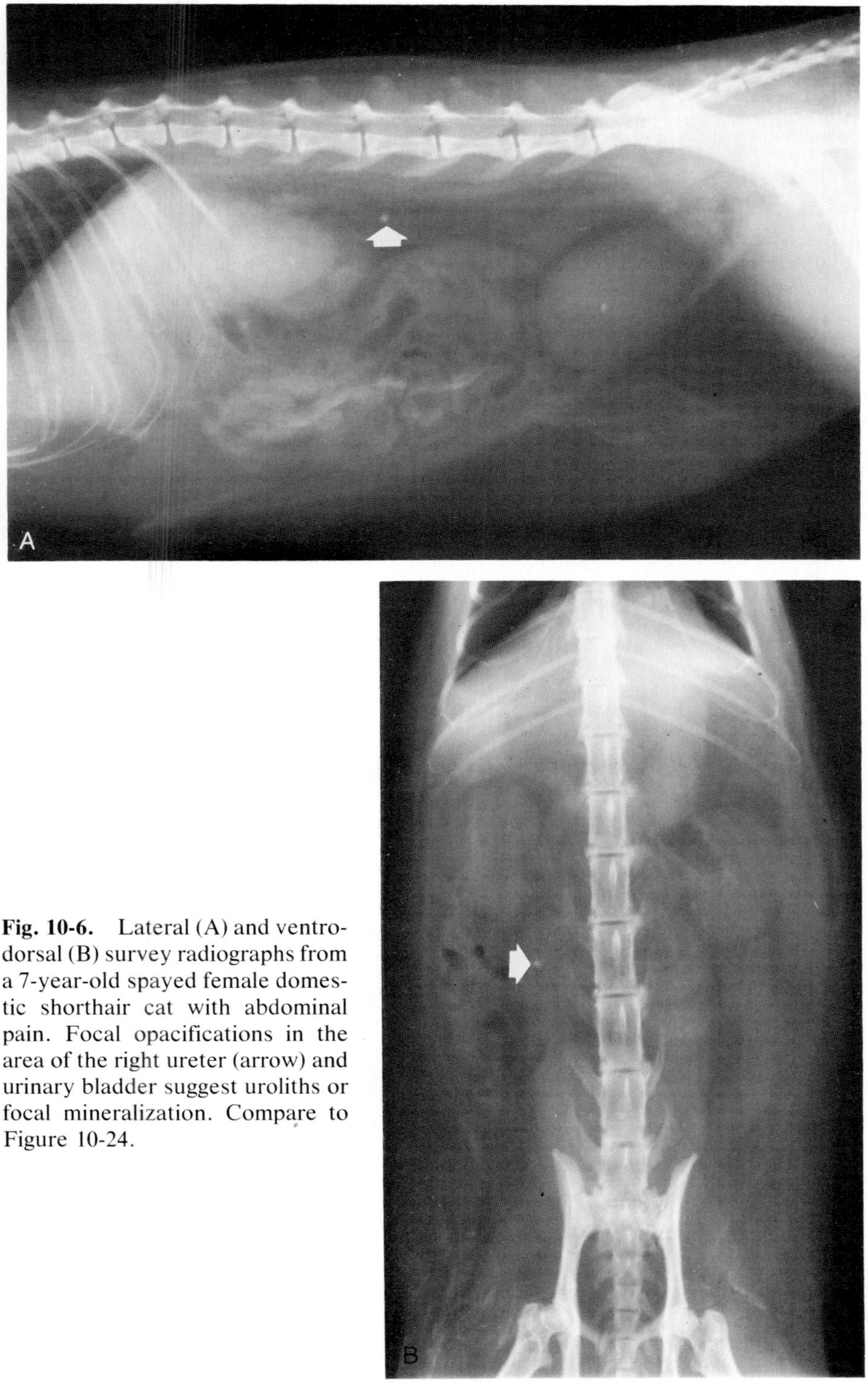

Fig. 10-6. Lateral (A) and ventrodorsal (B) survey radiographs from a 7-year-old spayed female domestic shorthair cat with abdominal pain. Focal opacifications in the area of the right ureter (arrow) and urinary bladder suggest uroliths or focal mineralization. Compare to Figure 10-24.

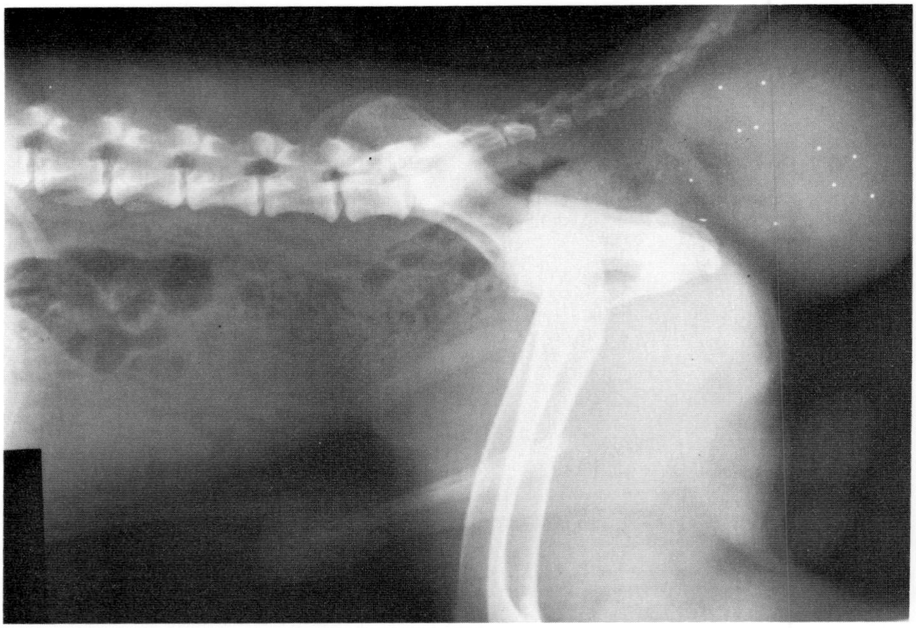

Fig. 10-7. A lateral survey radiograph from an 8-year-old male mixed breed dog with a history of a soft tissue mass elevating the tail head and abdominal straining. The absence of the urinary bladder silhouette on the survey radiograph is suggestive of a perineal hernia, which was confirmed at surgery.

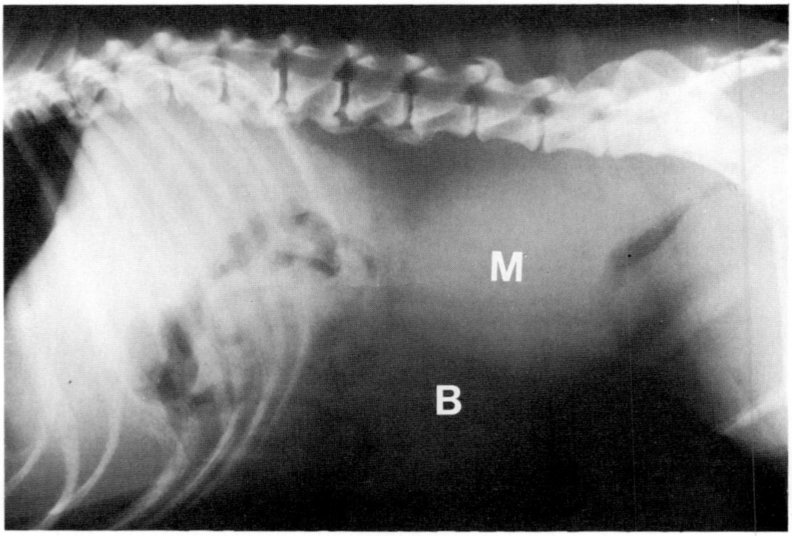

Fig. 10-8. Lateral survey radiograph from a 5-year-old male boxer dog with depression, anorexia, and vomiting of several weeks duration. Physical findings included superficial lymphadenopathy and a palpable abdominal mass. Aspiration biopsy indicated mast cell sarcoma. Cranioventral displacement of the urinary bladder (B) by enlarged sublumbar lymph nodes (M) is evident on the lateral survey radiograph.

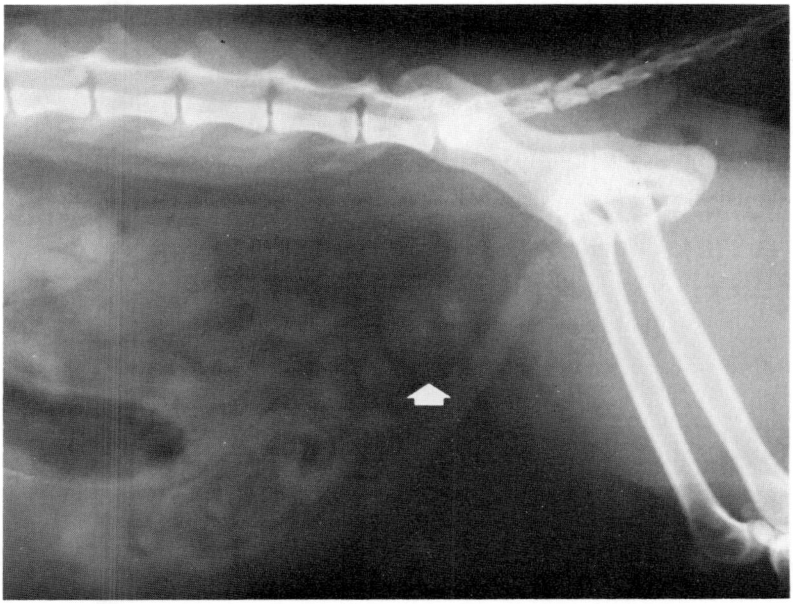

Fig. 10-9. Lateral survey radiograph from a 5-year-old male domestic shorthair cat with hematuria of 1 year duration. Two cystic uroliths and an abnormal bladder shape suggestive of a diverticulum (arrow) are encountered radiographically. Compare to Figure 10-30.

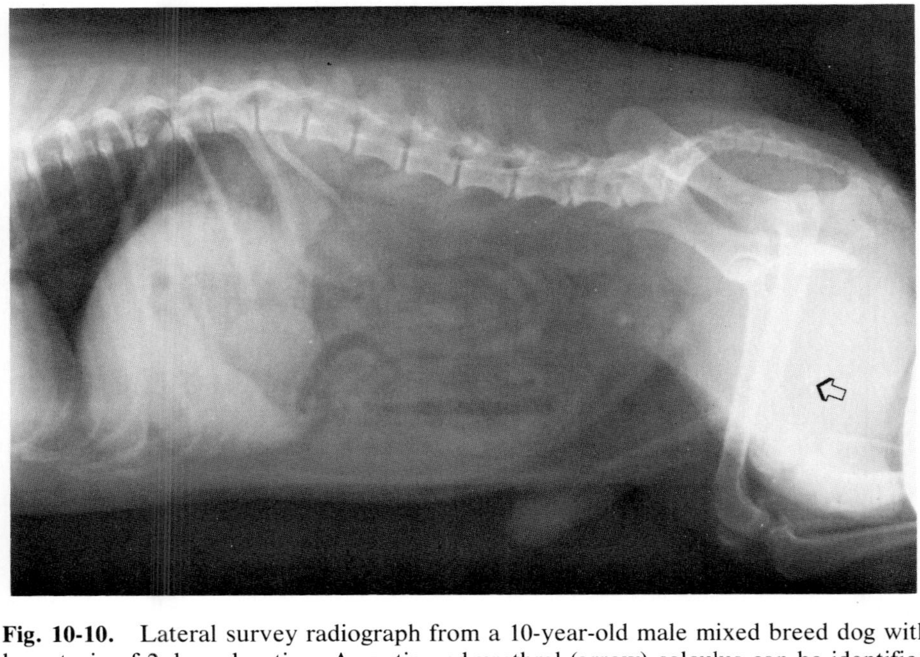

Fig. 10-10. Lateral survey radiograph from a 10-year-old male mixed breed dog with hematuria of 2 days duration. A cystic and urethral (arrow) calculus can be identified radiographically.

Table 10-1. Radiographic Characteristics of Common Uroliths

Predominant Mineral Type	Degree of Radiopacity	Shape
Cystine	+ to + +	Smooth; usually small; round to oval
Oxalate	+ + + +	Rough; round or oval
Phosphate (struvite)	+ + to + + + +	Smooth; round or faceted; sometimes assume shape of renal pelvis, ureter, bladder, or urethra
Phosphate (apatite)	+ + + +	Smooth; round or faceted
Urate	+ to + +	Smooth; round or oval
Silica	+ + to + + + +	Typically jackstone

(Osborne CA, Klausner JS: War on urolithiasis: Problems and solutions. Scientific Proceedings of the American Animal Hospital Association, South Bend, IN, 1978.)

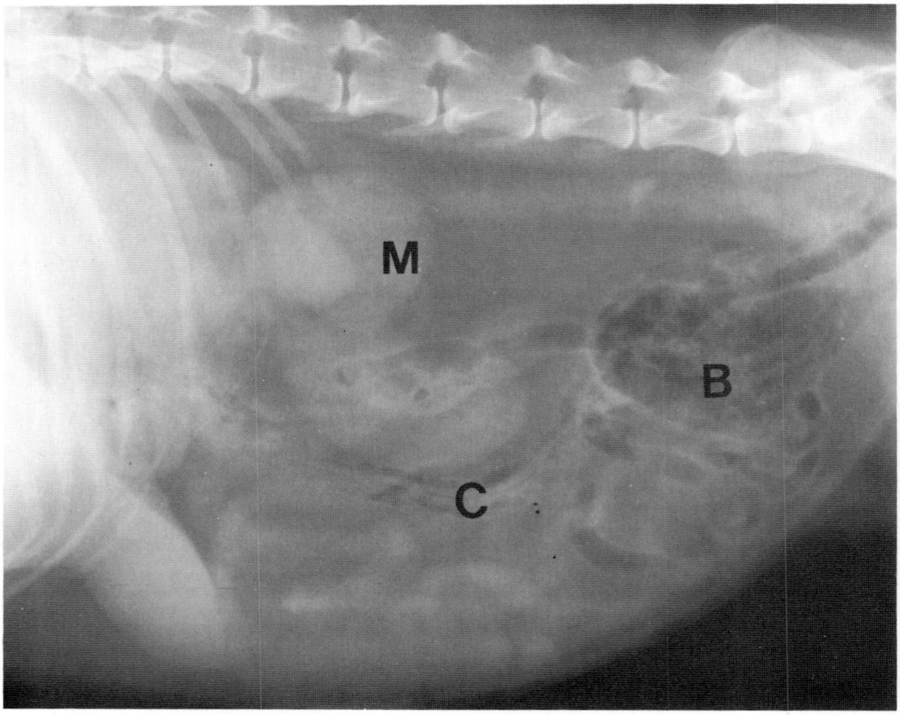

Fig. 10-11. A lateral survey radiograph of a 10-year-old female samoyed dog with a history of hematuria and dysuria. Gas within the urinary bladder (B) wall and lumen (emphysematous cystitis) and within the wall of the descending colon (C) (emphysematous colitis) are encountered radiographically. Hepatomegaly and a soft tissue mass (M) associated with the caudal pole of the right kidney are also encountered. Postmortem findings verified the existence of a functional adrenal cortical tumor which resulted in emphysematous cystitis and colitis, hepatomegaly, and ascending pyelonephritis.

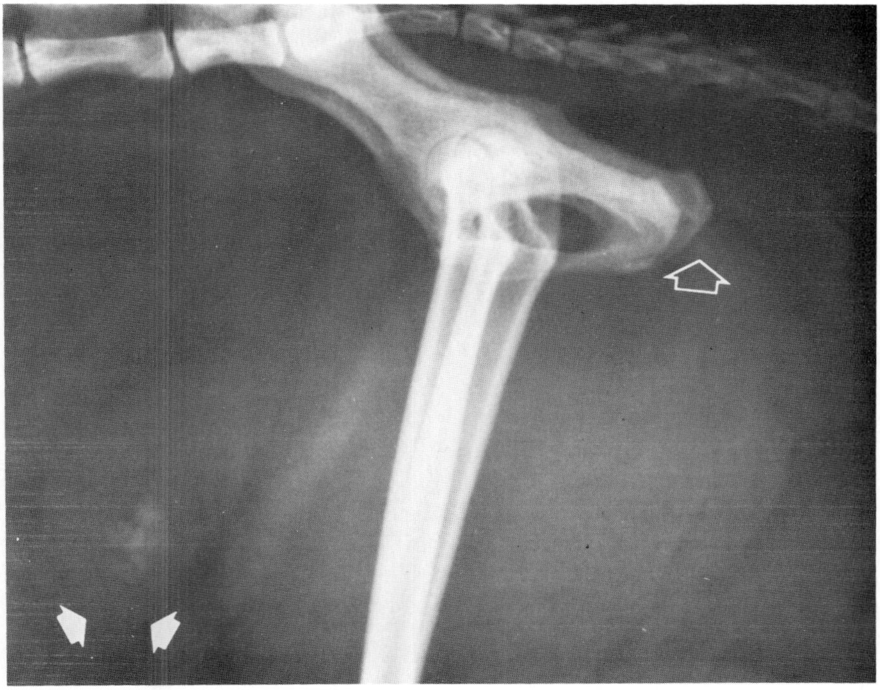

Fig. 10-12. Lateral survey radiograph from a 5-year-old neutered male domestic shorthair cat with dysuria and stranguria. A wedge-shaped protruding density from the cranioventral bladder margin is suggestive of a diverticulum (closed arrow). Multiple cystic uroliths and a solitary urethral urolith (open arrow) are illustrated. Compare to Figure 10-46. (Johnston GR, Feeney DA, Osborne CA: Urethrography and cystography in cats. Part II. Abnormal radiographic anatomy and complications. Comp Cont Vet Ed 4:931, 1982.)

tinguishing characteristics are listed in Table 10-1. Dystrophic calcification of the wall of the urinary bladder may be encountered on survey radiographs and may be secondary to inflammatory polypoid cystitis and neoplasia.[19,25] Superimposed radiopacities over the urinary bladder may be artifactual and caused by intestinal contents, nipples, prepuce, or foreign material in the skin or abdominal wall. Superimposed radiopacities can be further defined radiographically by taking additional abdominal radiographs in lateral, ventrodorsal, or oblique recumbencies.

Radiolucencies associated with the urinary bladder are less common and may be iatrogenic or secondary to infectious disease. Free gas within the bladder lumen may be secondary to catheterization or cystocentesis. The gas bubble will appear round, smooth, and freely movable when viewed on the lateral and ventrodorsal radiograhs. With emphysematous cystitis, gas is located within the wall and/or lumen of the urinary bladder and may appear as radiolucent coalescing lines following the contour of the urinary bladder wall (Fig. 10-11).

Emphysematous cystitis may be iatrogenic and secondary to traumatic catheterization in association with inflammatory, infectious, noninfectious, or neoplastic disease or may be primary and related to a gas-forming bacterium. Emphysematous cystitis may be encountered secondary to diabetes mellitus, Cushing's disease, and Clostridial infections.[26,27]

Urethra. The urethra of dogs and cats is a fibromuscular tubular conduit connecting the urinary bladder to the exterior and functions as a passageway for voiding bladder contents to the exterior. The urethra of male and female dogs and cats cannot be defined on survey radiographs because the fluid density of the urethra cannot be differentiated from other caudal abdominal and intrapelvic soft tissue densities. In obese dogs and cats, the proximal urethra originating at the bladder neck may be identified on a lateral survey radiograph. The urethra is amenable to radiographic evaluation using special contrast procedures because of its tubular nature. Radiopaque densities are commonly associated with the urethra of male and female dogs and cats.[26,28,29] The penile urethra in the area of the os penis is the most common site of urethral obstruction in male dogs (Fig. 10-10).[19] The penile urethra is also a common site of obstruction in male cats, but other sites have been reported (Fig. 10-12).[29] Urethral obstruction caused by uroliths is less common in female dogs and cats but has been reported (Fig. 10-4).[26,28,29]

CONTRAST RADIOGRAPHY

Contrast Agents

Contrast uroradiography will provide the clinician with additional anatomical and functional information not obtained by survey radiography. Contrast uroradiographic special procedures are simple, inexpensive, and relatively safe techniques that can be employed for evaluation of the kidneys, ureters, urinary bladder, and urethra.

Positive Contrast Agents. The positive contrast agents most frequently used for evaluation of the upper or lower urinary tract include organic iodinated benzoic acid derivatives. Sodium and meglumine, diatrizoates, and iothalamates are the current contrast agents most frequently used for evaluation of the urinary system.[5,9,24] Barium sulfate has been advocated as a positive contrast agent for evaluation of the urinary bladder because of its superior coating properties.[30] Complications of the use of barium sulfate are rare but have been reported to include barium casts and interstitial fibrosis secondary to vesicoureteral reflux.[31] Barium sulfate may also serve as a nidus for formation of uroliths.[32] Granulomatous disease may occur secondary to a ruptured urinary bladder or urethra if barium sulfate escapes into the peritoneal cavity.[33–38] However, the risk of potential complications associated with barium sulfate cystography may be overstated. The use of barium sulfate as a cystographic agent in normal male dogs indicated only a mild nonprogressive inflammatory reaction to the urinary bladder and kidneys.[39] Sodium and meglumine diatrizoates and iothalamates are aqueous iodinated contrast agents which will provide mucosal coating in areas of urothelial ulcerations and attached blood clots.[19] Organic iodinated contrast agents should be used as 5 to 10 percent solutions to minimize inflammatory bladder diseases caused by higher concentrations.[40] Inorganic iodide solutions of 10 percent concentrations should be avoided because of the greater irritation to the urinary bladder compared to organic iodide compounds.[41]

Negative Contrast Agents. Air, nitrous oxide, carbon dioxide, and oxygen are negative contrast agents that can be used for evaluation of the lower urinary tract. The advantage of air is that it is inexpensive and readily available. In cases of urothelial ulcerations and tears, air should be avoided because of a possibility of vascular embolization.[42,43] Carbon dioxide, nitrous oxide, and oxygen have a higher solubility coefficient in plasma than does air and should be utilized as negative contrast agents in suspected cases of urothelial ulcerations or tears.

Contrast Agent Influence on Clinical Laboratory Data. Procedures using contrast agents for evaluation of the upper and/or lower urinary tract may provide considerable information relative to the structure and function of these organs; they may also influence clinical laboratory data obtained from these organs for up to 24 hours following their use. Elevations in the specific gravity of the urine have been reported following the use of intravenous positive contrast agents.[44] Aqueous iodinated positive contrast agents may also influence in vitro studies used for quantitative and qualitative assessment of urinary tract pathogens.[45] Positive contrast agents can also influence the structure of cells exfoliated in the urine. Because of the influence of positive contrast agents on clinical laboratory data, urine samples must be collected prior to radiographic special procedures utilized for evaluation of the upper or lower urinary tract.

Complications. ***Positive Contrast Agents.*** Positive contrast agents are well tolerated because of their low toxicity. Few reports of complications have been reported. Because of the hypertonicity of the positive contrast agents, a local, reversible, inflammatory reaction may result if undiluted, highly concentrated volumes of positive contrast agents are allowed to come in contact with the mucosa of the urinary bladder for a prolonged period of time.[40] Systemic reactions to positive contrast agents have been infrequently reported in the veterinary literature.[46] The escape of aqueous iodinated contrast agents into the vascular plexus in the lamina propria in the event of urothelial tears may result in vascular embolization but should not be considered a serious complication because these agents are approved for use in vascular studies.

Negative Contrast Agents. The complications associated with negative contrast agents are rare. Vascular embolization of air secondary to urothelial tears during negative contrast or double contrast cystography have been reported.[42,43] If urothelial tears are suspected, a negative contrast agent such as carbon dioxide, nitrous oxide, or oxygen, which have a higher solubility coefficient in plasma and will reduce the likelihood of fatal vascular embolization

Table 10-2. Technique for Excretory Urography

1.	Routine patient preparation
	a. 24 hr without food; water ad libitum
	b. Cleansing enema at least 2 hr before radiography
2.	Assess hydration status; proceed only if it is normal
3.	Obtain survey radiographs
4.	Infuse contrast medium intravenously via the cephalic or jugular vein as rapidly as possible (bolus injection)
	a. Dose: 400 mg iodine/lb body weight
	b. Contrast medium: sodium iothalamate or sodium diatrizoate
5.	Make abdominal radiographs in the following sequence:
	a. Ventrodorsal views at 5 to 20 sec, 5 min, 20 min, and 40 min postinjection for general assessment
	b. Lateral view at 5 min postinjection for general assessment
	c. Oblique views at 3 to 5 min postinjection for ureteral termination in urinary bladder
	d. Lateral and ventrodorsal views at 30 to 40 min postinjection to observe urinary bladder if retrograde cystography is contraindicated or impossible

(Feeney DA, Barber DL, Johnston GR, et al: The excretory urogram: Techniques, normal radiographic appearance and misinterpretation. Comp Cont Vet Educ, 4:233, 1982.)

should be utilized. Iatrogenic emphysematous cystitis without fatal vascular embolization during double contrast cystography has been reported in cats.[26]

Contrast Evaluation of the Kidneys and Ureters

The indications for survey radiography in evaluation of the kidneys also apply to contrast evaluation of the kidneys and ureters. Information from survey radiographs on the size, shape and number, margination, location, and radiographic density of the kidneys and ureters may further justify contrast evaluation of these structures.

Excretory Urography. Because of the limitations of survey radiography, especially in patients with poor radiographic contrast and detail of the abdomen, excretory urography is indicated and will provide additional anatomical information and permit qualitative assessments of renal and ureteral function. Excretory urography (intravenous pyelography, intravenous urography) is a relatively simple, inexpensive technique that can be used to verify the location of upper urinary tract disease and to assess reversibility. Excretory urography cannot quantitatively assess renal function but can be used to assess relative renal function and has been reported as a technique for interpretation of the pathophysiologic mechanisms of renal disease.[46] Excretory urography can be performed in both azotemic and nonazotemic patients if the patient is adequately hydrated. In patients with severe renal failure, it may be necessary to increase the dose of contrast media to provide adequate visualization of the kidneys.

Prior to excretory urography, the patient should be prepared as was described for survey radiography. The technique of excretory urography is described in Table 10-2. Contrast media recommended for excretory urography include sodium and/or meglumine iothalamate and diatrizoate, given in bolus injection intravenously.[46–50] The dosage of contrast media recommended for excretory urography is 400 mg of iodine per pound (0.45 kg) of body weight injected into a preplaced intravenous catheter in the cephalic or jugular vein.[46,47,49] Maintenance of the intravenous catheter for 10 to 15 minutes post-injection is recommended for a readily available route to the circulatory system in event of a hypotensive reaction to the contrast media. Film sequences recommended for excretory urography include a ventrodorsal radiograph taken immediately after injection and right lateral and ventrodorsal radiographs obtained after 5, 10, 20, and 40 minutes.[46,47,49] Additional radiographs taken at earlier time sequences may be necessary for evaluation of ureteral termination. Patients with renal failure may require additional radiographs 1 to 2 hours post-injection. Normal canine and feline excretory urograms are illustrated in Figures 10-13 and 10-14.

Renal angiography is a special radiographic procedure where an angiography catheter is placed in or adjacent to the renal arteries.[51] Contrast media injection of the renal artery will provide detailed anatomical information about the renal architecture not defined by excretory urography. Renal angiography is an invasive procedure that requires general anesthesia and catheter placement in the abdominal aorta by selective catheterization of the femoral artery. Additional equipment required for renal angiography include image intensification fluoroscopy and a rapid film changer. Because of the specialization required and the equipment needed to perform renal angiography, this technique is not feasible for the general practitioner.

Renal ultrasonography is a noninvasive technique that uses high-frequency sound waves directed towards the kidney.[52] Echoes are reflected at tissue interfaces. These echoes are reconstructed into a two-dimensional image. Renal ultrasonography requires special equipment and considerable expertise but will provide information on renal architecture that cannot be obtained by excretory urography. Because of the noninvasiveness of renal ultrasonography, this technique is well suited to patients that are at risk for general anesthesia.

Normal Radiographic Findings. ***Kidneys.*** The normal radiographic findings encountered with excretory urography relative to quantitative appearance of the canine and feline kidney are listed in Table 10-3. Additional information relative to the number, size, shape, and location of the kidneys was previously described under survey radiography.

The two phases of excretory urogram are the nephrographic and pyelographic phases.[46,47] Opacification of the functional renal parenchyma is defined as the nephrogram phase of the excretory urogram. Opacification of the renal pelvis, renal pelvic pseudodiverticula, and ureters is termed the pyelographic phase. During the nephrographic phase, the kidneys are homogeneous except for the very early vascular and tubular phase of the nephrogram, in which the cortex appears more radiopaque than the medulla (Fig. 10-13 and 10-14).[46] The pyelographic phase that follows the nephrographic phase is less radiopaque than the nephrogram (Fig. 10-13 and 10-14). Each phase of the excretory urogram should be interpreted separately and subsequently compared to serial radiographs obtained during the excretory urogram.

The dynamic functional aspects of the excretory urogram are obtained from

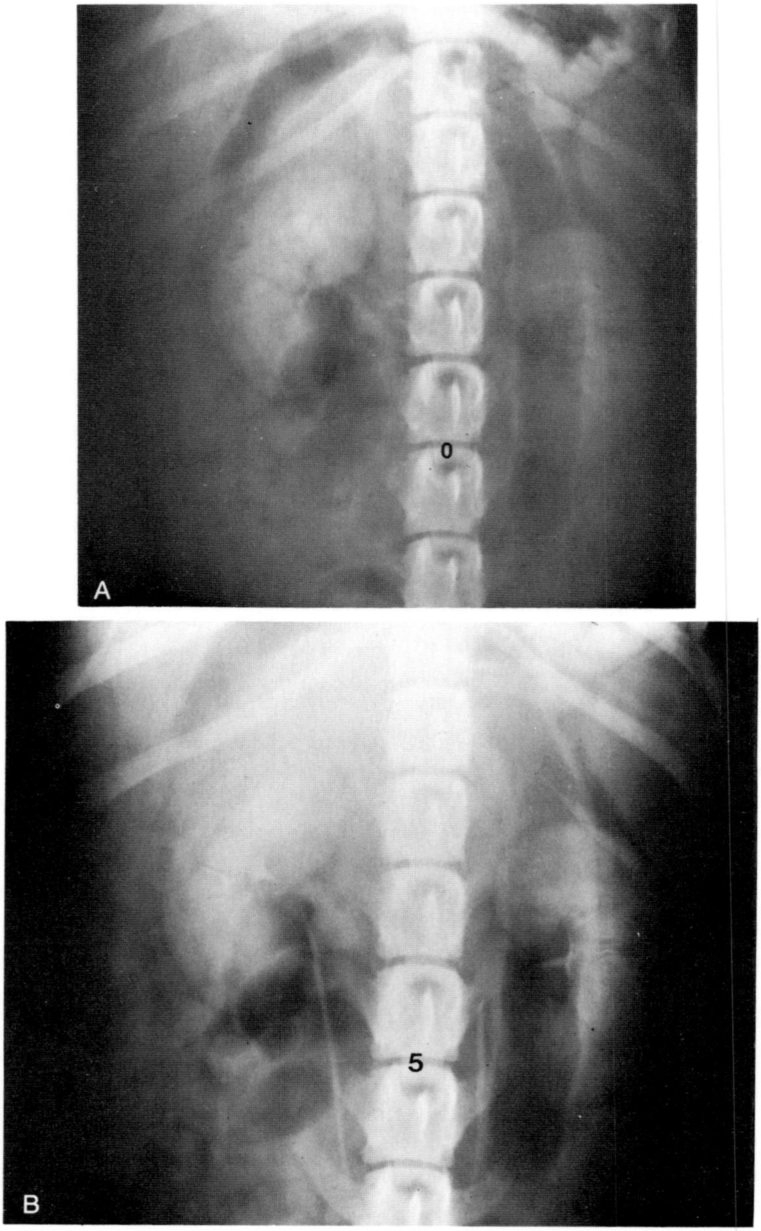

Fig. 10-13. Normal canine excretory urogram obtained 15 sec (labeled 0) (A), 5 min (B), (*Figure continues.*)

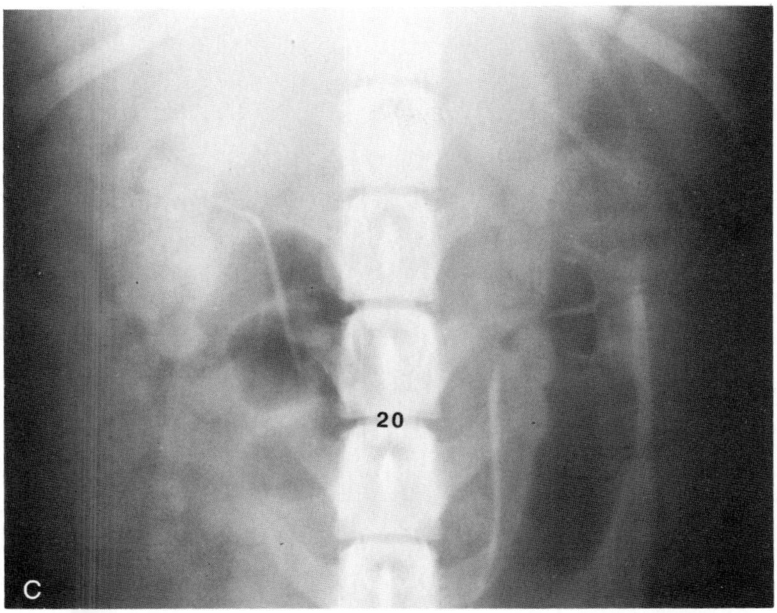

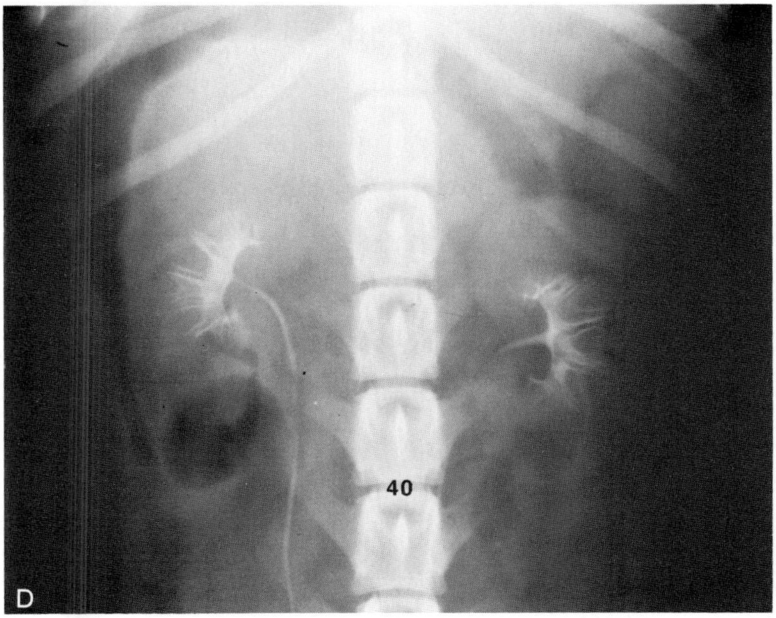

Fig. 10-13 (*continued*). 20 min (C), and 40 min (D) after the intravenous injection of contrast medium.

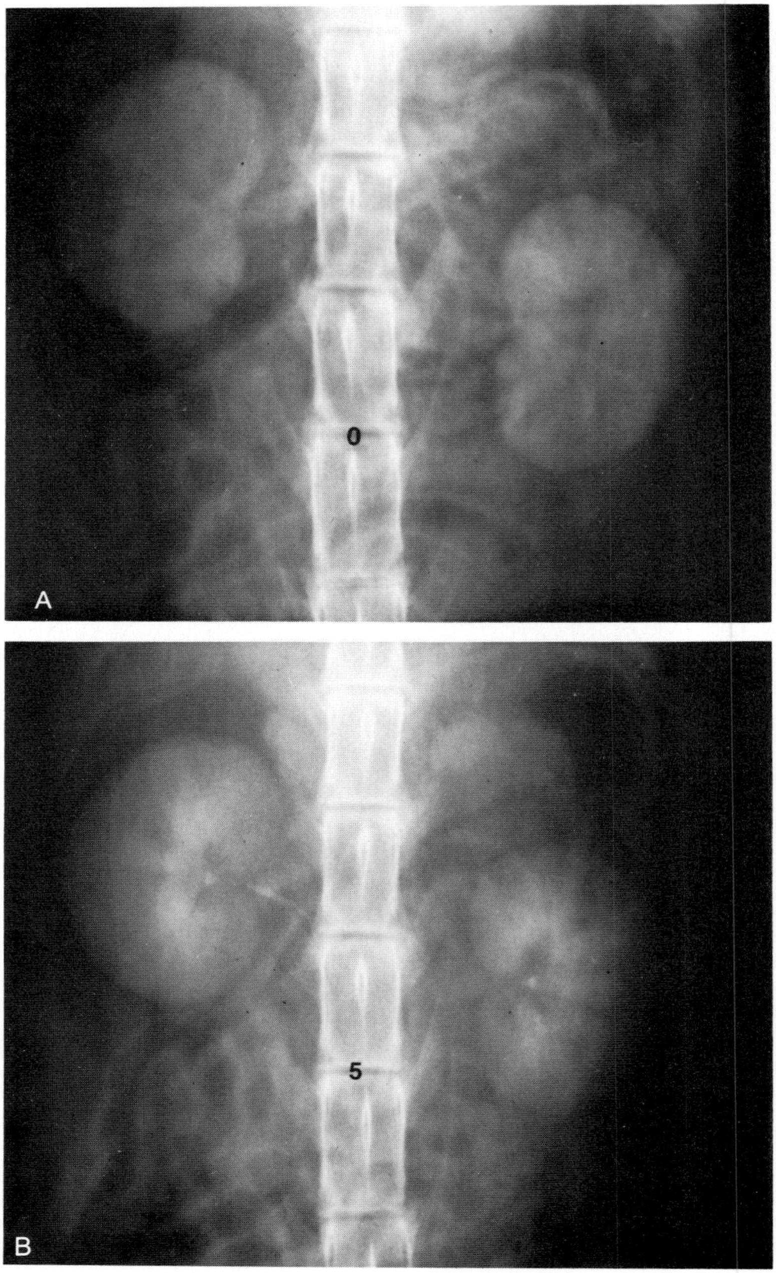

Fig. 10-14. Normal feline excretory urogram obtained 15 sec (labeled 0) (A), 5 min (B), (*Figure continues.*)

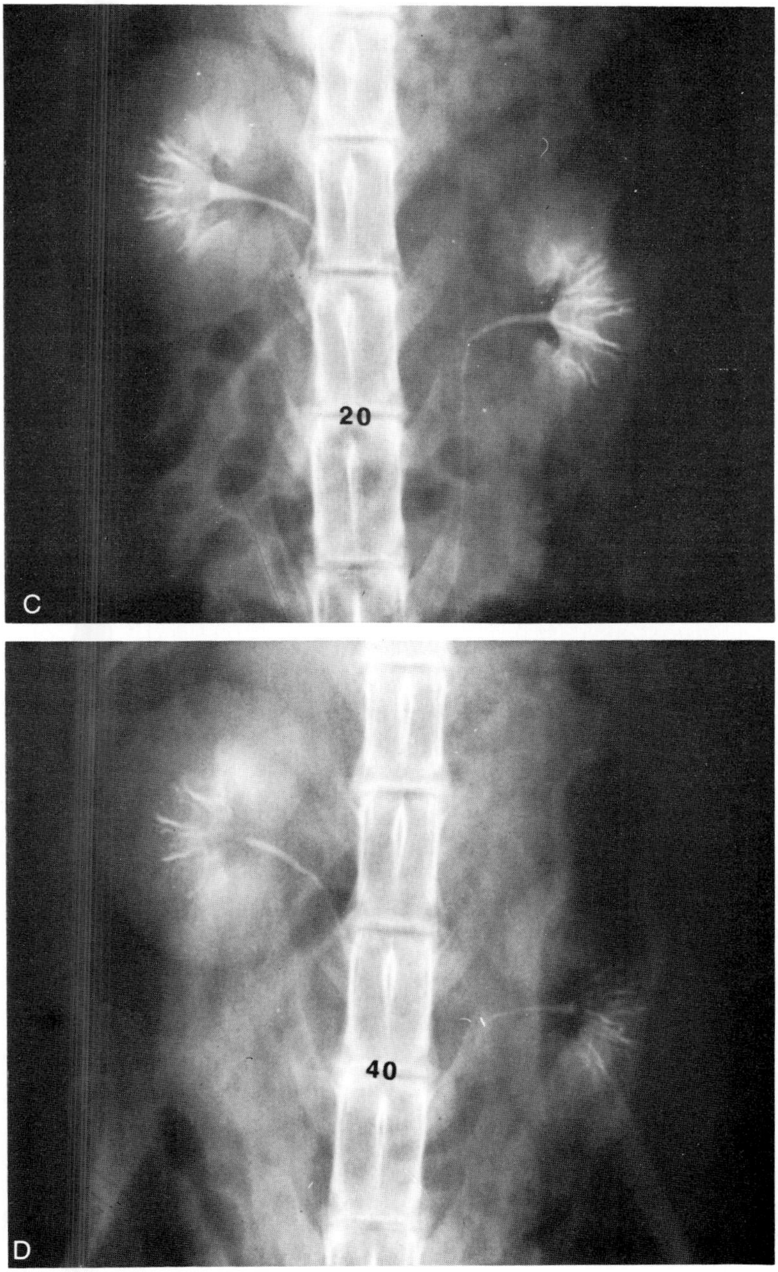

Fig. 10-14 (*continued*). 20 min (C), and 40 min (D) after the intravenous injection of contrast medium.

Table 10-3. Quantitative Appearance of Normal Canine and Feline Excretory Urograms

Structure	Measurement[a]	Value[b]
Kidney	Length	Dog 3.00 ± 0.25 × L-2 2.50 to 3.50 × L-2 Cat 2.4 to 3.0 × L-2 4.0 to 4.5 cm
	Width	Dog 2.00 ± 0.20 × L-2 Cat 3.0 to 3.5 cm
Renal pelvis	Width	Dog 0.03 ± 0.017 × L-2 (generally ≤ 1.0 mm) Cat Not reported
Pelvic diverticula	Width	Dog 0.02 ± 0.005 × L-2 (generally ≤ 1.0 mm) Cat Not reported
Proximal ureter	Width	Dog 0.07 ± 0.018 × L-2 (generally ≤ 2.5 mm) Cat Not reported
Distal ureter	Width	Not reported in dogs or cats

[a] Measurements apply only to the VD view.
[b] L-2 = the length of the body of the second lumbar vertebral body as visualized on the ventrodorsal view.

(Modified from Feeney DA, Barber DL, Johnston GR, et al: The excretory urogram: Techniques, normal radiographic appearance and misinterpretation. Comp Cont Vet Educ, 4:233, 1982.)

assessment of the nephrographic opacification and the subsequent fading of renal opacification on serial radiographs.[46,53] The normal nephrogram should be most dense 10 to 30 seconds following the bolus injection of the contrast media. In subsequent serial radiographs obtained following the injection of contrast media, the nephrographic opacification will progressively decrease. Less than 25 percent of normal dogs will have a detectable nephrogram 2 hours following the injection of contrast media. The pyelographic phase of the excretory urogram should be consistently dense, and the diameter of the ureters should vary with time due to peristalsis. The degree of nephrographic and pyelographic opacification obtained on the initial ventrodorsal radiograph and subsequently compared to the nephrographic and pyelographic phases of the excretory urogram on serial radiographs is used as a qualitative estimate of renal function.[46,53,54] In general, decreased renal function will result in a decreased opacification of the nephrographic and pyelographic phase of the excretory urogram.

Ureters. Since the ureters cannot be identified by survey radiography,

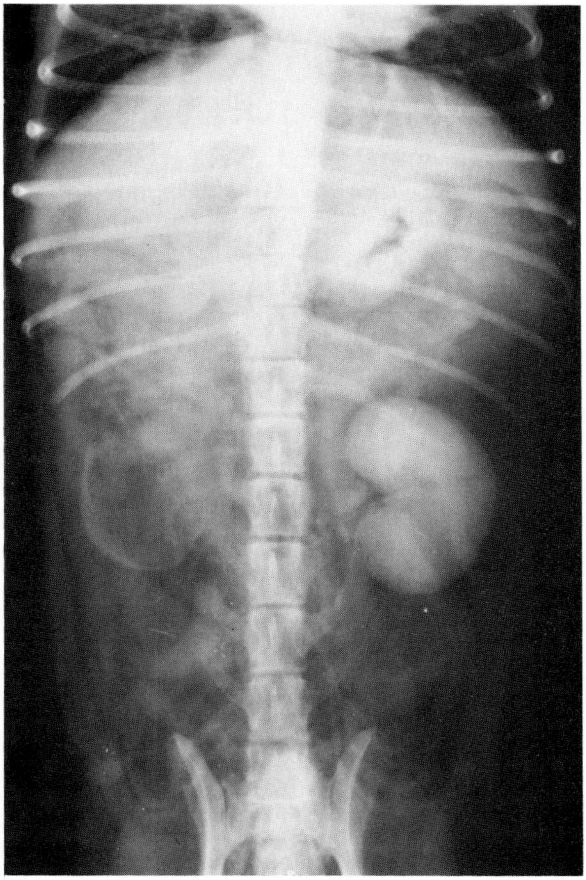

Fig. 10-15. Ventrodorsal radiograph of the nephrographic phase of an excretory urogram from a 12-year-old male miniature schnauzer dog with hematuria. A cortical rim of opacification to the right kidney is encountered radiographically and is suggestive of hydronephrosis. A nephrectomy revealed a transitional cell carcinoma causing renal pelvic obstruction.

excretory urography is required to visualize them. There are normally two ureters in dogs and cats, but they may vary in size (Table 10-3). They are tubular, with segmentation caused by peristaltic contractions for propulsion of urine from the renal pelvis to the urinary bladder. The ureters are primarily retroperitoneal but become intraperitoneal as they approach the trigone of the urinary bladder. The normal radiographic appearance of the ureters in excretory urography in dogs and cats is illustrated in Figures 10-13 and 10-14.[46–50] Functional assessment of the ureters can only be obtained by evaluation of serial radiographs during excretory urography. Complete opacification of the ureter from the renal pelvis to the trigone of the urinary bladder may be abnormal and related to poor ureteral peristalsis, ureteral obstruction, or abnormal renal solute diuresis.

Abnormal Radiograhic Findings. ***Kidneys.*** *Number.* Renal agenesis, aplasia, or nephrectomy must be suspected with the absence of opacification of a kidney on excretory urography.[1,2,55] Unilateral renal agenesis or nephrectomy will result in compensatory hypertrophy of the nonaffected kidney.

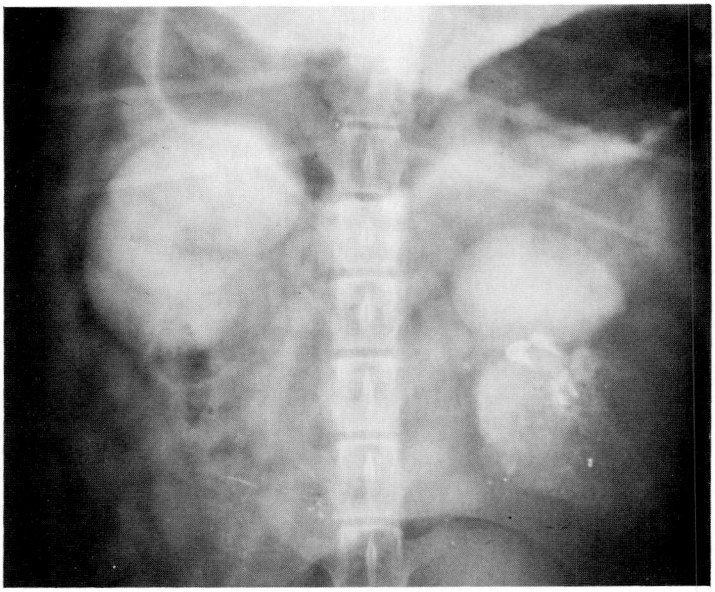

Fig. 10-16. Ventrodorsal radiograph from the nephrographic phase of an excretory urogram in the dog described in Figure 10-5B. Minimal opacification of the caudal pole of the left kidney and associated mineralizations were caused by a hemangioma. (Johnston GR, Feeney DA, Osborne CA; Radiographic findings in urinary tract infection. Vet Clin North Am 9:749, 1979.)

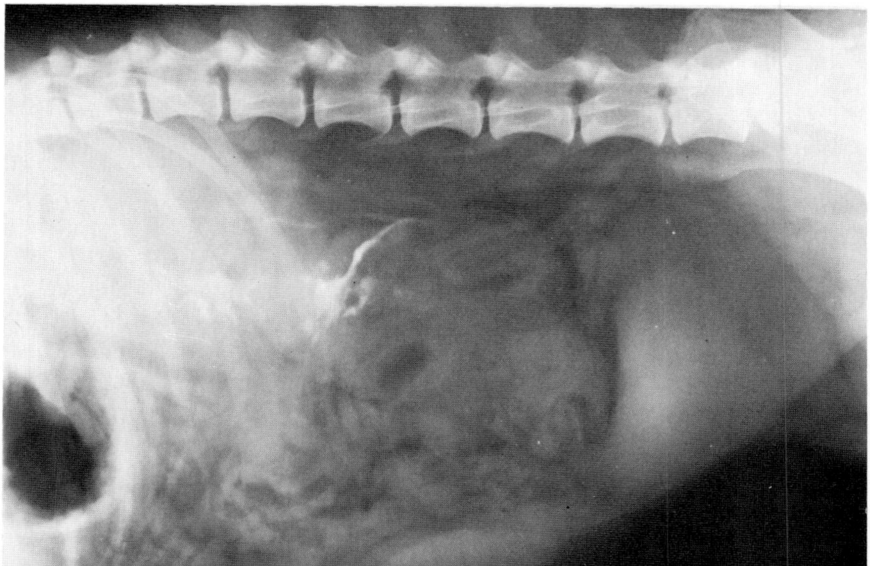

Fig. 10-17. Lateral radiographs of the pyelographic phase of an excretory urogram from the dog described in Figure 10-3. Deformity of the left renal pelvic and extraluminal compression of the urinary bladder were caused by a renal adenocarcinoma.

Table 10-4. Possible Structural Nephrographic Opacification Patterns[a] Associated with Certain Renal Diseases

Uniform opacification	
	Normal
	Compensatory hypertrophy
	Acute glomerular and/or tubulointerstitial disease
	Perirenal pseudocysts
	Hypoplasia
	Others?
Focal, nonuniform opacification	
	Neoplasm
	Hematuria
	Cyst
	Single infarct
	Hydronephrosis
	Abscess
	Others?
Multifocal, nonuniform opacification	
	Polycystic disease
	Multiple infarcts
	Acute pyelonephritis
	Chronic generalized glomerular and/or tubulointerstitial disease
	Feline infectious peritonitis
	Infiltrative neoplasia
	Others?
Nonopacification	
	Aplasia/agenesis
	Renal artery obstruction
	Nephrectomy or nonfunctional renal parenchyma
	Insufficient or extravascular contrast medium injection
	Others?

Bilateral conditions are fatal.

[a] Best identified on radiographs exposed 5–20 sec or 5 min after contrast medium injections. Do not overinterpret corticomedullary separation on early postinjection radiographs.

(Feeney DA, Johnston GR: Radiographic evaluation of the urinary tract in dogs and cats. In Thrall D (ed): Textbook of Veterinary Diagnostic Radiology. WB Saunders, Philadelphia, in press.)

Congenital anomalies may result in renal duplication or consolidation (horseshoe kidney).[10,56,57] The inability to identify a renal silhouette may be related to hypoplasia in association with renal failure and may require additional diagnostic techniques.

Size, shape, margination. The size, shape, and margination of the kidneys as defined by excretory urography should be used as roentgen signs in formulating a list of gamuts for subsequent consideration as differential diagnoses. The gamut approach of abnormal roentgen signs encountered during excretory urography is not pathognomonic for a disease entity. Subsequent investigative techniques including a surgical biopsy are necessary for a definitive diagnosis.

A large, regularly shaped, smoothly marginated kidney can be encountered with compensatory hypertrophy, infiltrative neoplasm, hydronephrosis, renal amyloidosis, glomerulonephritis, solitary renal cyst, and perirenal pseudocyst (Fig. 10-15).[1,2,4,58] Excretory urography will provide additional information on the architecture of the kidney by opacifying the functional renal parenchyma

Table 10.5. Pyelographic Appearance of Some Common Diseases of the Kidney

Pyelonephritis		
	Acute	
		Pelvic dilation
		Proximal ureteral dilation
		Absent or incomplete filling of diverticula
	Chronic	
		± Pelvic dilation with irregular borders
		Proximal ureteral dilation
		Short, blunt diverticula
Hydronephrosis:		
		Pelvic dilation
		Dilation of pelvic diverticula (note: diverticula may not be distinguishable if pelvic dilation is severe)
		Ureteral dilation
Neoplasia:		
	Of renal parenchyma:	
		Distortion or deviation of renal pelvis, with or without dilation
		Distortion or deviation of pelvic diverticula
	Of renal pelvis:	
		Distortion or dilation of renal pelvis
		Filling defects in renal pelvis
Uroliths:		
		Filling defects in renal pelvis
		Uroliths usually radiolucent compared to contrast medium
		May be changes as seen in pyelonephritis
		± Pelvic dilation

(Feeney DA, Barber DL, Osborne CA: Advances in canine excretory urography. In 30th Gaines Veterinary Symposium. Gaines Dog Research Center, White Plains, NY, 1981.)

and subsequently allowing identification of focal or diffuse nonfunctional areas. A sharp delineation between a well-perfused region of a kidney and a well-defined focal nonfunctional portion to that kidney would suggest a more benign abnormality such as a renal cyst.[59] An abnormal, poorly defined margin between a well-perfused region and a nonperfused kidney segment might indicate a neoplastic infiltrate (Fig. 10-16).

Large, irregularly shaped kidneys with rough margins of a focal, multifocal, or diffuse nature may be encountered secondary to neoplasia, renal abscesses, hematomas, polycystic kidneys, feline infectious peritonitis, or perirenal pseudocyst (Fig. 10-17).[1,2,4,58,60–66]

Kidneys of normal size, shape, and margination may be diseased, and differential diagnoses should include amyloidosis, glomerulonephritis, and acute pyelonephritis.[67,68] Kidneys of normal size but with irregular shapes may result from focal or multifocal diseases. Focal variations in renal shape may be related to renal infarction, inflammation, or abscessation.[69] Multifocal to diffuse abnormalities in renal shape and margination may be due to chronic pyelonephritis or polycystic renal disease.[70]

Small kidneys with regular shape and smooth margins may suggest renal hyperplasia but can result from endstage glomerulonephritis, amyloidosis, or familial renal diseases with specific breed predilections.[71-80] Small kidneys with irregular shapes and marginations can result from end-stage renal disease from

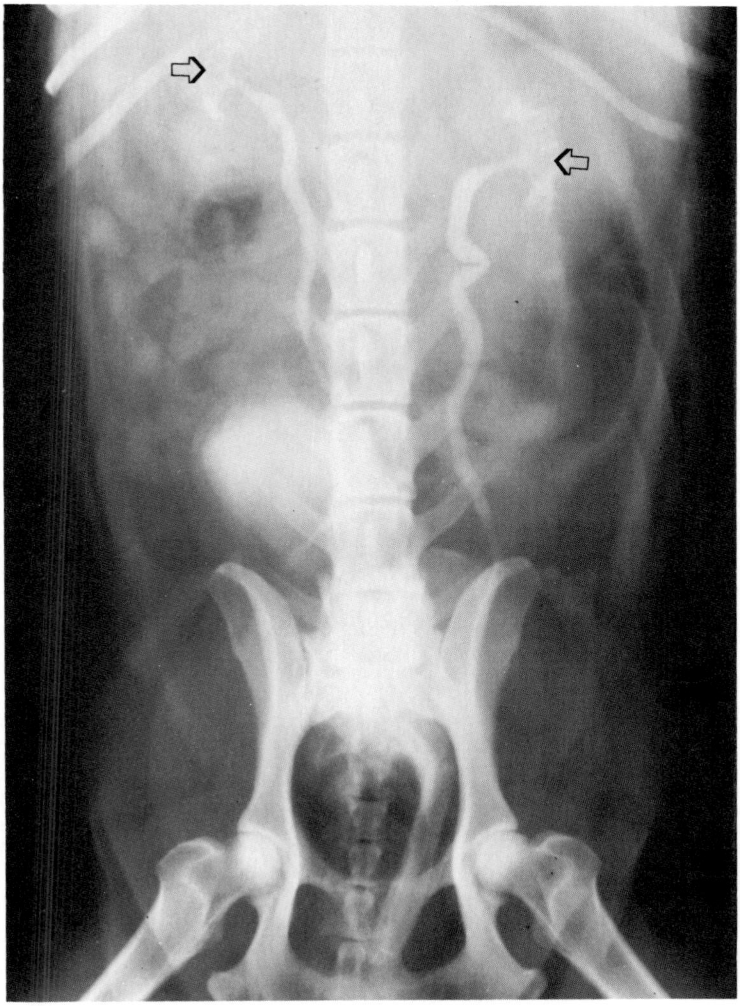

Fig. 10-18. Ventrodorsal radiograph of the pyelographic phase of an excretory urogram described in Figure 10-5A. Bilateral deformity of the renal pelvis characterized by blunting and clubbing of the pseudodiverticula of the renal pelvis and bilateral filling defects of the renal pelvis (arrows) are consistent with a radiographic diagnosis of renal pelvic calculi and pyelonephritis.

a variety of causes. Poor visualization of the kidneys during excretory urography is often a reflection of poor renal function and may provide limited information on renal size, shape, and marginations. Patients with end-stage renal disease will frequently have poor retroperitoneal and peritoneal contrast, which makes further identification of the kidney difficult during survey and contrast urography.

Location. The normal location of the kidneys in a dog and cat was pre-

Table 10-6. Possible Nephrographic Opacification Sequences Associated with Certain Renal Disease Processes

A. Good initial opacification followed by progressively decreasing opacity: normal
B. Fair to good initial opacification followed by progressively increasing opacity:
    Systemic hypotension due to radiocontrast agents
    Acute renal obstruction (including precipitated Tamm-Horsfall mucoprotein in renal tubules)
    Contrast medium-induced renal failure
    Others
C. Fair to good initial opacification followed by persistent opacity:
    Acute renal tubular necrosis
    Contrast medium-induced renal failure
    Systemic hypotension due to radiocontrast agents
    Others
D. Poor initial opacification followed by progressively decreasing opacity:
    Primary polyuric renal failure
    Inadequate contrast medium dose
    Others
E. Poor initial opacification followed by progressively increasing opacity:
    Acute extrarenal obstruction
    Systemic hypotension existing prior to contrast medium administration
    Renal ischemia (arterial or venous)
    Others
F. Poor initial opacification followed by persistent opacity:
    Primary glomerular dysfunction (chronic)
    Severe generalized renal disease

(Feeney DA, Barber DL, Osborne CA: Functional aspects of the nephrogram in excretory urography: A review. Vet Radiol 23:42, 1982.)

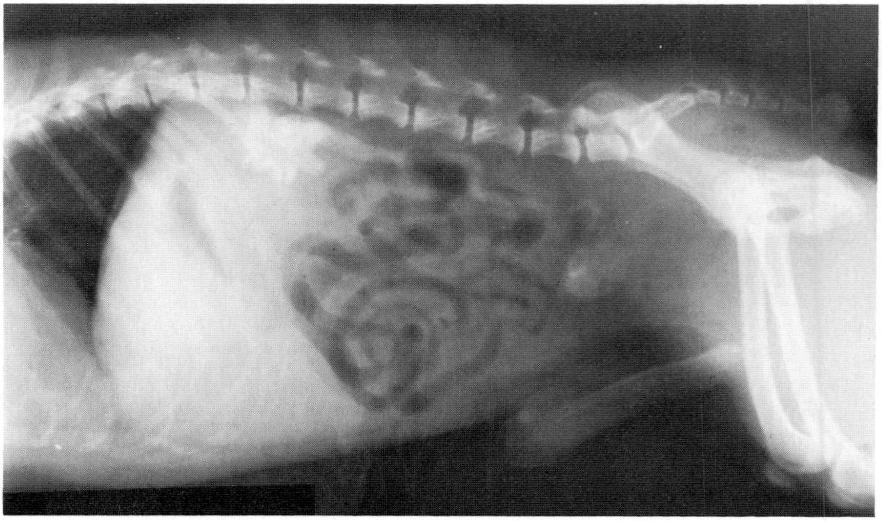

Fig. 10-19. Lateral radiograph of the pyelographic phase of an excretory urogram from an 11-year-old shipperkee dog with dysuria. Unilateral renal pelvic and ureteral dilation and nonopacification of the contralateral kidney were caused by a transitional cell carcinoma infiltrating the trigone of the urinary bladder. Compare to Figure 10-39B.

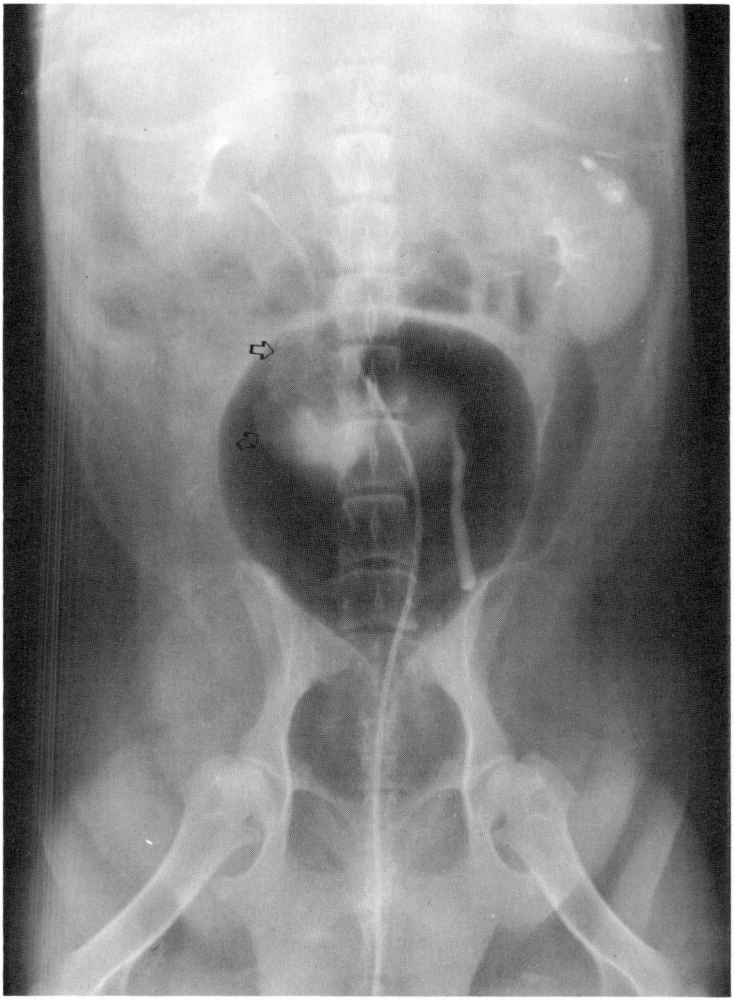

Fig. 10-20. Ventrodorsal radiograph of the pyelographic phase of an excretory urogram performed concurrently with a pneumocystogram from a 7-year-old spayed female basset hound with hematuria and dysuria. An attached filling defect in the urinary bladder (arrows) and a deformed renal pelvis are encountered radiographically. The bladder filling defect was caused by a transitional cell carcinoma. The deformity to the renal pelvis was caused by pyelonephritis.

viously defined under survey radiography. Renal ectopia is a cause of abnormal kidney location and has been described in the dog and the cat.[4,81,82] Thoracic and intraabdominal locations have been encountered. Renal ectopia may be associated with a degree of functional impairment of the ectopic kidney. Displacement of the kidney by adjacent mass lesions may result in an abnormal

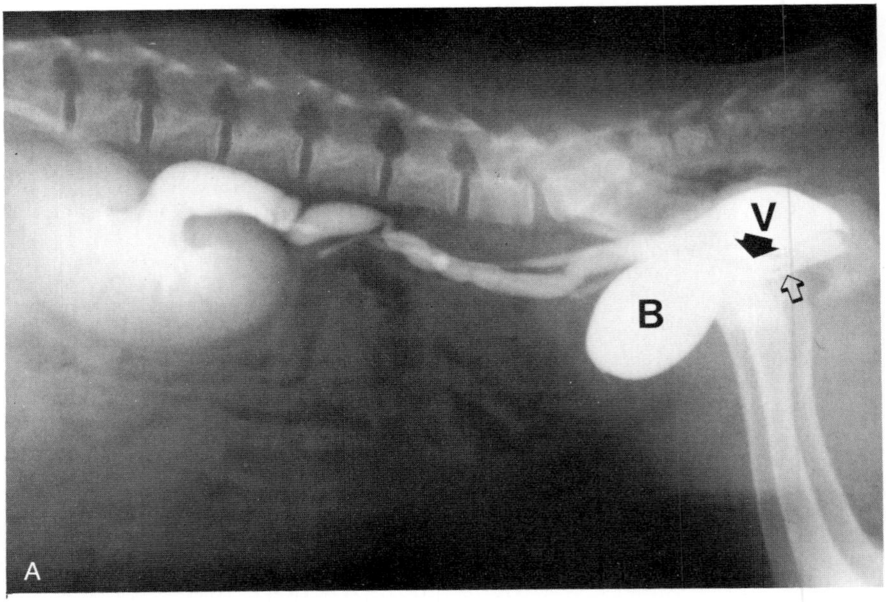

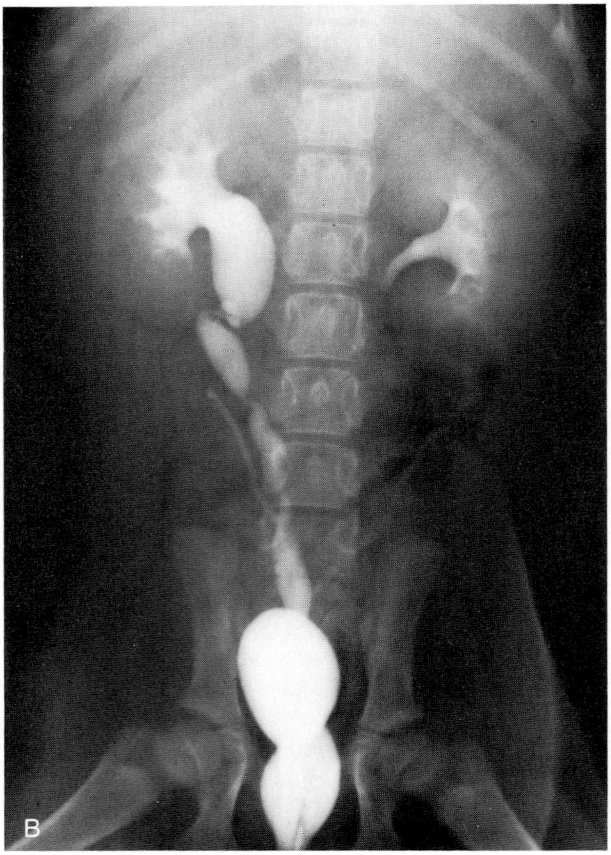

Fig. 10-21. Abnormal site(s) of termination to the ureters are the most common abnormality associated with ureteral location. Lateral (A) and ventrodorsal (B) radiographs of an excretory urogram obtained following retrograde vaginography on a 10-month-old female Siberian husky with urinary incontinence. The urinary bladder (B), vagina (V), urethra (open arrow), and ectopic ureter (black arrow) terminating in the distal urethra are identified on the lateral radiograph. Note the dilated left and right ureters and renal pelves on the ventrodorsal radiograph. Opacification of the left and right uterine horns can be identified on the lateral and ventrodorsal radiographs. (*Figure continues.*)

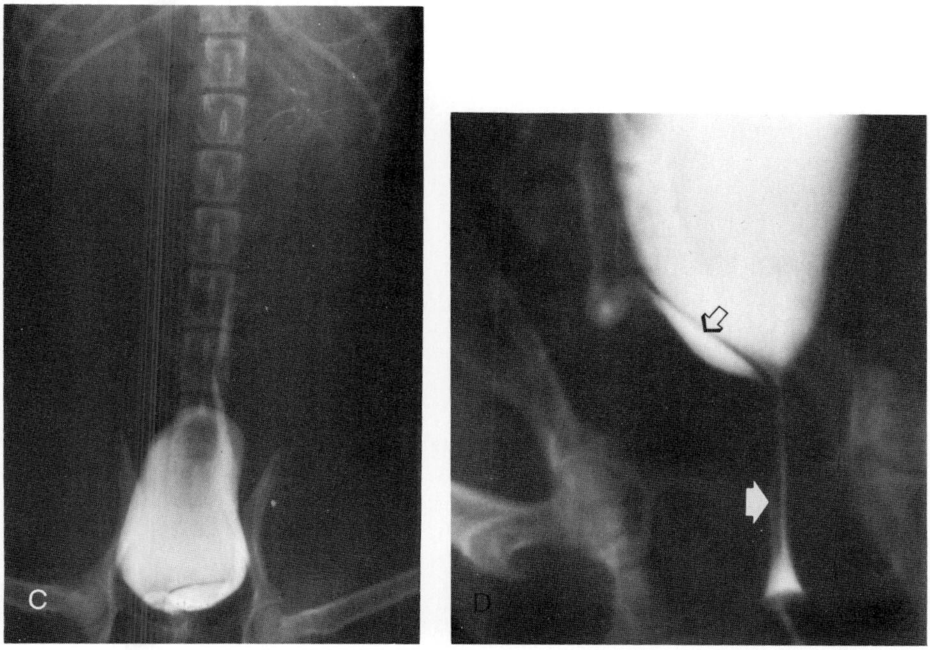

Fig. 10-21 (*continued*). (C) Ventrodorsal oblique radiograph of an excretory urogram from a 4-year-old spayed female mixed breed dog with urinary incontinence. (D) A positive contrast radiograph urethocystogram from same dog as in C. A dilated distal left ureter with intravesical ureteral dilation (open arrow) is caused by an ectopic left ureterocele that terminates in the distal urethra (closed arrow).

location. Adrenal, ovarian, hepatic, and splenic masses and gastric distention may result in displacement of the kidneys (Fig. 10-11).

Radiographic Density. Abnormal radiographic densities, radiolucent or radiopaque, and either focal or diffuse, associated with renal silhouettes has been described under survey radiography. Excretory urography causes uniform opacification of the kidneys because of the accumulation of radiographic contrast media within the renal tubules, renal vessels, and renal pelvis. Causes of focal, multifocal, or diffuse alterations in opacification of the nephrographic or pyelographic phase of the excretory urography are listed in Tables 10-4 and 10-5 and Figure 10-18.

Function. Abnormal roentgen signs may be encountered in the degree of nephrographic opacification and its subsequent fading on sequential radiographs. Causes for alterations in nephrographic opacification are listed in Table 10-6. Differential diagnoses considered because of abnormal nephrographic opacification require further investigations by renal biopsy for a definitive diagnosis and prognosis.

Ureters. *Number*. Renal diseases associated with agenesis and aplasia will

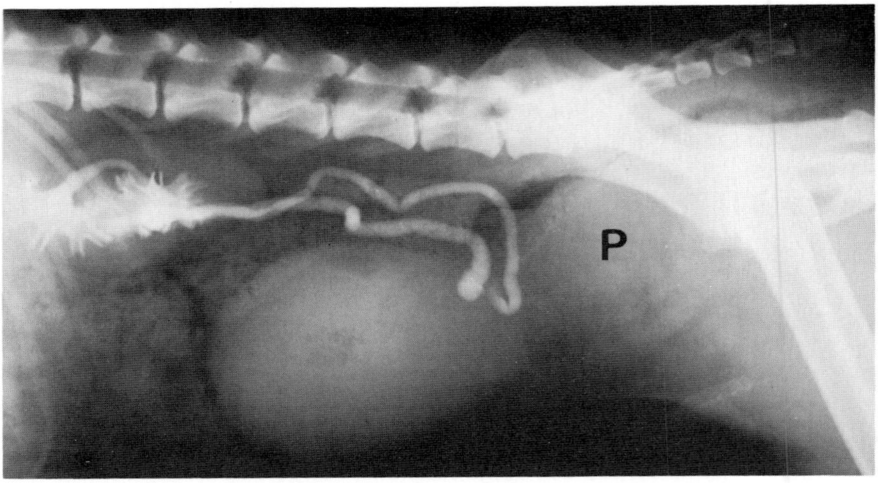

Fig. 10-22. Lateral radiograph of the pyelographic phase of an excretory urogram from a 3-year-old mixed breed dog with a palpable caudal abdominal mass. Dilation of the renal pelves and ureters and cranial displacement of the urinary bladder were caused by enlargement of the prostate gland (P) due to hyperplasia and inflammation. (Johnston GR, Feeney DA, Osborne CA: Radiographic findings in urinary tract infection. Vet Clin North Am 9:749, 1979.)

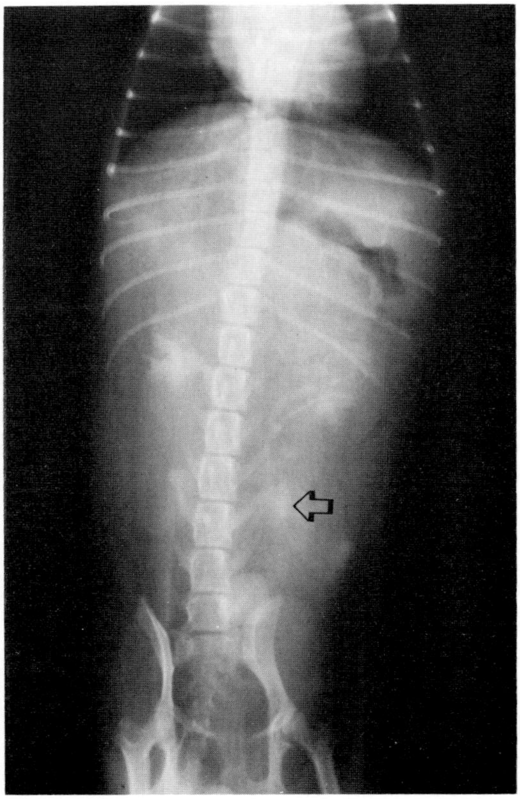

Fig. 10-23. Ventrodorsal radiograph from the pyelographic phase of an excretory urogram of the dog described in Figure 10-4. Unilateral left-sided ureteral rupture with retroperitoneal effusion of contrast media is illustrated (arrow).

result in the absence of opacification of the associated ureter. Duplication of the ureter has been described in dogs.[56]

Size, shape, margination. Roentgen signs associated with abnormal ureteral size, shape, and margination can be used to formulate a list of gamuts for ureteral diseases.

Diffuse enlargement of the ureters with a smooth mucosal margination and/or enlargement of the renal pelvis, with associated deformity of the renal pelvic diverticula, is most likely related to ureteroectasia secondary to obstruction, atony, or infection (Fig. 10-18, 10-19, 10-20, 10-21, and 10-22).[46,48,67,83,84] Ureteral dilatation secondary to chronic vesicoureteral reflux may be a cause for diffuse ureteral enlargement. Ureteral ectopica may result in diffuse dilatation of the abnormal ureter and has been reported in dogs and cats (Fig. 10-21). Focal ureteral enlargement with smooth margination has been reported secondary to ureteroceles and diverticula (Fig. 10-21C and D).[87–89]

Focal to diffuse ureteral enlargement with roughened, irregular mucosal patterns may be suggestive of ureteral fibrosis secondary to chronic inflammatory disease. A focal mucosal irregularity to the renal pelvis or ureter may be secondary to primary or metastatic neoplasia.

Small ureters with smooth, regular margins are most likely the result of an inadequate dosage of contrast media.

Location. Termination of the ureter at any site other than the trigone of the urinary bladder is considered an ectopic location (Fig. 10-21).[85,86] The most common site of abnormal ureteral termination is the vagina, followed by the urethra, bladder neck, and uterus. An abnormal size, shape, and margination to the affected ureter is frequently encountered and was previously described. Displacement of the termination of the distal ureter may be secondary to abdominal mass lesions. Prostatomegaly and uterine stump granulomas may result in displacement of the distal ureter and subsequent extraluminal compression (Fig. 10-22).

Radiographic density. Opacification of the ureters, as defined by excretory urography, was previously described under normal radiographic findings. Air within the ureteral lumen may be secondary to vesicoureteral reflux and will be described under cystography. Loss of retroperitoneal contrast secondary to ureteral trauma can be identified by excretory urography because of the retroperitoneal pooling of positive contrast medium (Fig. 10-23). Abnormal radiographic densities associated with the ureters on survey films can be further defined as intraluminal, mural, or extraluminal during excretory urography (Figs. 10-5, 10-18, and 10-24). Intraluminal filling defects encountered during excretory urography may result from uroliths and blood clots (Fig. 10-18). Mural and extraluminal compressive lesions secondary to neoplastic or inflammatory disease will frequently result in a focal dilation proximal to the site of obstruction (Fig. 10-22). Excretory urography will provide additional information on the size, shape, and margination of intraluminal, mural, or extraluminal lesions and functional impairment to the normal flow of urine from the renal pelvis to the urinary bladder. Failure to identify a segment of the ureter

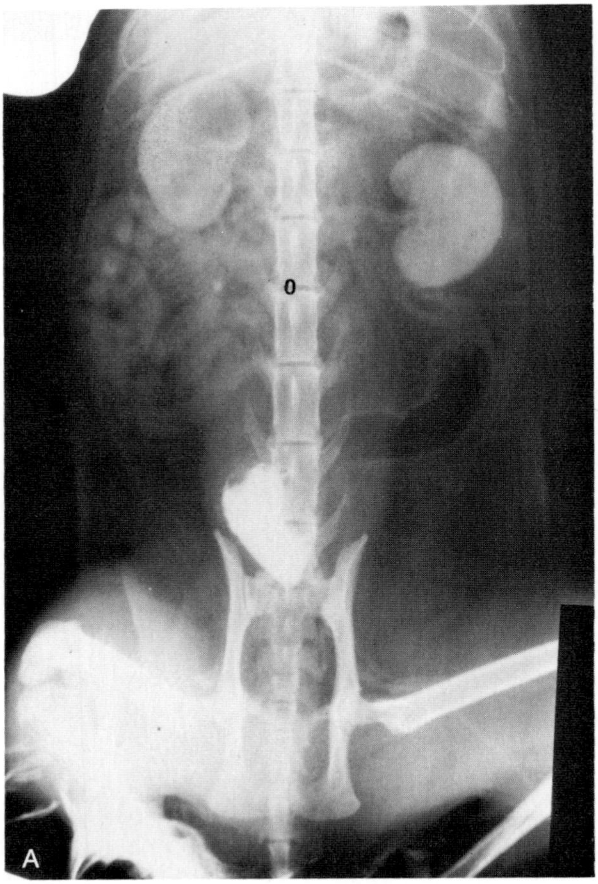

Fig. 10-24. Ventrodorsal radiographs of the pyelographic phase of an excretory urogram from the cat described in Figure 10-6. Radiographs obtained 15 sec (labeled 0) (A), (*Figure continues.*)

on a single radiograph should not be considered normal unless verified on subsequent serial radiographs.

Function. Ureteral atony and hypotonia may be encountered radiographically and are secondary to ureteral inflammation, paraureteral inflammation, trauma or ureteral obstruction (Figs. 10-18 through 10-22).[46,48,68,83,84,90] Assessment of the function of the ureter must be assessed by evaluating size, shape and margination of serial radiographs obtained during excretory urography.

Technical and Interpretative Pitfalls. The technical and interpretative pitfalls encountered during excretory urography are listed in Table 10-7.

Contrast Evaluation of the Urinary Bladder

Contrast radiographic evaluations of the urinary bladder are simple, inexpensive, and relatively low-risk, and can provide information on the site(s) of involvement and the magnitude of lower urinary tract disease. The indica-

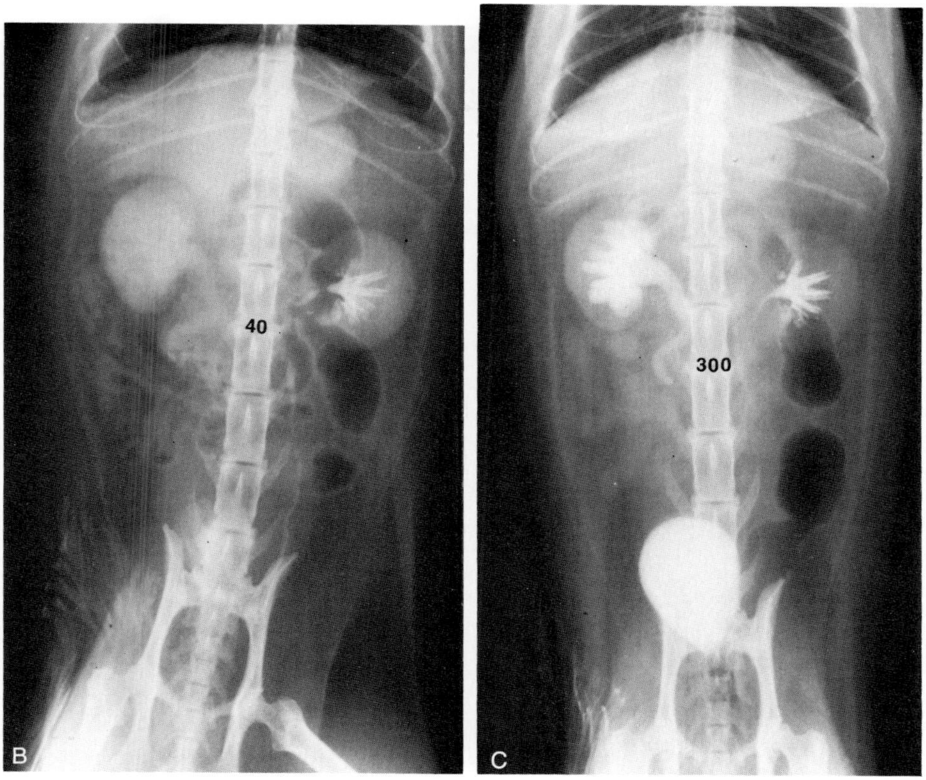

Fig. 10-24 (*continued*). 40 min (B), and 5 hr (300 min) (C) after the intravenous injection of contrast medium indicates ureteral and renal pelvic dilation and early hydronephrosis caused by the ureteral obstruction from a urolith.

tions for cystography are derived from the clinical signs and information obtained on survey abdominal radiographs. Clinical indications for cystography include hematuria, dysuria, and pollakiuria.[10,12,19] Radiographic indications include abnormal densities associated with the urinary bladder, nonvisualization of the urinary bladder, caudally located abdominal masses, and abnormal shape to the urinary bladder.[19,91]

Patient preparation for cystography is identical to the procedure described for the survey radiography and excretory urography and includes withholding food for 24 hours and a cleansing water enema 2 to 3 hours prior to cystography. Sedation or light general anesthesia is usually required to facilitate catheterization.[19,24]

Techniques. The technique of cystography is listed in Table 10-8 and illustrated in Figures 10-25, 10-26, and 10-27.[19,21,24,91]

Pneumocystography. Negative contrast cystography is a procedure whereby negative contrast media is infused into the urinary bladder to provide better radiographic evaluation (Fig. 10-25). The volume of injection will vary

Table 10-7. Common Pitfalls of Uroradiography

- I. Survey radiography
  - A. Radiopacities mistaken for radiopaque uroliths
    - 1. Opaque material in intestinal lumen
    - 2. Nipples of abdominal mammary glands
    - 3. Mineralization of renal parenchyma
    - 4. Deep circumflex iliac artery
    - 5. Prepuce of male dog
    - 6. Mineralization of lesions in tissues of body wall, vessels, or lymph node
    - 7. Polypoid or pedunculated cutaneous nodules
    - 8. Osseous metaplasia of transitional epithelium
  - B. Radiolucencies mistaken afor uroliths or abscesses caused by gas-forming bacteria
    - 1. Intestinal gas over urinary bladder
    - 2. Rectal gas over prostate
    - 3. Subcutaneous emphysema over genitourinary tract
    - 4. Iatrogenic intraluminal bladder gas owing to catheterization or cystocentesis
  - C. Failure to identify calculi
    - 1. Calculi superimposed over bony structures
    - 2. Inadequate radiographic contrast between calculi and soft tissue
    - 3. Small size of calculi
    - 4. Failure to evaluate the entire urinary tract
- II. Excretory urography
  - A. Inadequate radiopacity of excretory pathway because of technical errors
    - 1. Inadequate dose of contrast medium, especially with renal dysfunction
    - 2. Perivascular injection of contrast medium
    - 3. Rate of administration of contrast medium too slow
    - 4. Inadequate iodine concentration in contrast medium
  - B. Overinterpretation of normal findings
    - 1. Ureteral peristalsis mistaken for strictures
    - 2. Peak ureteral distention mistaken for ureteral dilation
    - 3. False-positive protein reactions caused by iodine-containing contrast medium interpreted as significant
    - 4. Alteration of urine specific gravity caused by excretion of contrast medium
    - 5. Incomplete filling of renal pelvic diverticula misinterpreted as evidence of disease
    - 6. Superposition of gas-filled bowel over kidneys mistaken for radiolucent renal parenchymal filling defects (i.e., cysts, abscesses)
  - C. Underinterpretation of abnormal findings
    - 1. Dilated renal pelvis interpreted as normal
    - 2. Irregular renal outline interpreted as superposed intestine
  - D. Complications caused by contrast medium
    - 1. Allergic
      - a. Urticaria
      - b. Pruritus
      - c. Laryngospasm, bronchospasm[a]
    - 2. Anaphylactic
      - a. Collapse
      - b. Shock
      - c. Hysteria[a]
    - 3. Toxic
      - a. Acute renal shutdown, predisposed by dehydration[a]
      - b. Osmotic nephrosis[a]
- III. Cystography
  - A. Positive contrast cystography
    - 1. Technical pitfalls. Use of:
      - a. Not enough positive contrast medium to distend bladder lumen
      - b. Excessively concentrated positive contrast medium
    - 2. Interpretative pitfalls
      - a. Thickened bladder wall associated with partial bladder distention mistaken for cystitis or neoplasia
      - b. Free luminal filling defects
      - c. Normal or abnormal vesicoureteral reflux

(*continued*)

Table 10-7 (*continued*).

- 3. Complications
  - a. Traumatic catheterization
  - b. Iatrogenic infection
  - c. Bladder rupture
  - d. Vascular embolization[b]
  - e. Adverse reactions to positive contrast medium
    - (1) Systemic (see IID1 and 2)
    - (2) Local—reversible inflammation of the urothelium
- B. Negative contrast cystography
  - 1. Technique pitfalls. Use of:
    - a. Not enough negative contrast medium to distend bladder lumen
    - b. Inadequate radiographic contrast to demonstrate free luminal filling defects
  - 2. Interpretative pitfalls
    - a. Thickened bladder wall associated with partial bladder distention mistaken for inflammation or neoplasia
    - b. Free luminal filling defects
    - c. Normal or abnormal vesicoureteral reflux
- C. Double contrast cystography
  - 1. Technical pitfalls. Use of:
    - a. Not enough negative contrast medium to distend bladder lumen
    - b. Too much positive contrast medium
  - 2. Interpretative pitfalls
    - a. Thickened bladder wall associated with inadequate bladder distention mistaken for inflammation or neoplasia
    - b. Free luminal filling defects
    - c. Normal or abnormal vesicoureteral reflex
    - d. Complications (see IIIA3a–d)

IV. Urethrography
- A. Positive contrast urethrography
  - 1. Technical pitfalls. Use of:
    - a. Too little contrast medium to fill urethra
    - b. Excessive concentration of positive contrast medium which obscures luminal defects
    - c. Incorrect type of positive contrast medium
    - d. Inadequate vesical hydrostatic volume and pressure
  - 2. Interpretative pitfalls
    - a. Incomplete filling associated with use of too little contrast medium mistaken for urethral obstruction
    - b. Free luminal filling defects
    - c. Urethral peristalsis, spasms, or voluntary contraction mistaken for strictures
  - 3. Complications
    - a. Traumatic catheterization
    - b. Iatrogenic infection
    - c. Urethrovascular reflux of contrast medium, diluent, and urethral bacteria
    - d. Bladder rupture
- B. Negative contrast urethrography
  Because of the superiority of positive contrast urethrography over negative contrast urethrography, we do not routinely recommend this procedure.
- C. Double contrast urethrography
  Because of the adequacy of positive contrast urethrography, we do not routinely recommend this procedure.

[a] Adverse reactions have been cited in man.

[b] If contrast media other than recommended organic iodine-containing agents are used, vascular embolization may become a problem.

(Johnston GR, Feeney DA, Osborne CA: Radiographic findings in urinary tract infection. Vet Clin North Am 9:749, 1979.)

Table 10-8. Techniques of Cystography

A. Negative contrast cystography (pneumocystography)
   1. Aseptically catheterize the urinary bladder
   2. Remove residual urine
   3. Infuse negative contrast media (air, CO_2, NO_2) until bladder is maximally distended as determined by digital palpation
   4. Expose lateral and ventrodorsal radiographs
   5. Remove bladder contents

B. Double contrast cystography
   1. Same as A1–3 above for pneumocystography
   2. Infuse undiluted positive contrast medium in a volume appropriate to the size of the animal
      a. Cats: 0.5–1.0 ml
      b. Dogs:
         1. less than 25 lb: 1–3 ml
         2. >25 lb <75 lb: 3–6 ml
         3. >75 lb: 6–12 ml
   3. Same as A4 and A5 above for pneumocystography

C. Positive contrast cystography
   1. Same as A1, 2 above for pneumocystography
   2. Infuse a 5 to 10% solution of positive contrast media until bladder is maximally distended as determined by digital palpation.
   3. Same as A4, 5 above for pneumocystography

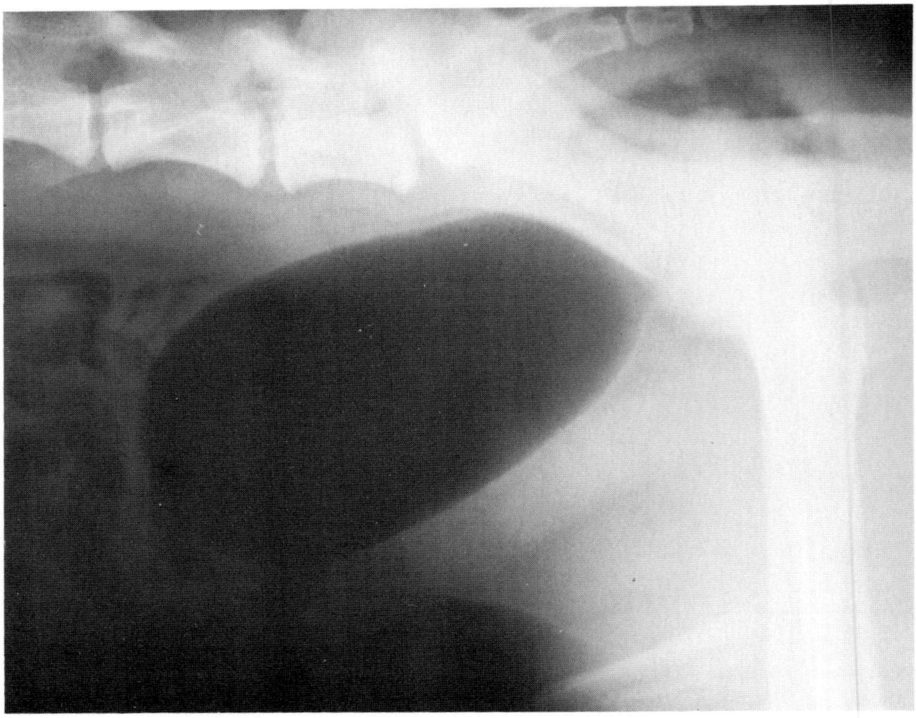

Fig. 10-25. Lateral radiograph of a pneumocystogram of a normal 3-year-old male malamute. (Johnston GR, Feeney DA, Osborne CA: Radiographic findings in urinary tract infection. Vet Clin North Am 9:749, 1979.)

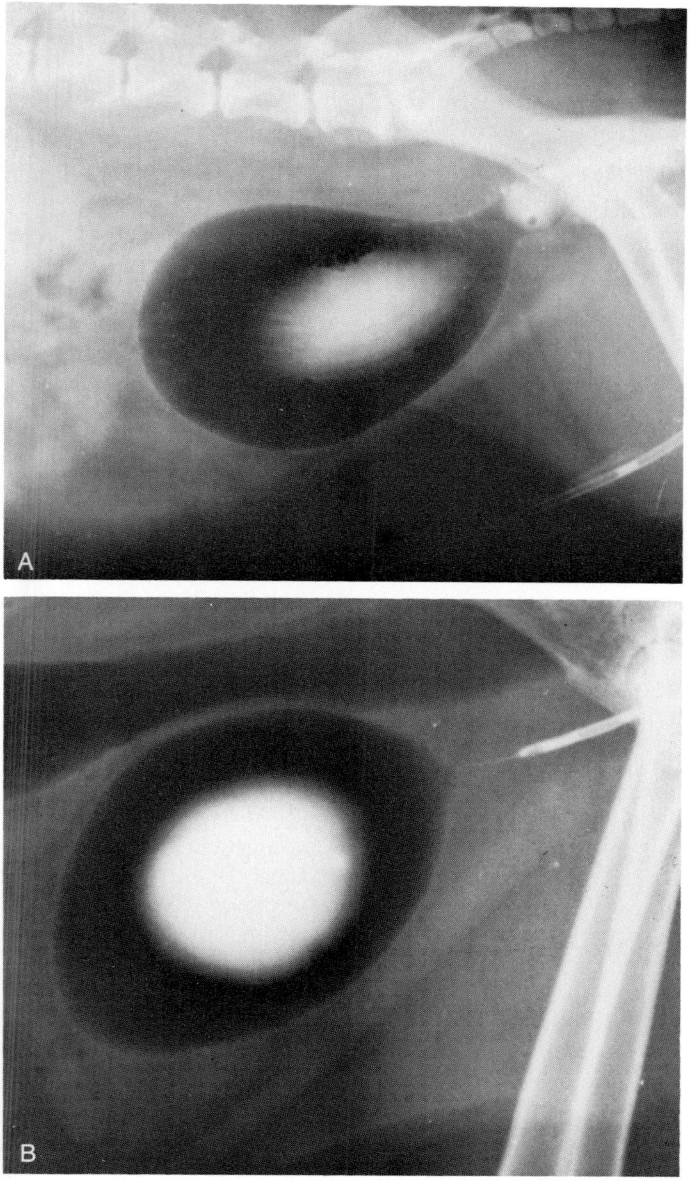

Fig. 10-26. Lateral radiographs of normal double contrast cystograms from a 12-year-old miniature schnauzer (A) and a 14-year-old spayed domestic shorthair cat (B). The positive contrast medium in the double contrast cystogram on the dependent side should have a smooth interface with the mucosa of the urinary bladder. The thickness of the urinary bladder wall should be uniform if the urinary bladder is adequately distended. Radiolucent filling defects at the periphery of the contrast puddle in Figure 10-26A are the result of air bubbles of variable size. (A from Johnston GR, Feeney DA, Osborne CA: Radiographic findings in urinary tract infection. Vet Clin North Am 9:749, 1979; B from Johnston GR, Feeney DA, Osborne CA: Urethrography and cystography in cats. Part I. Techniques, normal radiographic anatomy, and artifacts. Comp Cont Vet Ed 4:823, 1982.)

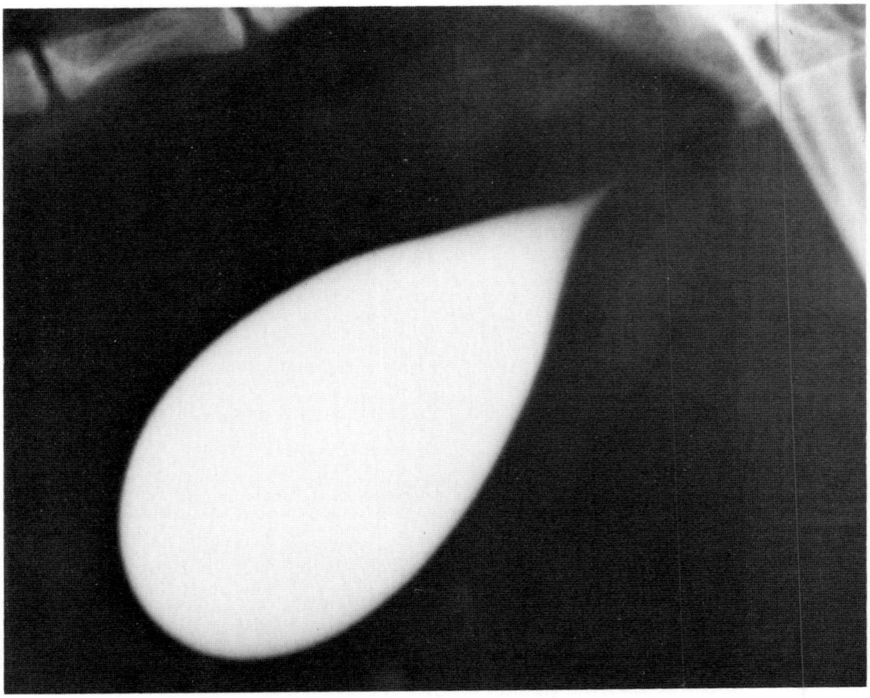

Fig. 10-27. Lateral radiograph of a normal positive contrast cystogram from a 2-year-old neutered male domestic shorthair cat. The shape of the feline urinary bladder will vary depending on the degree of distension. Note smooth mucosal margin and tear-shaped configuration. (Johnston GR, Feeney DA, Osborne CA: Urethrography and cystography in cats. Part I. Techniques, normal radiographic anatomy, and artifacts. Comp Cont Vet Ed 4:823, 1982.)

considerably, depending upon the patient's size, clinical signs, and the duration of lower urinary tract disease.[19,91] In general the urinary bladder should be palpated to ensure adequate urinary bladder distention.[24] Lateral and ventrodorsal radiographs should be obtained following infusion of the negative contrast media. Additional oblique radiographs may be necessary for evaluation of focal lesions. The selection of the negative contrast agent (air, carbon dioxide, nitrous oxide, or oxygen) should be based on the clinical signs and the presence of macroscopic hematuria.

The advantage of pneumocystography is that it is relatively simple to perform, fast, and inexpensive.[19] Its major disadvantage is that it provides poor mucosal detail and will not demonstrate small intraluminal filling defects.[19] An additional disadvantage of pneumocystography with air is the potential for fatal vascular embolization described previous.

Double contrast cystography. Double contrast cystography is better than pneumocystography and positive contrast cystography for demonstrating mucosal disease, mural lesions, and free luminal or attached filling defects (Fig. 10-26).[19] Double contrast cystography uses both positive and negative contrast agents. It can be performed following excretory urography or positive contrast cystography. In this procedure the positive contrast medium is removed from the urinary bladder and the negative contrast medium then infused. Barium sulfate has been recommended for double contrast cystography because of its superior mucosal coating capabilities compared to aqueous iodinated compounds.[30] The aqueous iodinated compounds previously described as positive contrast agents have the advantage of being sterile, individually packaged, and readily available. They have inferior mucosal coating capabilities compared to barium sulfate, but have been reported to adhere to mucosal ulcerations/erosions and attached blood clots.[19,26]

Positive contrast cystography. Positive contrast cystography is a procedure whereby positive contrast medium is infused into the urinary bladder (Fig. 10-27). A 10 to 15 percent solution of aqueous iodinated contrast medium is recommended. Positive contrast cystography is the procedure of choice for locating the urinary bladder and demonstrating the site or sites of bladder tears or rupture.[19] The major disadvantage of positive contrast cystography is masking of free luminal filling defects.[19]

Technical and interpretative pitfalls and complications. The technical and interpretative pitfalls and complications of cystography are listed in Table 10-7. A more detailed description of the complications of cystography is beyond the scope of this manuscript but have been described.[24,26,92]

Normal Radiographic Findings. ***Number, Size and Shape.*** The size and shape of the urinary bladder is influenced by the distention of the bladder and its relationship to adjacent structures. The normal size and shape of the bladder were described under survey radiography can be reviewed in Figs. 10-25, 10-26, and 10-27.[19,24]

Location. The location of the urinary bladder will vary depending on its degree of distention in dogs and cats (Figs. 10-25, 10-26, 10-27). The location relative to the degree of distention was described under survey radiography.[19,24]

Radiographic density. The radiographic density of the bladder lumen and its contents encountered during cystography will be influenced by the choice of contrast medium. Radiopacities or radiolucencies encountered on survey radiographs may be further defined by cystography.[19,24,26]

Mucosal surface. The mucosal surface encountered by cystography should be smooth and well defined where the contrast media interfaces the urinary bladder wall (Figs. 10-25, 10-26, and 10-27).[19,24]

Mural thickness. The normal thickness of the urinary bladder wall in dogs and cats is approximately 1 mm and should be uniform on both the lateral and ventrodorsal radiographs if the urinary bladder is adequately distended (Figs. 10-25, 10-26, and 10-27).[19,24]

Vesicoureteral reflux. Vesicoureteral reflux is the retrograde migration of bladder contents into the ureter through a normal or impaired vesicoureteral junction.[93,94,95] Vesicoureteral reflux may be encountered during cystography, appearing as positive and/or negative contrast medium linearly located along

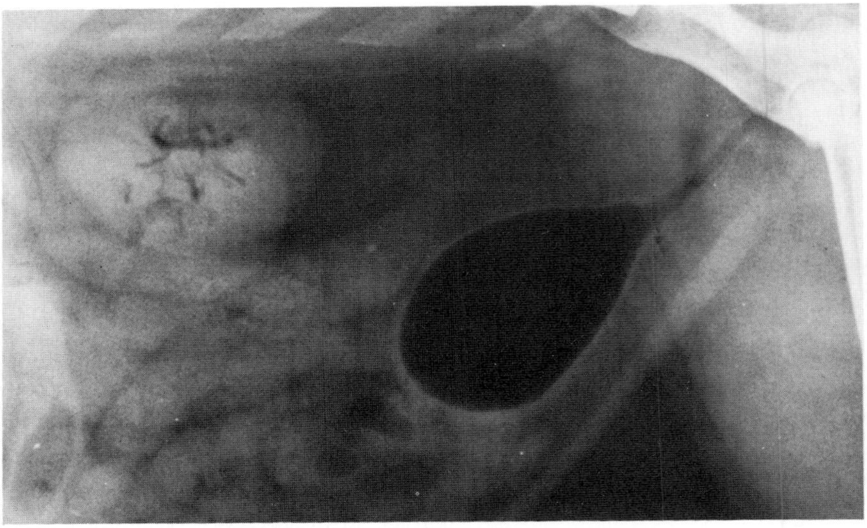

Fig. 10-28. Bilateral vesicoureteral reflux (VUR) was encountered during pneumocystography on an 8-year-old male domestic shorthair cat with dysuria. VUR may be encountered in normal dogs and cats and may be age-dependent or related to positioning, degree of bladder distension, anesthesia/sedation, or the presence of urinary tract disease. Compare to Figure 10-29. (Johnston GR, Feeney DA, Osborne CA: Urethrography and cystography in cats. Part I. Techniques, normal radiographic anatomy, and artifacts. Comp Cont Vet Ed 4:823, 1982.)

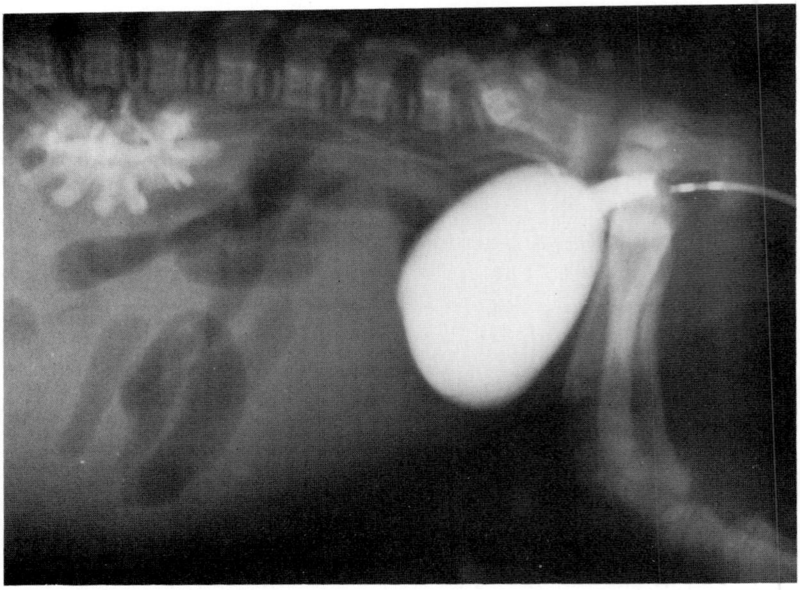

Fig. 10-29. Lateral radiograph of a positive contrast retrograde urethrocystogram in a normal 8-week-old female beagle. Bilateral vesicoureteral reflux of the positive contrast medium into the ureters and renal pelves are encountered. (Johnston GR, Feeney DA, Osborne CA: Radiographic findings in urinary tract infection. Vet Clin North Am 9:749, 1979.)

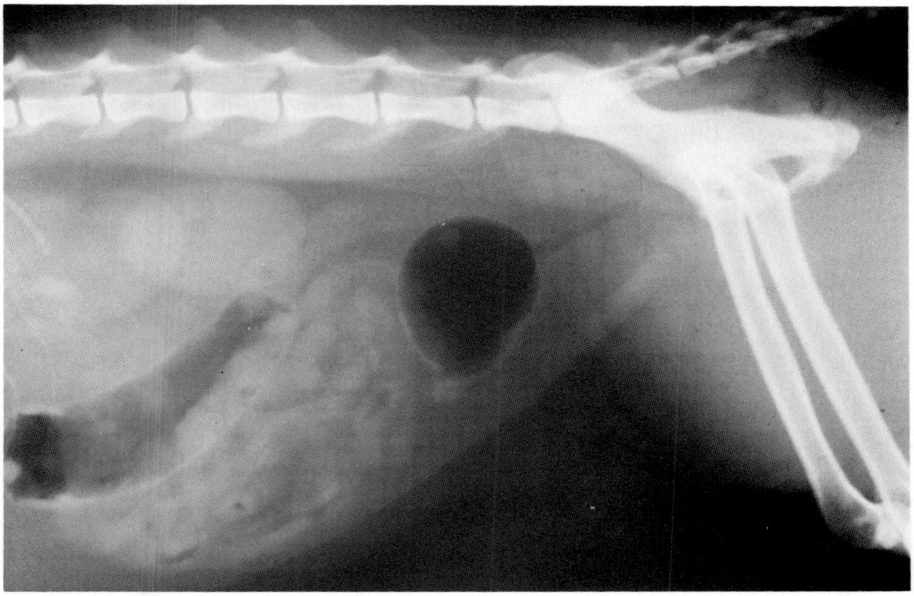

Fig. 10-30. Lateral radiograph of a pneumocystogram from the cat described in Fig. 10-9. A well-defined diverticula and two uroliths are illustrated. Urachal diverticula may have a variable appearance and may be "nipple-shaped" (Fig. 10-46) or "cyst-like" (Fig. 10-31).

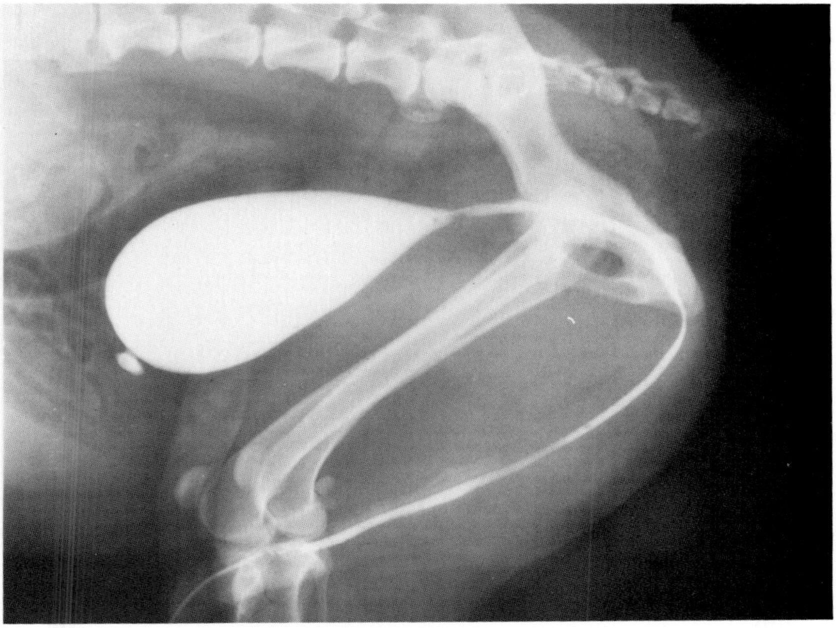

Fig. 10-31. Lateral radiograph of a positive contrast retrograde urethrocystogram from a 10-year-old male Labrador retriever with hematuria. A well-defined "cyst-like" diverticulum is encountered. *E. coli* was cultured from the urine. Diverticula may predispose to urinary tract infection by causing urine stasis.

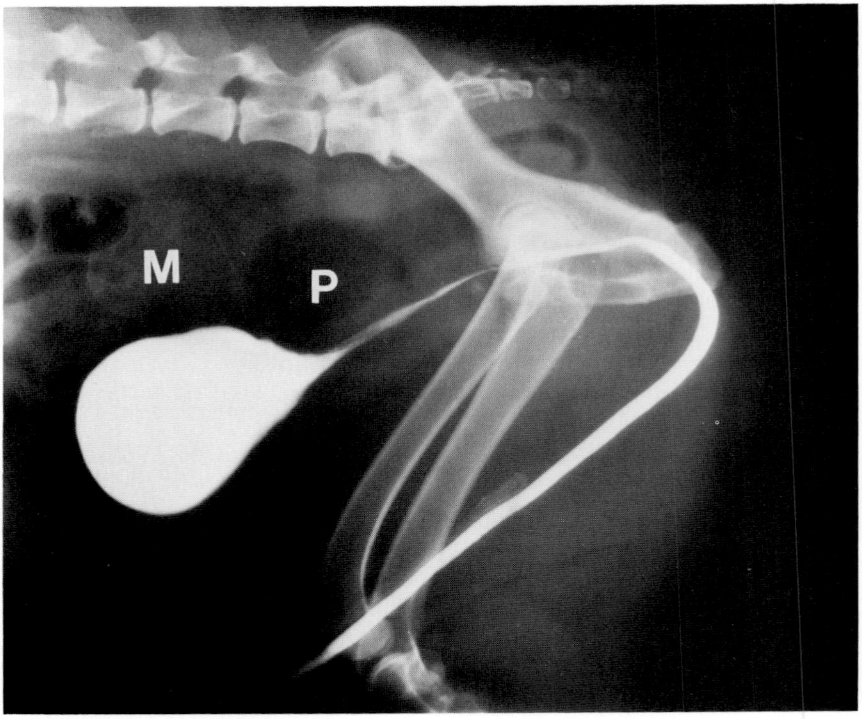

Fig. 10-32. Lateral radiograph of a positive contrast retrograde urethrocystogram from a 9-year-old male Boxer dog with hematuria. Cranial and ventral urinary bladder displacement by a gas filled prostatic abscess (P) and a calcified nonprostatic cystic mass (M) are illustrated radiographically and were confirmed by surgical biopsy.

the sublumbar area from the bladder trigone to the renal pelvis (Fig. 10-28). Reflux may occur to varying distances into the ureter(s) with a variable degree of ureteral and renal pelvic distention. Vesicoureteral reflux may also be encountered during antegrade or retrograde cystourethrography and during manual compression of the urinary bladder.[24,96,97]

Vesicoureteral reflux may be normal and has been reported to be age-dependent in young dogs (Fig. 10-29).[98] It may also depend on positioning, degree of bladder distention, depth of anesthesia, and the type of chemical restraint.[94,99,100] The incidence of vesicoureteral reflux in young dogs has been reported to be 80 percent up to 3 months of age and then to decline to 10 percent in older dogs.[93] The higher incidence of vesicoureteral reflux in younger dogs may be related to a shorter intravesical ureter relative to the diameter of the ureter in the younger animal.[93] Vesicoureteral reflux may be abnormal and related to urinary bladder infection, lower urinary tract obstruction, neurologic bladder disease, and congenital anomalies of the vesicoureteral junction.[94,101,102] Some urinary tract pathogens may produce a neural toxin which may predispose to vesicoureteral reflux and subsequent ascending ureteritis, pyelitis, and pyelonephritis.[103,104]

Abnormal Radiographic Findings. ***Number, Size, and Shape.*** Abnormalities such as soft tissue masses in the caudal abdomen encountered on survey radiographs may be further characterized by contrast cystography. Abnormalities of urinary bladder shape on survey radiographs may be related to artifactual superimposition of a fluid-filled bowel loop, inadequate urinary bladder distention, or congenital or acquired diverticular (Figs. 10-30 and 10-31).

Location. Abnormal urinary bladder location caused by caudal abdominal masses and abdominal, linguinal, or perineal hernias may be further characterized by cystography (Fig. 10-32).

Radiographic density. Abnormal radiographic densities associated with the urinary bladder can be further characterized by cystography as being intraluminal, extraluminal or mural (Figs. 10-30 and 10-32).

Mucosal pattern. Mucosal proliferation can occur during inflammatory, infectious, noninfectious, or neoplastic disease,[19,26] and will give the radiographic appearance of mucosal irregularity. Radiographically, mucosal irregularity appears as a roughened irregular outline to the mucosal surface of the urinary bladder (Fig. 10-33). Inadequate distention of the urinary bladder is a common technical pitfall and will result in focal, multifocal, or diffuse mucosal irregularity. Mucosal irregularity is not pathognomonic for any specific disease and may be encountered with inflammatory, noninfectious, infectious, or neoplastic disease.[19,26]

Mucosal ulcerations and erosions may be encountered radiographically in association with mucosal irregularity and are characterized by the adherence of positive contrast media to the mucosal surface during double contrast cystography. (Figs. 10-33, 10-34, and 10-35).[19,26]

Mural lesions. Thickening of the urinary bladder wall may be artifactual and related to inadequate urinary bladder distention or may indicate focal, multifocal, or diffuse bladder wall disease caused by inflammatory cell infiltrates, hemorrhage, edema, fibrosis, or neoplasm.[19,24,26] Because of the nonspecificity of the cause of bladder wall thickening, it must be evaluated in the light of history, disease duration, laboratory data, and cytology. Dogs and cats with lower urinary tract disease may have no radiographic abnormalities on contrast cystography. Focal bladder wall thickening is frequently encountered with lower urinary tract disease in dogs and cats and may be related to inflammatory, infectious, noninfectious, or neoplastic disease (Figs. 10-28, 10-33, and 10-35). Focal ventral bladder wall thickening may also be related to inadequate urinary bladder distention.[24] Diffuse bladder wall thickening may be encountered in cats and dogs with acute or chronic lower urinary tract disease from inflammatory or neoplastic origin (Figs. 10-36 and 10-37). Prolonged urinary bladder distention during urethral obstruction in male dogs and cats may result in hemorrhage, edema, and inflammation within the urinary bladder wall, which will result in diffuse mural thickening (Fig. 10-37). However, the distensibility of the urinary bladder in obstructed male cats is greater than in cats with chronic

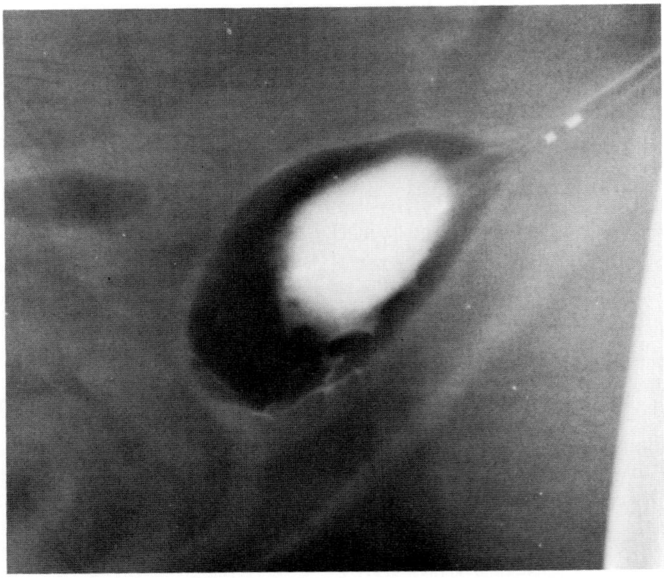

Fig. 10-33. Mucosal irregularity, contrast coating the urinary bladder wall, and cranioventral bladder wall thickening are encountered on a lateral radiograph of a double contrast cystogram from an 8-year-old spayed female Siamese cat with heamturia and dysuria of one week duration. Mucosal irregularity is frequently encountered in dogs and cats with acute or chronic lower urinary tract disease secondary to neoplastic, infectious or noninfectious diseases. (Johnston GR, Feeney DA, Osborne CA: Urethrography and cystography in cats. Part II. Abnormal radiographic anatomy and complications. Compend Contin Educ Pract Vet 4:931, 1982.)

cystitis, because fibrosis to the bladder wall results in poor distensibility. Diffuse bladder wall thickening has also been reported secondary to inadequate urinary bladder distention.[24]

Luminal filling defects. Luminal filling defects within the urinary bladder will result in abnormal filling of the urinary bladder because the defects occupy a portion of the bladder lumen and result in displacement of positive and/or negative contrast media.[19,26] Filling defects may be attached or free luminal. The most common intraluminal urinary bladder filling defects of dogs and cats are air bubbles, uroliths, sebaceous or mucous plugs, and blood clots (Figs. 10-26A, 10-34, 10-37, 10-38). The differential radiographic characteristics of free luminal filling defects are listed in Table 10-9.

Attached filling defects. Attached filling defects differ from free luminal defects in that they are attached to the wall of the urinary bladder. Some free luminal defects such as blood clots and uroliths may also be attached to the bladder wall (Fig. 10-30). Because of their bladder wall attachment, filling defects will project into the lumen of the urinary bladder to varying degrees. Additional attached filling defects include submucosal hematomas, abscesses,

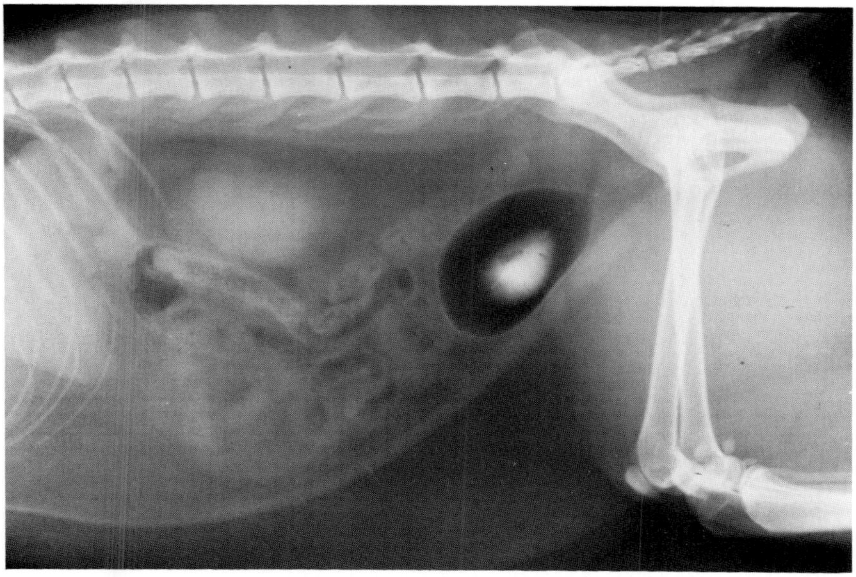

Fig. 10-34. Lateral radiograph of a double contrast cystogram from a 5-year-old male domestic shorthair cat with hematuria and dysuria and a stricture at the site of a prior perineal urethrostomy. Contrast coating of the cranial ventral mucosa of the urinary bladder and two free luminal filling defects are encountered. Contrast coating of the mucosa may be encountered secondary to erosions, ulcerations of the bladder mucosa, and attached blood clots. The two free luminal filling defects in the urinary bladder lumen are most likely blood clots.

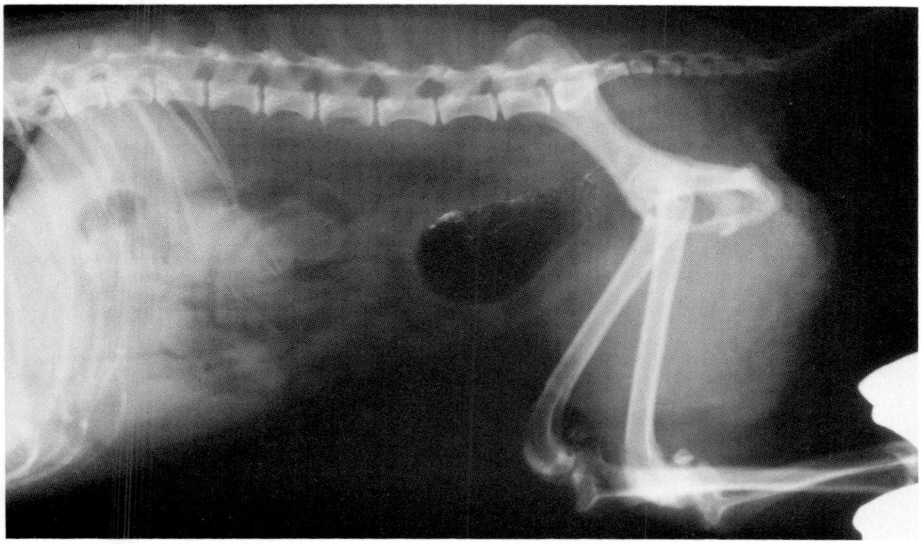

Fig. 10-35. Contrast coating of the bladder mucosa and thickening of the bladder wall and urethra were encountered during double contrast cystography on an 8-year-old female Miniature Poodle with hematuria and dysuria secondary to a transitional cell carcinoma. Compare to Figures 10-33, 10-34, 10-36 and 10-37.

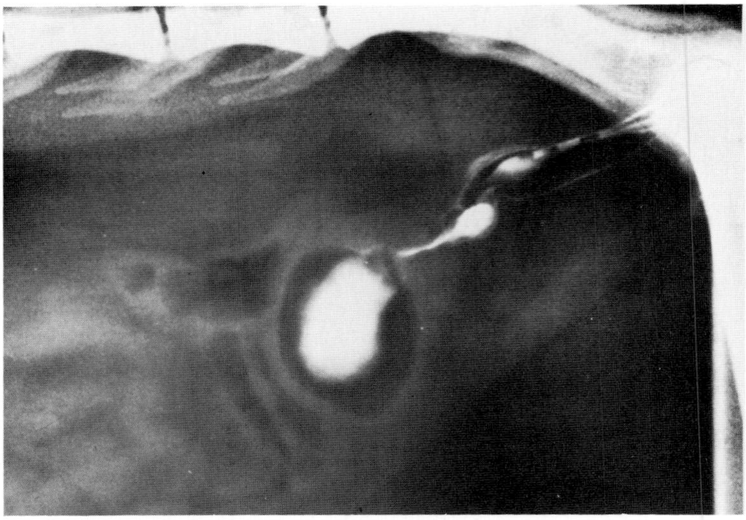

Fig. 10-36. Lateral double contrast cystogram on an adult neutered male domestic shorthair cat with chronic hematuria and dysuria. Diffuse thickening of the bladder wall and nondistensibility were secondary to chronic inflammatory cystitis. Multifocal to diffuse bladder wall thickening can be secondary to neoplastic, infectious, or noninfectious bladder disease. Compare to Figures 10-35 and 10-37.

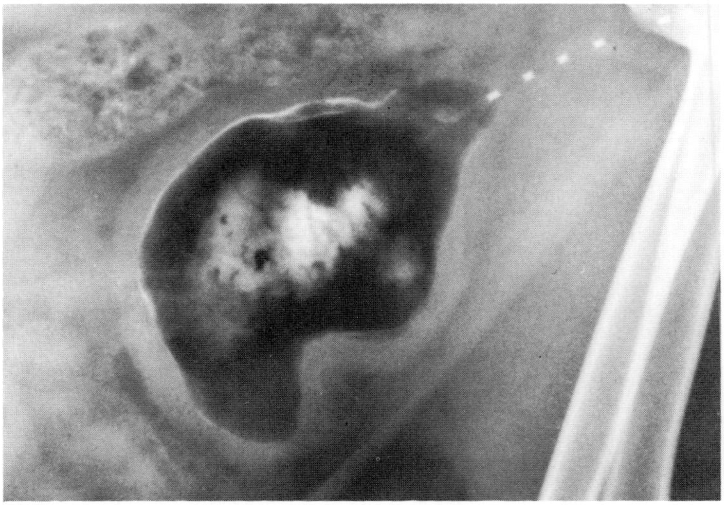

Fig. 10-37. Diffuse mural thickening, contrast coating of the bladder mucosa, and multiple free luminal blood clots, mucous plug, and/or uroliths with a bladder wall invagination are present on a double contrast cystogram from a 3-year-old neutered male domestic shorthair cat 4 days following relief for urethral obstruction. A catheterized urine sample was positive for *Proteus mirabilis*. A chronic, necrotic, transmural cystitis was diagnosed at necropsy. (Johnston GR, Feeney DA, Osborne CA: Urethrography and cystography in cats. Part II. Abnormal radiographic anatomy and complications. Comp Cont Vet Ed 4:931, 1982.)

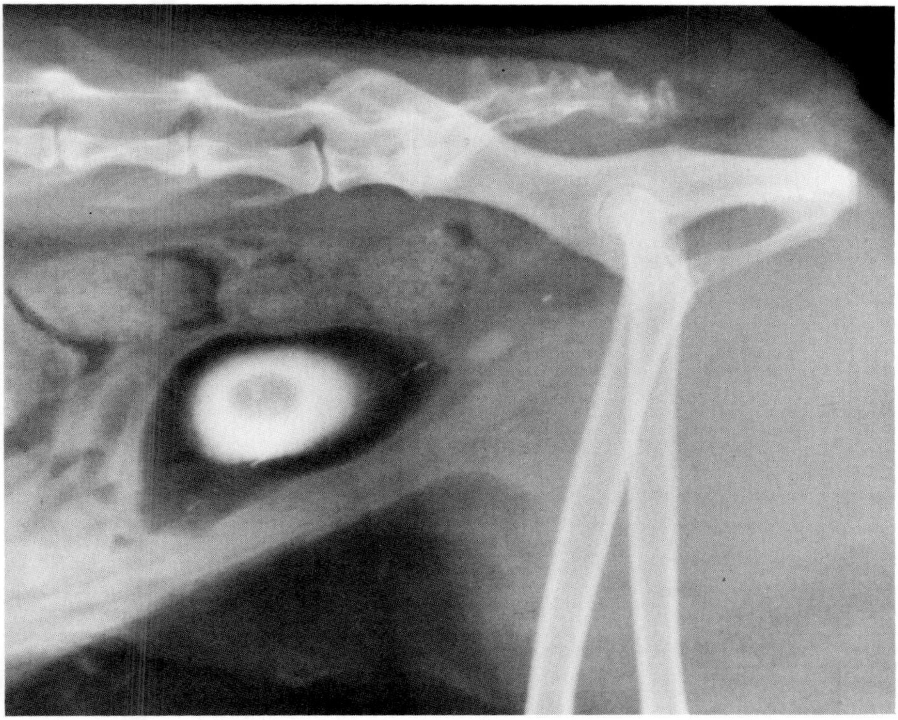

Fig. 10-38. A lateral radiograph of a double contrast cystogram from a 4-year-old female Manx cat with recurrent hematuria and dysuria. A urachal diverticulum, a solitary free luminal cystic calculus, and a urethral calculus are identified. Compare to Figure 10-45.

granulomas, and inflammatory and neoplastic polypoid lesions (Figs. 10-20, 10-39A, B and C). The radiographic density of attached filling defects is variable and is related to the radiographic density of the contrast media surrounding the filling defect. Filling defects surrounded by positive contrast media will be more radiolucent than ones surrounded by negative contrast media (Figs. 10-38 and 10-39C). An attached filling defect does not indicate a poor prognosis (Fig. 10-39C). A definitive diagnosis can only be obtained by considering the history, physical findings, clinical laboratory data, and cytology. The differential features of inflammatory polypoid cystitis and neoplastic polypoid lesions are described in Table 10-10.

Luminal communicating patterns: vesical diverticula. Urinary bladder diverticula can be congenital or acquired.[105] Remnants of the urachus have been reported in dogs and cats and may predispose to stasis of urine and urinary tract infection.[26,105] The most common location of congenital urachal diverticula is cranioventral and is best defined on the lateral cystogram (Figs. 10-30,

Table 10-9. Differential Radiographic Characteristics of Intraluminal Filling Defects of the Urinary Bladder

Radiographic Criteria	Air Bubbles	Calculi	Sebaceous or Mucous Plugs	Blood Clots
Size	Small to large	Small to large	Small	Small to large
Numbers	Single, multiple coalescent	Single or multiple	Single or multiple	Single or multiple
Shape	Commonly round; if coalescing, ovoid or polyhedral	Spheroidal, ovoid, polygonal, pumpkin seed	Spheropidal, ovoid, polygonal, linear	Spheroidal, ovoid, polygonal, linear
Margination	Smooth and distinct	Smooth or irregular, distinct or indistinct	Smooth or irregular, distinct or indistinct	Indistinct and irregular
Location	Commonly at periphery of contrast puddle; if large and coalescing, anywhere	Center of contrast puddle or attached to bladder wall	Center of contrast puddle or attached to bladder wall	Center of contrast puddle or attached to bladder wall
Density				
Survey radiography	Radiolucent	Water-dense (radiolucent) calculi: nondetectable Radiopaque calculi: radiopaque or nondetectable (if small)	Nondetectable	Nondetectable
Pneumocystography	Radiolucent	Water-dense calculi: nondetectable or radiopaque (if attached) Radiopaque calculi: radiopaque	Nondetectable	Nondetectable or radiopaque (attached)
Double contrast cystography	Radiolucent	Water-dense calculi: radiolucent Radiopaque calculi: radiolucent	Radiolucent	Radiolucent
Positive contrast urethrocystography	Radiolucent	Water-dense calculi: radiolucent or nondetectable Radiopaque calculi: radiolucent or nondetectable	Nondetectable	Nondetectable

(Johnston GR, Feeney DA, Osborne CA: Urethrography and cystography in cats. Part II. Abnormal radiographic anatomy and complication. Comp Cont Vet Ed 4:931, 1982.)

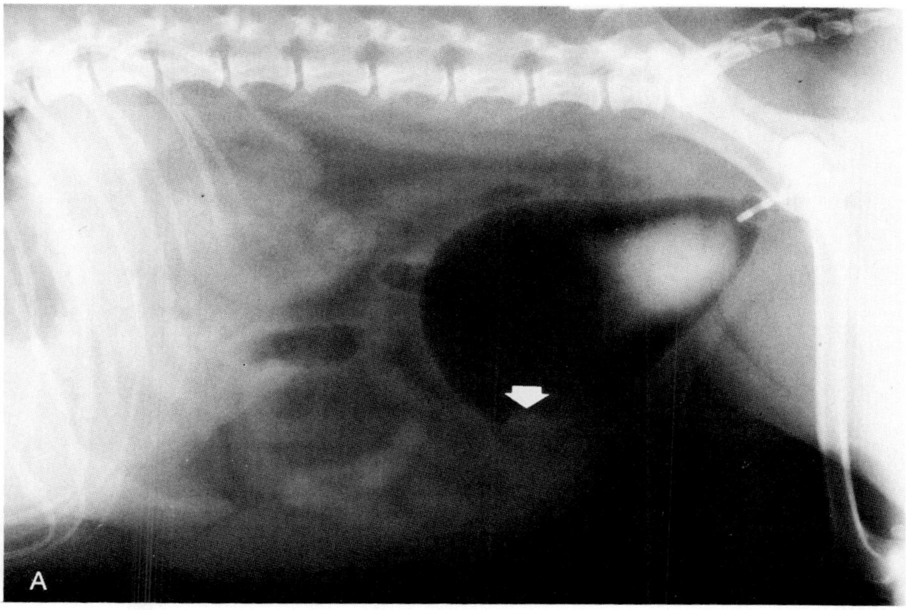

Fig. 10-39. Attached polypoid filling defects of the urinary bladder in dogs and cats may be encountered radiographically and can be caused by hematomas, abscesses, granulomas, or inflammatory or neoplastic diseases. (A) A lateral radiograph of a double contrast cystogram from an 8-year-old female mixed breed dog with urinary tract infection. An attached filling defect on the cranioventral urinary bladder wall is identified (arrow). Minimal bladder wall thickening of the wall adjacent to the mass would suggest a benign lesion. Surgical biopsy indicated the mass to be a benign lesion. (*Figure continues.*)

10-31, and 10-38). Urachal diverticula are variable in shape and may appear nipple shaped (Fig. 10-38), or cystic (Fig. 10-31). They may be associated with attached or free luminal uroliths (Fig. 10-30),[26,105] and may also be encountered secondary to bladder trauma.[24,105] Serial radiography is recommended for differentiating pseudodiverticula caused by spasms of the urinary bladder from true urachal diverticula. Urachal diverticula are encountered in dogs and cats with lower urinary tract disease. The significance of diverticula in cats as a predisposing factor for lower urinary tract disease with sterile urine is unknown. The incidence of urachal diverticula in cats without a history of lower urinary tract disease is also unknown. Positive contrast cystography and positive contrast retrograde or antegrade urethrocystography are the techniques of choice for identification of urachal diverticula.

Vesicoureteral reflux. The radiographic appearance and significance of vesicoureteral reflux was previously described under normal radiographic findings.

Extraluminal mass lesions. Extraluminal mass lesions may be encountered

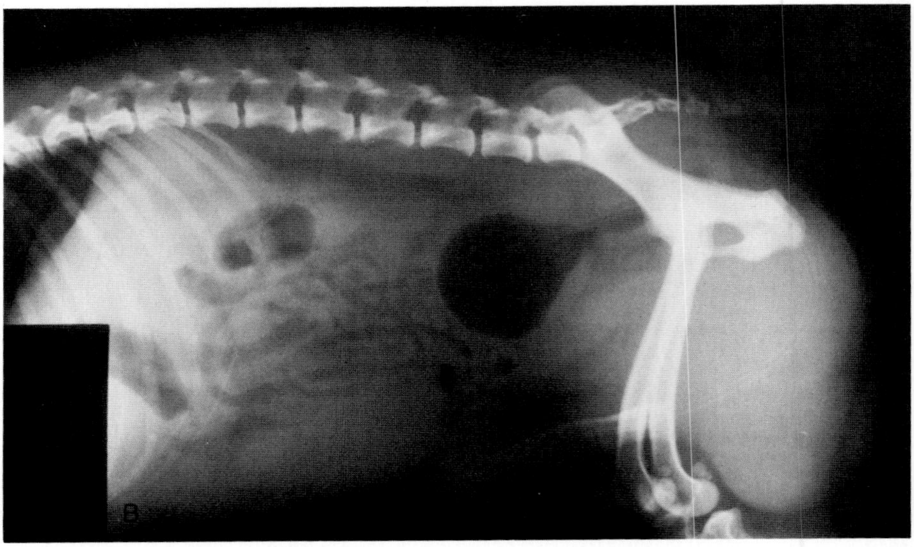

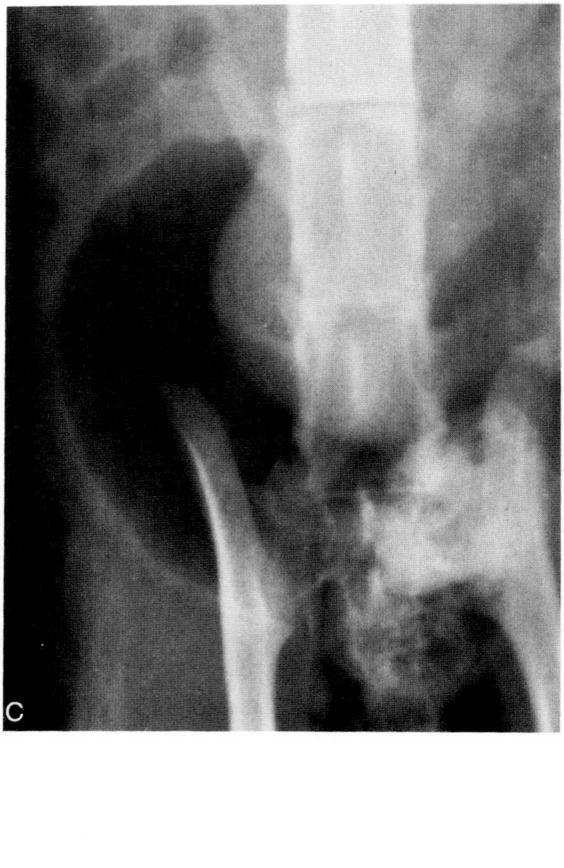

Fig. 10-39 (*continued*). (B) Lateral pneumocystogram from the dog described in Figure 10-19. Mural thickening of the bladder neck and trigone regions was caused by a transitional cell carcinoma with a minor intraluminal component. Note broad "shoulder" of transition from normal bladder wall to abnormal bladder wall. Compare to Figure 10-20, 10-39A, and 10-39C. (C) Ventrodorsal pneumocystogram from an 18-month-old neutered male Persian cat with lower urinary tract disease. The large soft tissue mass was histologically diagnosed as an ulcerative submucosal hematoma. Note shape of transition between normal and abnormal bladder wall. (Johnston GR, Feeney DA, Osborne CA: Urethrography and cystography in cats. Part II. Abnormal radiographic anatomy and complications. Comp Cont Vet Ed 4:931, 1982.)

Table 10-10. Differentiation of Attached Luminal Filling Defects of the Urinary Bladder

Radiography Criteria	Inflammatory Polyp	Neoplastic Polyp
Size	Small to large	Small to large
Number	Single or multiple	Single or multiple
Shape	Often symmetric, occasionally nonsymmetric	Often symmetric, occasionally nonsymmetric
Transition from normal to abnormal	Often sharp and distinct	Often gradual and distinct
Thickening of adjoining bladder wall	+ to + +	+ to + + + +
Location	Anywhere	Anywhere
Intraluminal component	Prominent intraluminal filling defect with mineral mural component	Prominent intraluminal filling defect with or without minimal mural component
Density	Soft tissue (fluid)	Soft tissue (fluid): uncommonly calcified

(Johnston GR, Feeney DA, Osborne CA: Radiographic findings in urinary tract infection. Vet Clin North Am 9:749, 1979.)

during cystography and are caused by diseases of adjacent structures. Uterine stump granulomas, prostatic cysts and sublumbar abscesses may result in extraluminal compression of the urinary bladder (Fig. 10-8 and 10-32).[19,106] Extraluminal mass lesions may result in compromise of the vesicoureteral junction or bladder neck–urethral junction (Fig. 10-22). Extension of an inflammatory process to involve the wall and lumen of the urinary bladder has been reported secondary to an ovarian stump abscess.[106] Extraluminal compressive lesions may require additional radiographic procedures to characterize their location and relationship to the urinary bladder. Barium enemas, contrast vaginography, and excretory urography may be required to rule out ureteral and bladder neck–urethral obstruction.

Contrast Evaluation of the Urethra

Contrast evaluation of the urethra should follow cystography to completely evaluate the lower urinary tract. Patients with clinical signs of lower urinary tract disease may have concurrent bladder and/or urethral disease.[19] The clinical indications for urethrography are identical to those for cystography and include, in addition, palpable periurethral masses, resistance to catheterization, and blood dripping from the prepuce.[91] Radiographic indications described for cystography may also indicate concurrent urethral disease.[19] Abnormalities encountered on survey radiographs associated with the urethra do not negate the requirement for urethrography since additional sites of involvement along the urethra may be subsequently defined. Multiple pelvic fractures and pelvic masses may require urethrography to rule out involvement of the urethra. Pneumourethrography and double contrast urethrography are not recommended because of inadequate contrast. Air should be avoided in patients with suspected urethral lacerations because of the potential for fatal vascular embolization. Patient preparation described for survey radiography is recommended for urethrography.

Table 10-11. Techniques of Urethrography

A. Retrograde contrast urethrocystography
   1. Aseptically catheterize the urinary bladder
   2. Remove residual urine
   3. Infuse a 5–10% solution of positive contrast medium until the bladder is maximally distended as determined by digital palpation
   4. Fill lumen of catheter with a 1:2 dilution of positive contrast medium
   5. Secure balloon-tipped catheter inside the external urethral orifice by inflating the balloon cuff
   6. Inject an appropriate amount of positive contrast medium
      a. Cats: 3 ml
         Dogs:
         1. Less than 25 lb: 7–10 ml
         2. >25 lb <75 lb: 10–15 ml
         3. >75 lb: 15–20 ml
   7. Expose lateral and ventrodorsal recumbent radiographs towards the end of injection of positive contrast medium
   8. Remove bladder contents

B. Antegrade cystourethrography
   1. Use appropriate chemical restraint
   2. Fill the urinary bladder with a 5–10% solution of positive contrast medium by one of the following techniques:
      a. Excretory urography
      b. Catheterization
      c. Transabdominal infusion via a 3 inch 22-gauge spinal needle
   3. The maximum degree of bladder distention should be employed to initiate spontaneous micturation
   4. With spontaneous micturation, remove catheter and expose lateral recumbent radiograph during voiding
   5. Without spontaneous micturation following maximum bladder distention, remove catheter and induce micturation by external bladder compression with the aid of a wooden spoon and expose lateral recumbent radiograph during voiding
   6. Remove bladder contents

Techniques. ***Antegrade (Voiding) Cystourethrography.*** The technique of antegrade (voiding) cystourethrography is described in Table 10-11. Antegrade cystourethrography is recommended on patients that are difficult to catheterize or are a high-risk population for urinary tract infection. Antegrade cystourethrography may demonstrate vesicoureteral reflux and congenital anomalies of the urinary bladder and urethra that may not be demonstrated by retrograde urethrography. Antegrade cystourethrography is more difficult to perform than retrograde urethrocystography and subsequently should be reserved for those cases where retrograde urethrocystography fails to provide a diagnosis. The technique of antegrade urethrocystography requires light anesthesia or sedation and gradual infusion of the urinary bladder until the detrusor reflex is initiated.[19,24] Technical difficulties encountered during antegrade cystourethrography may be related to the degree of sedation/anesthesia.[24] A normal antegrade cystourethrogram in a male cat is illustrated in Figure 10-40.

Retrograde urethrocystography. Retrograde urethrocystography is a simple, inexpensive technique that can be used to evaluate urethral structure. Balloon tipped catheters are recommended for retrograde urethrocystography to seal the distal urethra and ensure retrograde infusion of a continuous column of contrast medium.[19,24,107] The use of non-balloon urethral or ureteral cath-

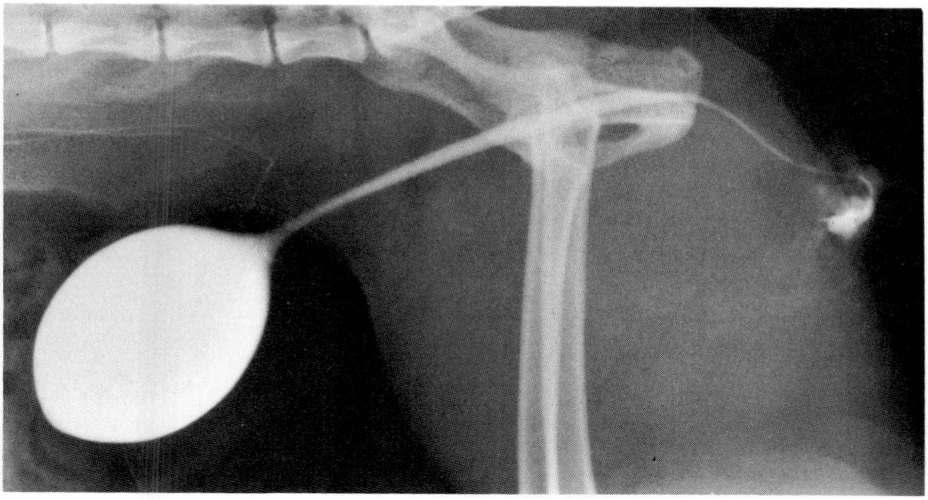

Fig. 10-40. Normal male feline positive contrast antegrade (voiding) cystourethrogram performed by external bladder compression using a wooden spoon. Note the bilateral vesicoureteral reflux. Compared to normal retrograde urethrocystogram in a male cat in Figure 10-41C. (Johnston GR, Feeney DA: Localization of feline urethral obstruction. Vet Clin North Am 14:555, 1984.)

eters for retrograde urethrography may result in paracatheter reflux and incomplete filling of the proximal portions of the urethra.[24,107] The technique of retrograde urethrocystography should include maximum distention of the urinary bladder prior to retrograde infusion of contrast medium through the urethral lumen. The technique of maximum-distention urethrocystography is described in Table 10-11 and is recommended to provide a sufficient level of intravesical hydrostatic pressure to ensure maximum distention of the urethral lumen.[108] Normal retrograde urethrocystograms for male and female dogs and cats are illustrated in Figures 10-41A, B, C, and D.

Prostatic Urethrography. The technique of maximum-distention urethrocystography is recommended for prostatic urethrography because it provides a maximal distention of the lumen of the prostatic urethra.[108] A balloon-tipped catheter located in the penile urethra is recommended over a non-balloon catheter in the prostatic urethra because retrograde infusion of contrast media into a non-balloon catheter in the prostatic urethra may not adquately distend the lumen of the prostatic urethra. Lateral and ventrodorsal radiographs are recommended for evaluation of the prostatic urethra. Additional oblique films may be necessary to prevent superposition of the penile urethra on the prostatic urethra on ventrodorsal radiograph.

Technical and Interpretative Pitfalls and Complications. The technical and interpretative pitfalls and complications associated with antegrade cystourethrography and retrograde urethrocystography are listed in Table 10-7.

Normal Radiographic Findings. ***Canine.*** The male canine urethra is com-

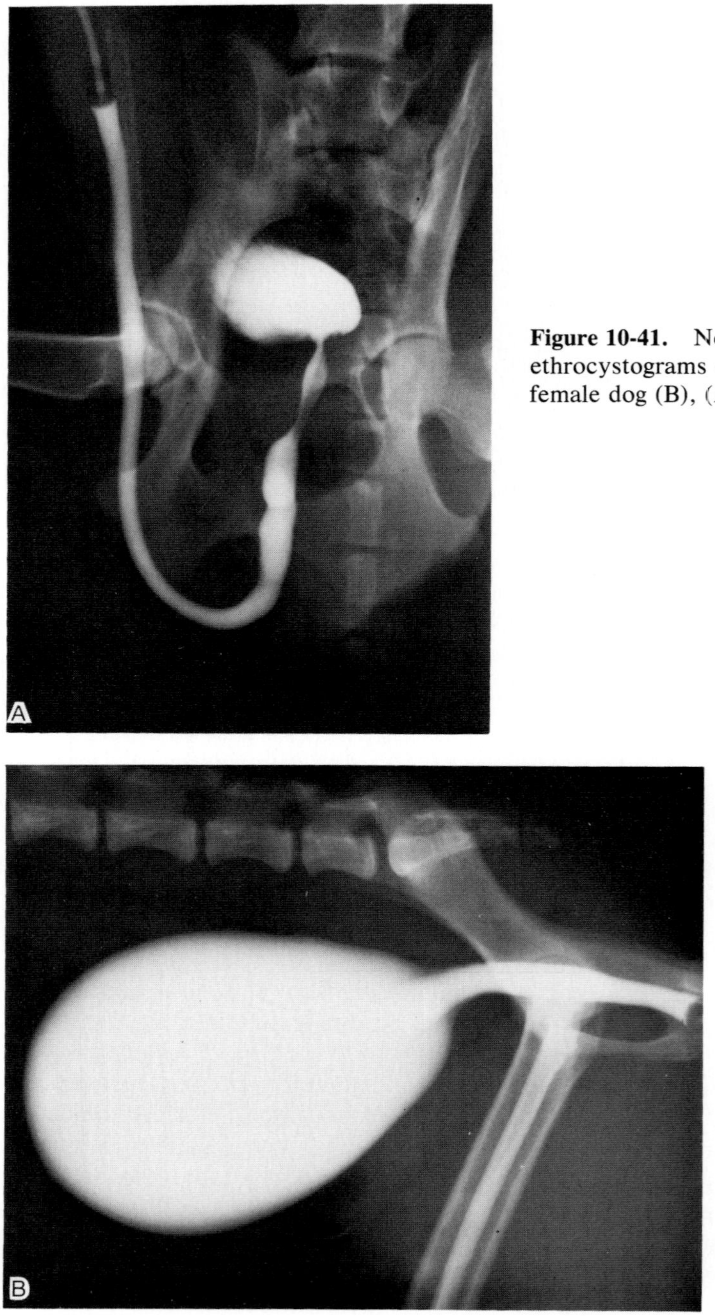

Figure 10-41. Normal retrograde urethrocystograms on a male dog (A), female dog (B), (*Figure continues.*)

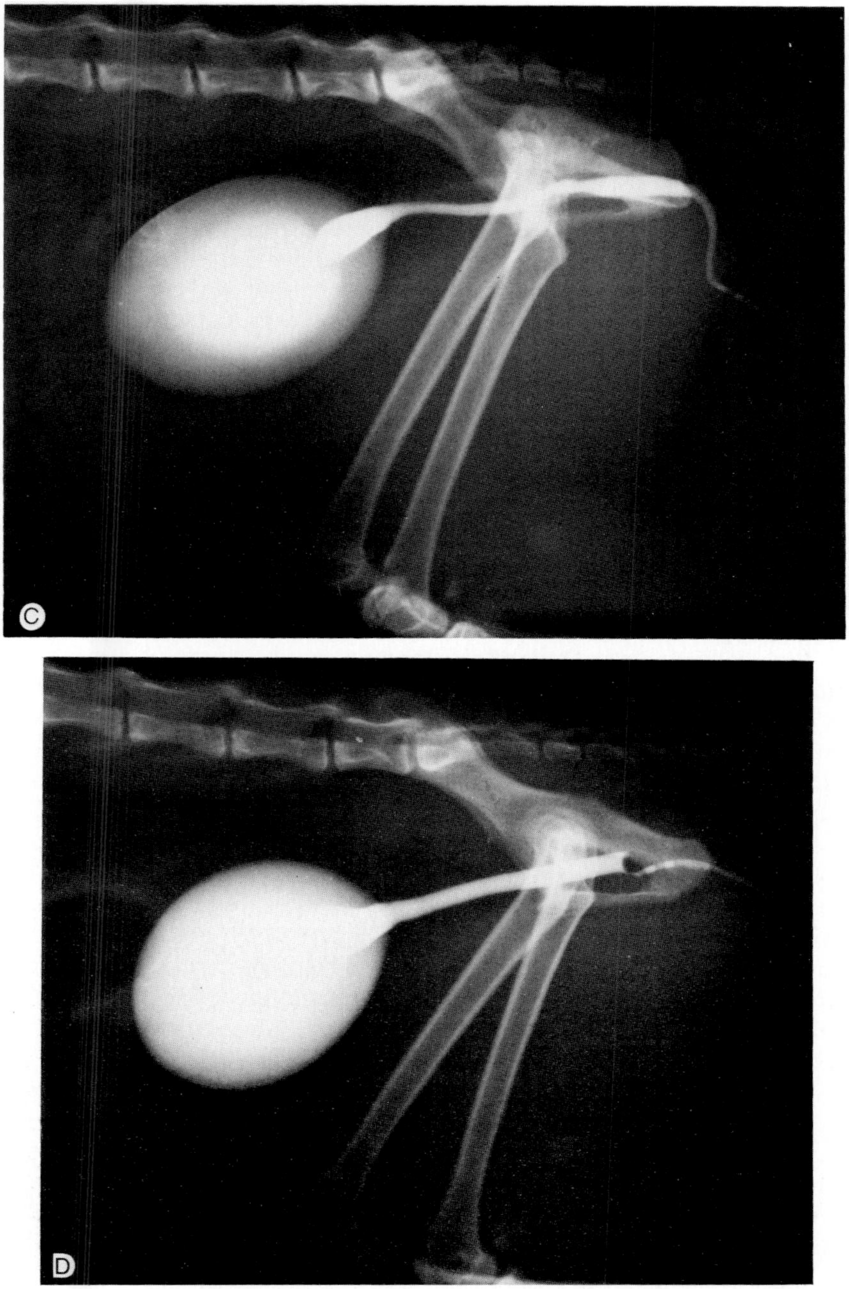

Fig. 10-41 (*continued*). male cat (C), and female cat (D). (Johnston GR, Feeney, DA, Osborne CA: Radiographic findings in urinary tract infection. Vet Clin North Am 9:749, 1979.)

posed of three regions: prostatic, membranous, and penile (Fig. 10-41A).[19,107] The prostatic urethra is spindle-shaped, with proximal and distal portions narrower than the middle portion. A linear filling defect may be encountered on the dorsal wall of the prostatic urethra and is the result of caliculus seminalis. The middle portion of the prostatic urethra is wider than the membranous or penile urethra.[108] The mucosal pattern of the prostatic urethra should be smooth. The membranous urethra connects the distal prostatic urethra with the penile urethra. The lumen of the membranous urethra varies in diameter, which may be caused by inadequate urinary bladder distention, peristalic contractions, or spasms of the smooth or skeletal muscle in the wall of the membranous urethra.[107] The penile urethra has a uniform diameter throughout its length, but variations may be encountered if the radiographic exposure occurs following the injection of contrast medium or if the peristalic contractions are encountered at the time of exposure. Variations in luminal diameter can be further evaluated by obtaining subsequent radiographs in lateral or ventrodorsal recumbency following an additional incremental infusion of contrast medium with radiographic exposure towards the end of injection.

The urethra of the female canine will have a variable diameter depending upon the degree of urinary bladder distention (Fig. 10-41B). Urethral displacement relative to the floor of the pelvis and urethral flexures may be encountered depending upon the degree of urinary bladder distention.

Feline. The male cat's urethra is composed of five regions: preprostatic, prostatic, postprostatic, bulbic, and penile.[7,24] Radiographically, these five regions cannot be individually identified (Fig. 10-41C).[24] The intrapelvic urethra from the ischial arch to the bladder neck urethral junction should have a uniform diameter if the urinary bladder is adequately distended. Variations in diameter in the area of the prostatic urethra may be encountered but can be ruled out from mural or extraluminal lesions following subsequent antegrade (voiding) cystourethrography.[24] The diameter of the penile urethra is variable, with maximum dimensions in the area of the ischial arch and subsequent gradual luminal narrowing to the external urethral orifice (Fig. 10-41C). Focal or regional narrowing of the urethral lumen may be associated with urethral spasms secondary to catheter location.[24] These pseudolesions can be further defined by performing antegrade cystourethrography.

The female cat's urethra is similar to the female dog's urethra and should have a uniform diameter from the bladder neck–urethral junction to the inflated balloon catheter if the urinary bladder is adequately distended (Fig. 10-41D).[24,207] Variations in urethral diameter may be related to inadequate urinary bladder distention or urethral spasms or peristalic contractions.[24]

Abnormal Radiographic Findings. ***Mucosal and Mural Lesions.*** The etiology for mucosal and mural lesions involving the urethra are nonspecific and include the causes previously described for mucosal and mural lesions for the urinary bladder. Mucosal and mural lesions may be focal or multifocal (Fig. 10-42). The significance of mucosal and mural lesions must follow careful consideration of the history, physical findings, and laboratory data. Mucosal and mural lesions may be related and occur secondary to prolonged use of in-

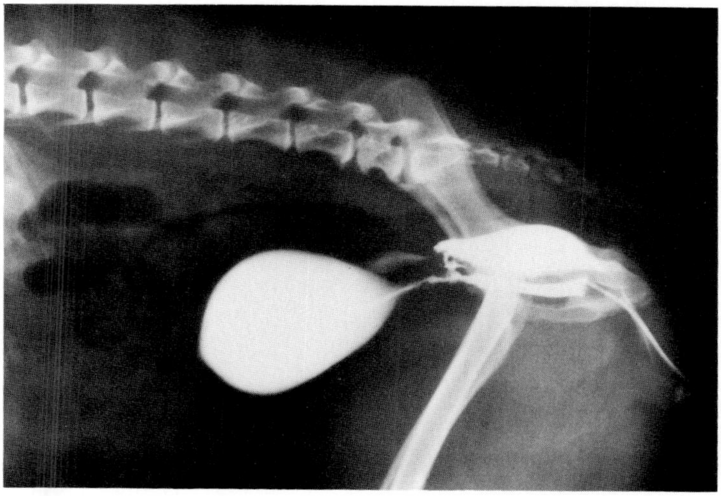

Figure 10-42. Lateral radiograph of a positive contrast retrograde urethrocystogram from a 10-year old female English setter with chronic hematuria and dysuria. Mucosal irregularity, nondistensibility of the proximal urethra, and a urethrovaginal fistula were caused by a transitional cell carcinoma of the proximal urethra.

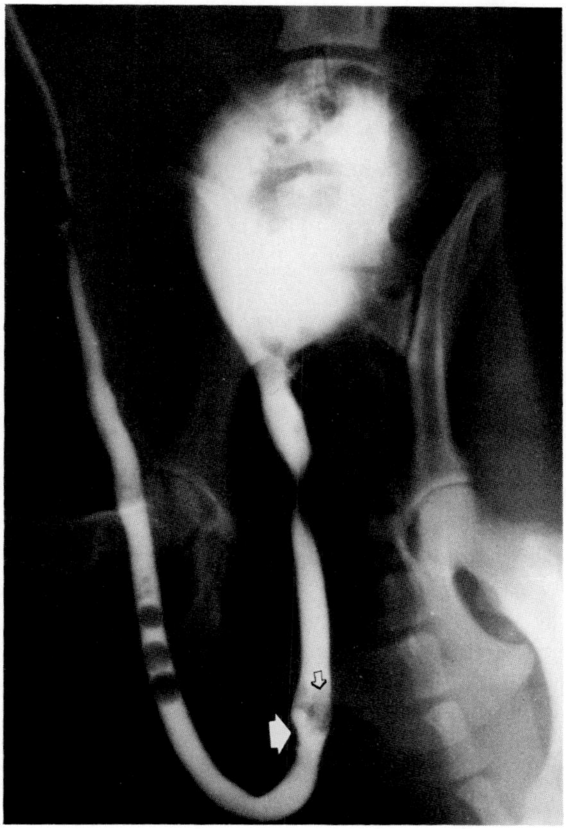

Fig. 10-43. Ventrodorsal oblique radiograph of a positive contrast retrograde urethrocysotgram from 12-year old male beagle with chronic hematuria and dysuria. Three large and several small air bubbles conforming to the lumen of the penile urethra are encountered. The irregular filling defect at the ischial arch is a blood clot (open arrow). The narrowed distal penile urethral lumen adjacent to the balloon catheter is caused by a urethral spasm or a peristatic contraction. Mucosal irregularity at the junction of the membranous and penile urethra (white arrow) was caused by catheter trauma. (Johnston GR, Feeney DA, Osborne CA: Radiographic findings in urinary tract infection. Vet Clin North Am 9:749, 1979.)

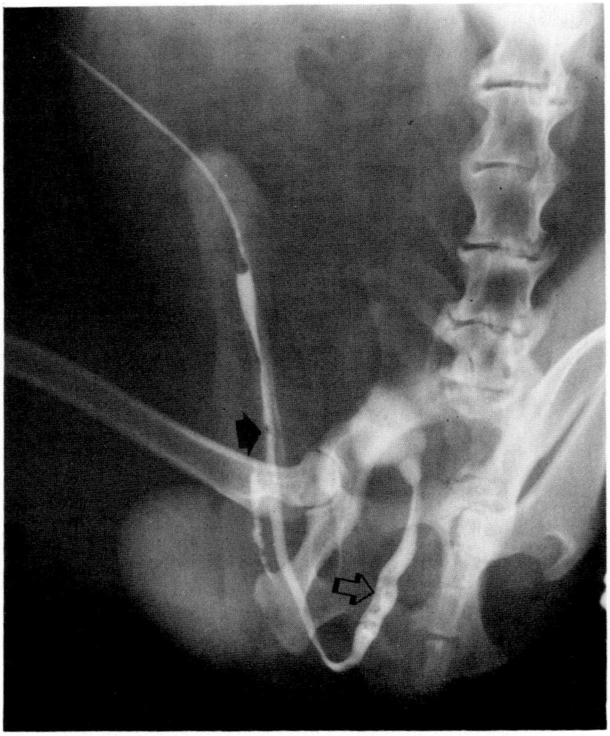

Fig. 10-44. Positive contrast retrograde urethrocystogram from a 6-year old male Irish setter with lower urinary tract disease. A solitary urethral calculus in the penile urethra (black arrow), periurethral escape of contrast media, periurethral soft tissue gas, and multiple filling defects including air bubbles and a blood clot (open arrow) in the membranous urethra are identified.

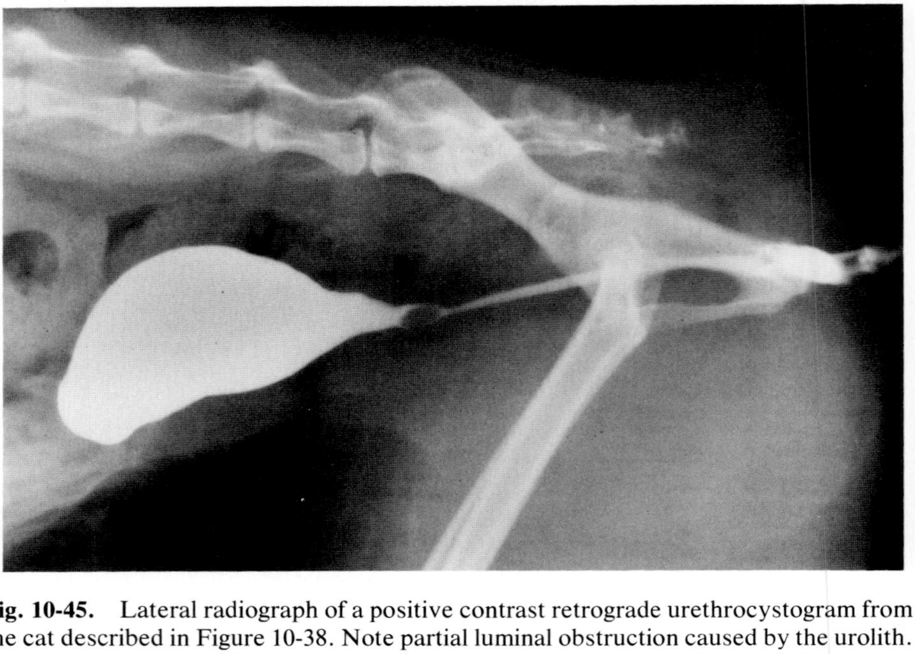

Fig. 10-45. Lateral radiograph of a positive contrast retrograde urethrocystogram from the cat described in Figure 10-38. Note partial luminal obstruction caused by the urolith. (Johnston GR, Feeney DA: Localization of feline urethral obstruction. Vet Clin North Am 14:555, 1984.)

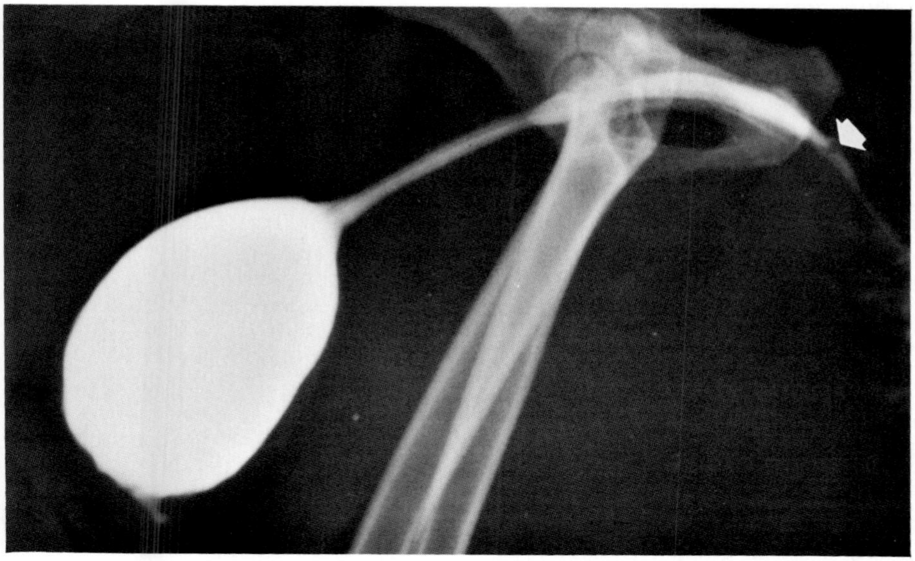

Fig. 10-46. Lateral radiograph of a positive contrast antegrade cystourethrogram from the cat described in Fig. 10-12. A thickened bladder wall, urachal diverticulum and a urethral calculus (arrow) are identified. Cystic urolith visible on the survey radiograph are obscured by the positive contrast medium. (Johnston GR, Feeney DA, Osborne CA: Urethrography and cystography in cats. Part II. Abnormal radiographic anatomy and complications. Comp Cont Vet Ed 4:931, 1982.)

dwelling catheters. Mucosal irregularity may be encountered in the area of the ischial arch of the penile urethra of the male dog secondary to iatrogenic catheter-induced urethral trauma (Fig. 10-43). Mucosal lesions can be differentiated from mural lesions by careful evaluation of the distensibility of the urethral lumen. A rigid, nondistensible urethral lumen with mucosal irregularity may indicate an infiltrate of inflammatory or neoplastic origin (Fig. 10-42). Luminal narrowing with or without mucosal irregularity may be encountered radiographically and can be caused by urethral spasms following catheterization or diffuse inflammatory disease following prolonged use of indwelling catheters (Figs. 10-43, 10-44).

Filling defects. Filling defects of the urethra may be attached or free luminal and include those previously described for the urinary bladder. The most common free luminal filling defects of the urethra include air bubbles, blood clots, uroliths, and sebaceous and mucous plugs (Figs. 10-43, 10-44, 10-45, and 10-46). The differential radiographic features of free luminal filling defects are described in Table 10-12. Uroliths may be free luminal or attached and are most frequently encountered in the ischial arch and proximal penile urethra in male dogs (Fig. 10-44). The most common site for urolith in male cats is the penile urethra (Fig. 10-46).[26] However, urethral obstruction proximal to the

Table 10-12. Differential Radiographic Characteristics of Intraluminal Filling Defects of the Urethra Encountered during Positive Contrast Urethrography

Radiographic Criteria	Air Bubbles	Calculi	Sebaceous or Mucous Plugs	Blood Clots
Size	Small about 5–10 mm	Small, about 5–10 mm	Small, about 5–10 mm	Small
Number	Single, multiple, or coalescent	Single or multiple	Single or multiple	Single or multiple
Shape	Round if smaller than urethral lumen; oval or polyhedral if coalescent	Spheroid, ovoid, polygonal, or pumpkin seed	Spheroid, ovoid, polygonal, or linear	Spheroid, ovoid, polygonal or linear
Margination	Smooth and distinct	Smooth or irregular, commonly distinct	Smooth or irregular, distinct or indistinct	Irregular and indistinct
Location	Anywhere	Commonly in membranous urethra (ischial arch) or penile urethra (os penis); may be attached or combined within a blood clot	Commonly in penile urethra in male cats; but may be located anywhere within urethra	Anywhere
Relationship to urethral lumen	Always conform to shape of urethral lumen	May cause focal distension if larger than urethral lumen; will conform to urethral lumen if small	Conform to shape of urethral lumen	Conform to shape of urethral lumen
Radiographic density	Radiolucent	Radiolucent	Radiolucent	Radiolucent

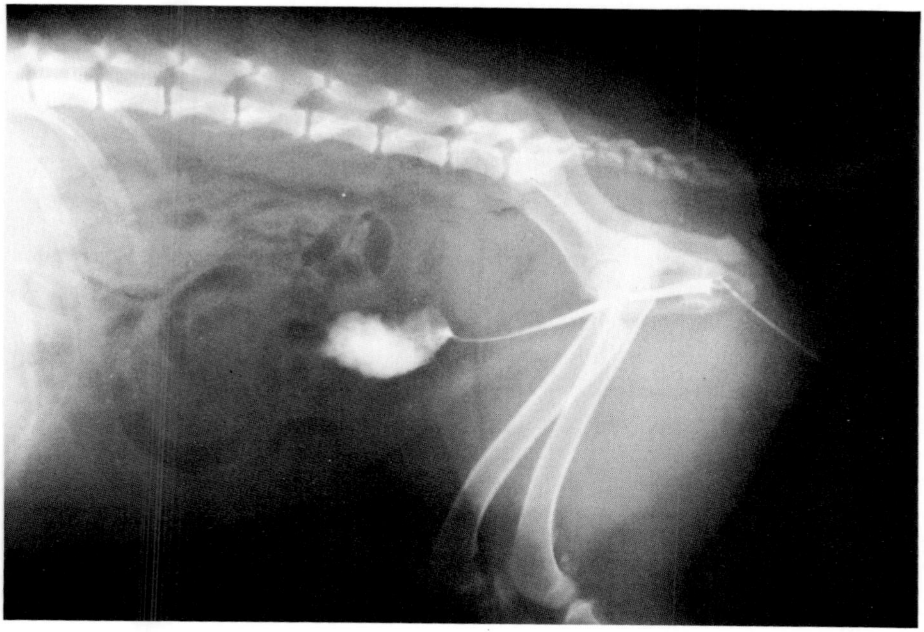

Fig. 10-47. Lateral radiograph of a positive contrast retrograde urethrocystogram from a 2-year-old female mixed breed dog with dysuria. Cranial ventral displacement of the urinary bladder and urethra were caused by a transmissible venereal sarcoma.

penile urethra may be encountered. Urethral calculi are less frequently encountered in the female dog and cat but they've been reported as a cause for urethral obstruction (Figs. 10-4 and 10-45).[26,28] Attached luminal filling defects include blood clots, uroliths, neoplasms, and inflammatory lesions secondary to surgery or trauma.

Extraluminal lesions. Extraluminal compressive lesions are less common but may cause luminal compression and displacement. Periurethral soft tissue masses from inflammatory or neoplastic origin, vaginal and uterine tumors, and uterine stump granulomas may result in urethral displacement and luminal compression (Figs. 10-32 and 10-47). Extraluminal compressive lesions will result in luminal displacement and luminal narrowing with a smooth mucosal pattern. Extraluminal compressive lesions of inflammatory or neoplastic origin may infiltrate the wall of the urethra and cause mural and mucosal lesions that result in luminal narrowing, mucosal irregularity, and nondistensibility of the urethral lumen.

Prostatic urethra. The normal radiographic appearance of the prostatic urethra has previously been described. The causes of mucosal and mural lesions listed for the urinary bladder and urethra also apply to the prostatic urethra. The distensibility of the prostatic urethra is variable and may be influenced by the degree of urinary bladder distention, catheter selection, and location. Mucosal irregularity without a rigid nondistensible lumen may be secondary to prostatic hypertrophy. Mucosal irregularity with a rigid nondistensible urethral lumen may be secondary to primary urethral tumors or prostatic neoplasia. Filling defects have been reported but are less frequent than in other areas of the urethra.[19] Extraluminal compressive lesions have a radiographic appearance similar to those previously described and may occur secondary to a prostatic cyst (Fig. 10-32). Prostatic reflux occurs when positive or negative contrast medium refluxes into the parenchyma of the prostate gland. The significance of urethroprostatic reflux is unknown, as it has been reported to occur in normal dogs and in dogs with inflammatory, infectious, noninfectious, and neoplastic diseases of the prostate gland.[109,110] Urethroprostatic reflux into large cystic masses may be encountered with prostatic cysts that communicate with the lumen of the prostatic urethra and congenital remnants of the uterine masculinus (Fig. 10-32). Consult the chapter on prostatic diseases for further information.

REFERENCES

1. Finco DR, Thrall DE, Duncan JR: The urinary system. p. 419. in Catcott EJ (ed): Canine Medicine. 4th Ed. Am Vet Pubns, Santa Barbara, CA, 1979
2. Finco DR, Barsanti JA, Crowell WA: The urinary system. p. 363. In Pratt PW (ed): Feline Medicine. Am Vet Pubns, Santa Barbara, CA, 1983
3. Grandage J: Some effects of posture of the radiographic appearance of the kidneys of the dog. J Am Vet Med Assoc, 166:165, 1975
4. Allan G: Radiology in the dx of kidney disease. Aust Vet Pract 12:97, 1982
5. Biery DN: Upper urinary tract. p. 481. In O'Brien TR (ed): Radiographic Diagnosis of Abdominal Disorders in the Dog and Cat: Radiographic Interpretation, Clinical Signs, Pathophysiology. WB Saunders Co, Philadelphia, 1978
6. Ellenport CR: Carnivore Urogenital Apparatus. p. 1576. In Getty R (ed): Anatomy of Domestic Animals. 5th Ed. WB Saunders Co, Philadelphia, 1975
7. Crouch JE: Text Atlas of Cat Anatomy. Lea & Febiger Co, Philadelphia, 1969
8. Finco DR, Stiles NS, Kneller SK, et al: Radiologic estimation of kidney size in the dog. J Am Vet Med Assoc, 159:995, 1971
9. Barrett RB, Kneller, SK: Feline kidney measurement. Acta Radiol 319(suppl):279, 1972
10. Osborne CA, Low DG, Finco DR: Canine and Feline Urology. WB Saunders Co, Philadelphia, 1972
11. Barsanti JA, Crowell, W: Renal amyloidosis. p. 1063. In Kirk RW (ed): Current Veterinary VII. WB Saunders Co, Philadelphia, 1980
12. Barber DL: Radiographic evaluation of a focal inflammatory renal lesion. J Am Anim Hosp Assoc 12:451, 1976
13. Senior DF: Parasites of the canine urinary tract. p. 1141. In Kirk RW (ed): Current Veterinary Therapy VII. WB Saunders Co, Philadelphia, 1980
14. Brace JJ: Perirenal cysts (pseudocysts) in the cat. p. 980. In Kirk RW (ed): Current Veterinary Therapy VIII. WB Saunders Co, Philadelphia, 1983

15. Barber DL, Rowland GN: Radiographically detectable soft tissue calcification in chronic renal failure. Vet Radiol 20:117, 1979
16. Hall MA, Osborne CA, Stevens JB: Hydronephrosis with heteroplastic bone formation in a cat. J Am Vet Med Assoc 160:857, 1972
17. Miller JB, Sande RD: Osseous metaplasia in the renal pelvis of a dog with hydronephrosis. Vet Radiol 21:146, 1980
18. Rendano VT, Taylor MJ, Robinette JD: Nephrocalcinosis in a dog. J Am Vet Med Assoc 15:26, 1974
19. Park RD: Radiology of the urinary bladder and urethra. p. 543. In O'Brien TR (ed): Radiographic Diagnosis of Abdominal Disorders in the Dog and Cat: Radiographic Interpretation, Clinical Signs, Pathophysiology. WB Saunders Co, Philadelphia, 1978
20. Evens HE, Christensen GC: Miller's Anatomy of the Dog. 2nd Ed. WB Saunders Co, Philadelphia, 1979
21. Kealy JK: Diagnostic Radiology of the Dog and Cat. WB Saunders Co, Philadelphia, 1979
22. Mahaffey MB, Barsanti JA, Barber DL, Crowell WA: Pelvic bladder in dogs without urinary incontinence. J Am Vet Med Assoc 184:1477, 1984
23. Nickel R, Schummer A, Seiferie E: The Viscera of the Domestic Mammals. 2nd Ed. Springer-Verlag, New York, 1979
24. Johnston GR, Feeney DA, Osborne CA: Urethrography and cystography in cats. Part I. Techniques, normal radiographic anatomy and artifacts. Compend Cont Vet ed 4:823, 1982
25. O'Brien TR: What is Your Diagnosis? J Am Vet Med Assoc 157:975, 1970
26. Johnston GR, Feeney DA, Osborne CA: Urethrography and cystography in cats. Part II. Abnormal radiographic anatomy and complications. Compend Cont Vet Ed 4:931, 1982
27. Root CR, Scott RC: Emphysematous cystitis and other radiographic manifestation of diabetes mellitus in dogs and cats. J Am Vet Med Assoc 158:721, 1971
28. Osborne CA, Abdullahi S, Klausner JS, et al: Non-surgical removal of uroliths from the urethra of female dogs. J Am Vet Med Assoc 182:47, 1983
29. Johnston GR, Feeney DA: Localization of feline urethral obstruction. Vet Clin North Am 14:555, 1984
30. Osborne CA, Jessen CR: Double contrast cystography in the dog. J Am Vet Med Assoc 159:1400, 1971
31. Brodeur AE, Goyer, RA, Melich W: A potential hazard of barium cystography. Radiology 85:1080, 1965
32. Doyle FH: Cystography on bladder tumors. A technique using steripaque and carbon dioxide. Br J Radiol 34:205, 1961
33. Cochran DQ, Almond CH, Shucart WA: An experimental study of the effects of barium and intestinal contents on the peritoneal cavity. Am J Roentgenol 89:883, 1963
34. Kay S, Choy SH: Results of intraperitoneal injection of barium sulfate contrast medium. Arch Pathol 59:388, 1955
35. Kleinsasser LJ, Warshaw, A.: Perforation of the sigmoid colon during barium enema. Ann Surg 4:560, 1952
36. Saunders AW, Kobernick SD: Fate of barium sulfate in the retroperitoneum. Am J Surg 93:907, 1957
37. Sisel RJ, Donovan AJ, Yellin AE: Experimental fecal peritonitis: Influence of barium sulfate or water-soluble radiographic contrast material on survival. Arch Surg 104:765, 1972

38. Zheutlin N, Lasser EC, Rigler LG: Clinical studies on effect of barium in the peritoneal cavity following rupture of the colon. Surgery 32:967, 1952
39. Feeney DA, Johnston GR, Tomlinson MJ, Osborne CA: Comparison of effects of sterilized, micropulverized barium sulfate suspension and meglumine iothalamate solution on the normal canine urinary tract following retrograde urethrocystography. Am J Vet Res 45:730, 1984
40. McAlister WH, Shockelford GD, Kissone J: The histologic effects of 30% Cystokon, Hypaque 25% and Renografin-30 in the bladder. Radiology 104:563, 1972
41. Breton L, Pennock PW, Valli VE: Effects of Hypaque 25% and sodium iodide 10% in the canine urinary bladder. J Am Vet Radiol Soc 19:116, 1978
42. Ackerman N, Wingfield WE, Corley EA: Fatal air embolization associated with pneumocystography. J Am Vet Med Assoc 160:1616, 1972
43. Zontine WJ, Andrews LK: Fatal air embolization as a complication of pneumocystography in two cats. J Am Vet Radiol Soc 19:8, 1978
44. Feeney DA, Osborne CA, Jessen CR: Effects of radiographic contrast media on results of the urinalysis with emphasis on specific gravity. J Am Vet Med Assoc 176:1378, 1980
45. Ruby AL, Ling GV, Ackerman N: Effects of sodium diatrizoate on the in vitro growth of three common canine urinary bacterial species. Vet Radiol 24:222, 1983
46. Feeney DA, Barber DL, Osborne CA: Advances in canine excretory urography. In Proceedings 30th Gaines Veterinary Symposium. Gaines Dog Research Center, White Plains, NY, 1981
47. Feeney DA, Barber DL, Johnston GR, Osborne CA: The excretory urogram: Techniques, normal radiographic appearance and misinterpretation. Compend Cont Vet educ 4:233, 1982
48. Kneller SK: Role of excretory urography in the dx of renal and ureteral disease. Vet Clin North Am 4:843, 1974
49. Feeney DA, Thrall DE, Barber DL, et al: Normal canine excretory urogram: Effects of dose, time and individual dog variation. Am J Vet Res 40: 1596, 1979
50. Bartels JE. Feline intravenous urography. J Am Anim Hosp Assoc 9:349, 1973
51. Barber DL: Renal angiography in veterinary medicine. J Am Vet Radiol Soc 16:187, 1975
52. Resnick MI, Sanders RC: Ultrasound in urology. Williams & Wilkins Co, Baltimore, 1979
53. Feeney DA, Barber DL, Osborne CA: Functional aspects of the nephrogram in excretory urography: A review. Vet Radiol 23:42, 1982
54. Thrall DE, Finco DR: Canine excretory urography: Is quantity a function of BUN? J Am Anim Hosp Assoc 12:446, 1976
55. Robinson GW: Uterus uncornius and unilateral renal agenesis. J Am Vet Med Assoc 147:516, 1965
56. O'Hardley P, Carrig PB, Unshaw R: Renal and ureteral duplication in a dog. J Am Vet Med Assoc 174:484, 1979
57. Osborne CA, Quast JF, Barnes DM, Shockner P: Congenital fusion of kidneys in a dog. Vet Med Small Anim Clin 67:39, 1972
58. Chastain CB, Grier RL: Bilateral retroperitoneal perirenal cysts in a cat. Feline Pract 5:51, 1975
59. Stowater JL: Congenital solitary renal cyst in a dog. J Am Anim Hosp Assoc 11:199, 1975
60. Caywood DD, Osborne CA, Johnston GR: Neoplasms of the canine and feline urinary tracts. p. 1203. In Kirk RW (ed): Current Veterinary Therapy VII. WB Saunders Co, Philadelphia, 1980

61. McKenna SC, Carpenter JL: Polycystic disease of the kidney & liver in the Cairn Terrier. Vet Pathol 17:436, 1980
62. Northington JW, Juliana MM: Polycystic kidney disease in a cat. J Small Anim Pract, 18:663, 1977
63. Rendano VT, Parker RB: Polycystic kidneys and peritoneal pericardial diaphragmatic hernia in a cat. J Small Anim Pract, 17:479, 1976
64. Crowell WA, Hubbell JJ, Riley JC: Polycystic renal disease in related cats. J Am Vet Med Assoc 175:286, 1979
65. Osborne CA, Johnson KH, Kurtz HJ, Hanlon GF: Renal lymphoma in the dog and cat. J Am Vet Med Assoc 158:2058, 1971
66. Batterschell D, Garcia JP, Renal lymphosarcoma in a cat. Mod Vet Pract 50:51, 1969
67. Fuller WJ: Subacute pyelonephritis with a unilaterally non-visualized pyelogram. J Am Anim Hosp Assoc 12:509, 1976
68. Barber DL, Finco DR: Radiographic findings in induced bacterial pyelonephritis in dogs. J Am Vet Med Assoc 175:1183, 1979
69. Barber DL: Radiographic evaluation of a focal inflammatory renal lesion. J Am Anim Hosp Assoc 12:451, 1976
70. Chalifoux A, Phaneuf JB, Oliver N, Gosselin J: Glomerular polycystic kidney disease in a dog. Can Vet J 23:365, 1982
71. Witcock BP, Patterson JM: Familial glomerulonephritis in Doberman Pinscher dogs. Can Vet J 20:244, 1979
72. Bernard MA, Valli VE: Familial renal disease in Samoyed dogs. Can Vet J 18:181, 1977
73. Burk RL, Barton CL: Renal failure and hyperparathyroidism in an Alaskan Malamute pup. J Am Vet Med Assoc 172:64, 1978
74. DiBartola SP, Chew J, Boyce JT: Juvenile renal disease in related Standard Poodles. J Am Vet Med Assoc 183:693, 1983
75. English PB, Winter H: Renal cortical hypoplasia in a dog. Aust Vet J 55:181, 1979
76. Chew DJ, DiBartola SP, Boyce JT, et al: Juvenile renal disease in Doberman pinscher dogs. J Am Vet Med Assoc 182:481, 1983
77. Finco DR, Kurtz HJ, Low DG, et al: Familial renal disease in Norwegian elkhound dogs. J Am Vet Med Assoc 156:747, 1970
78. O'Brien TD, Osborne CA, Yano BC, et al: Clincopathologic manifestations of progressive renal disease in Lhaso Apso and Shih Tzu dogs. J Am Vet Med Assoc 180:658, 1982
79. Finco DR: Congenital and inherited renal disease. J Am Anim Hosp Assoc 9:301, 1973
80. Lucke VM, Kelly DF, Darke PG, et al: Chronic renal failure in young dogs—possible renal dysplasia. J Small Anim Pract 21:169, 1980
81. Wells MJ, Coyne JA, Prince JL: Ectopic kidney in a cat. Mod Vet Pract 61:693, 1980
82. Johnson CA: Renal ectopia in a cat. J Am Anim Hosp Assoc 15:599, 1979
83. Rose JG, Gillenwater JY: Effects of obstruction on ureteral function. Urology 12:139, 1978
84. Rose JG, Gillenwater JY: Effect of chronic uretheral obstruction and infection upon ureteral function. Invest Urol 11:47, 1974
85. Faulkner RT, Osborne CA, Feeney DA: Canine and feline urethral ectopia. p. 1043. In Kirk RW (ed): Current Veterinary Therapy VIII. WB Saunders Co, Philadelphia, 1983

86. Owen RR: Canine urethral ectopia. J Small Anim Pract 14:407, 1983
87. Scott RC, Greene RW, Patnaik AK: Unilateral ureterocele associated with hydronephrosis in a dog. J Am Anim Hosp Assoc 10:126, 1974
88. Smith CW, Park RD: Bilateral ectopic ureteroceles in a dog. Canine Pract 1:28, 1974
89. Stowater JL, Springer AL: Ureterocele in a dog. Vet Med Small Anim Clin 74:1753, 1979
90. Selcer BA: Urinary tract trauma associated with pelvic trauma. J Am Anim Hosp Assoc 18:785, 1982
91. Park RD, Radiographic contrast studies of the lower urinary tract. Vet Clin North Am 4:863, 1974
92. Barsanti JA, Crowell W, Losonsky J: Complications of bladder distention during retrograde urethrography. Am J Vet Res 208:819, 1981
93. Christie BA: Incidence and etiology of vesicoureteral reflux in apparently normal dogs. Invest Urol 19:184, 1971
94. Christie BA: Vesicoureteral reflux in dogs. J Am Vet Med Assoc 162:772, 1973
95. Christie BA: Occurrence of vesicoureteral reflux and pyelonephritis in apparently normal dogs. Invest Urol 10:359, 1973
96. Vlahkis E, Hartman GW, Kelalis PP: Comparison of voiding cystourethhrography and expression cystourethrography. J Urol 106:414, 1971
97. Feeney DA, Osborne CA, Johnston GR: Vesicoureteral reflux induced by manual compression of the urinary bladder of dogs and cats. J Am Vet Med Assoc 182:795, 1983
98. Lenaghan D, Cussen LJ: Vescoureteral reflux in pups. Invest Urol 5:449, 1968
99. Woodward JR, Filardi G: Demonstration of vesicoureteral reflux under general anesthesia. J Urol 116:501, 1976
100. Timmons JW, Watts FB, Perlmutter AD: A comparison of awake and anesthesia cystography. p. 363. In Bergsma D, Duckett JW (ed): Urinary System Malformations in Children. Alan R Liss Inc, New York, 1976
101. Shopfner CE: Vescoureteral reflux. Radiology 95:637, 1970
102. Sommer JL, Roberts JA: Ureteral reflux resulting from chronic urinary tract infection in dogs: Long-term studies. J Urol 95:502, 1966
103. Grana L, Donnellan WL, Swenson O: Effects of gram-negative bacteria on ureteral structure and function. J Urol 99:539, 1968
104. Harrison L, Cass A, Cox C, Boyce W: Role of bladder infection in the etiology of vesicoureteral reflux in dog. Invest Urol 12:123, 1974
105. Klausner JS, Johnston GR, Osborne CA: Diverticula of the urinary bladder. p. 1093. In Current Veterinary Therapy VIII. RW Kirk (ed): WB Saunders Co, Philadelphia, 1983
106. Spackman C, Caywood D, Johnston GR, Feeney DA: Uterine stump granuloma: A complication of ovariohysterectomy in dogs. J Am Anim Hosp Assoc 20:449, 1984
107. Johnston GR, Jessen CR, Osborne CA: Retrograde contrast urethrography. p. 1189. In RW Kirk (ed): Current Veterinary Therapy VI. WB Saunders Co, Philadelphia, 1977
108. Feeney DA, Johnston GR, Tomlinson MJ, Osborne CA: Dimension of the prostate and membranous urethra during maximum distension retrograde urethrocystography in normal male dog. Vet Radiol 25:249, 1984

109. Feeney DA, Johnston GR, Tomlinson MJ, et al: Maximum distention retrograde urethrocystography in healthy male dogs. Occurrence and radiographic appearance of urethro-prostatic reflux. Am J Vet Res 45:948, 1984
110. Ackerman N: Prostatic reflux during positive contrast retrograde urethrography in the dog. Vet Radiol 24:251, 1983

Index

Page numbers followed by f represent figures; those followed by t represent tables.